Behavioral Problems in
Children and Adolescents

Behavioral Problems in Children and Adolescents

Second Edition

Editor

Jaydeep Choudhury
DNB (PED) MNAMS FIAP
Professor
Department of Pediatrics
Institute of Child Health
Kolkata, West Bengal, India

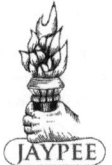

JAYPEE BROTHERS MEDICAL PUBLISHERS
The Health Sciences Publisher
New Delhi | London

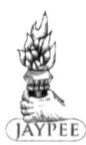 **Jaypee Brothers Medical Publishers (P) Ltd**

Headquarters
Jaypee Brothers Medical Publishers (P) Ltd
EMCA House, 23/23-B, Ansari Road, Daryaganj
New Delhi 110 002, India
Landline: +91-11-23272143, +91-11-23272703
+91-11-23282021, +91-11-23245672
Email: jaypee@jaypeebrothers.com

Corporate Office
Jaypee Brothers Medical Publishers (P) Ltd
4838/24, Ansari Road, Daryaganj
New Delhi 110 002, India
Phone: +91-11-43574357
Fax: +91-11-43574314
Email: jaypee@jaypeebrothers.com

Overseas Office
JP Medical Ltd
83, Victoria Street, London
SW1H 0HW (UK)
Phone: +44 20 3170 8910
Fax: +44 (0)20 3008 6180
Email: info@jpmedpub.com

Website: www.jaypeebrothers.com
Website: www.jaypeedigital.com

© 2024, Jaypee Brothers Medical Publishers

The views and opinions expressed in this book are solely those of the original contributor(s)/author(s) and do not necessarily represent those of editor(s) or publisher of the book.

All rights reserved. No part of this publication may be reproduced, stored or transmitted in any form or by any means, electronic, mechanical, photocopying, recording or otherwise, without the prior permission in writing of the publishers.

All brand names and product names used in this book are trade names, service marks, trademarks or registered trademarks of their respective owners. The publisher is not associated with any product or vendor mentioned in this book.

Medical knowledge and practice change constantly. This book is designed to provide accurate, authoritative information about the subject matter in question. However, readers are advised to check the most current information available on procedures included and check information from the manufacturer of each product to be administered, to verify the recommended dose, formula, method and duration of administration, adverse effects and contraindications. It is the responsibility of the practitioner to take all appropriate safety precautions. Neither the publisher nor the author(s)/editor(s) assume any liability for any injury and/or damage to persons or property arising from or related to use of material in this book.

This book is sold on the understanding that the publisher is not engaged in providing professional medical services. If such advice or services are required, the services of a competent medical professional should be sought.

Every effort has been made where necessary to contact holders of copyright to obtain permission to reproduce copyright material. If any have been inadvertently overlooked, the publisher will be pleased to make the necessary arrangements at the first opportunity.

Inquiries for bulk sales may be solicited at: jaypee@jaypeebrothers.com

Behavioral Problems in Children and Adolescents

First Edition: 2014

Second Edition: **2024**

ISBN: 978-93-5696-391-7

Dedicated to

(Late) Dr Tapan Kumar Ghosh
You dreamt of this book; I have done your unfinished work.

Contributors

Alafiya Nasrulla MS CCC-SLP
Speech and Language Pathologist
Ummeed Child Development Center
Mumbai, Maharashtra, India

Anjana Thadhani DNB DCH FCPS
PGD Developmental Neurology
Developmental Pediatrician
Consultant
Department of Pediatrics
KEM Hospital and Niramay Guidance Clinic
Mumbai, Maharashtra, India

Anjan Bhattacharya
DCH MRCP FRCPCH
Senior Consultant Developmental Pediatrician
Child Development Centre
Apollo Multispecialty Hospital, Kolkata
Director, Post Graduate Diploma in Early Intervention for Neurodevelopmental Disorders
CCPTR
Maulana Abul Kalam Azad University of Technology (MAKAUT)
Kolkata, West Bengal, India

Jai Ranjan Ram MD MRCPsych (UK) CCST in Child Psychiatry (UK)
Child Psychiatrist
Consultant Psychiatrist
Apollo Multispecialty Hospital and Mental Health Foundation
Kolkata, West Bengal, India

Jaydeep Choudhury
DNB (PED) MNAMS FIAP
Professor
Department of Pediatrics
Institute of Child Health
Kolkata, West Bengal, India

Jaydeb Ray MD (Ped) MD (Comm Med) DNB (Ped) DCH FIAP FNNF FIAMS
Principal and Professor of Pediatrics
Department of Pediatrics
Institute of Child Health
Kolkata, West Bengal, India

Jewel Chakraborty PhD (Scholar)
BPT MPT (Neuro) CMT C/SI (USC-USA)
Consultant Physiotherapist
Child Development Centre
Apollo Multispecialty Hospital
Kolkata, West Bengal, India

Ketan Bharadva
MD Fellowship in Neonatology
Consultant Pediatrician
Director
Neoplus ICU for Children
Surat, Gujarat, India

Mandira Roy
DNB (Ped) PGDDN (Kerala)
Assistant Professor
Department of Pediatrics
Santiniketan Medical College and Hospital
Bolpur, West Bengal, India

Contributors

Monidipa Banerjee DTM&H
DCH FRCPCH (UK) Diploma in Pediatric
Neurodisability
Specialist Pediatrician and
Medical Adviser
Children's Neurodevelopmental
Services West and Community
Pediatrics
Betsi Cadwaladr University Health
Board, Penrhosgarnedd Bangor
LL57 2NB, UK

Nandita Chatterjee
DCH DNB (Ped) PGDDN FNNF FIAP
Developmental Pediatrician
Professor and Head
Department of Pediatrics
MGM Medical College
Kishanganj, Bihar, India

Piyali Bhattacharya
DCH MD (Ped) FIAP FRCP (London)
Consultant Pediatrician
Department of General Hospital
Sanjay Gandhi Postgraduate
Institute of Medical Sciences
Lucknow, Uttar Pradesh, India

Preeti M Galagali MD PGDAP
Director and Consultant
Adolescent Health Specialist
Department of Pediatrics
Bengaluru Adolescent Care
and Counseling Centre
Bengaluru, Karnataka, India

Ranjana Chatterjee MD DCH
Retired Professor of Pediatrics
RG Kar Medical College
Kolkata, West Bengal, India

Saheli Misra DNB (Ped) MRCPCH
Professor
Department of Pediatrics
ESI-PGIMSR and ESIC Medical
College
Kolkata, West Bengal, India

Samir Hasan Dalwai
MD DNB FCPS DCH LLB
Director
Department of Developmental
Pediatrics
New Horizons Child Development
Center
Mumbai, Maharashtra, India

Shabina Ahmed MD FIAP
Founder Director
Assam Autism Foundation
Guwahati, Assam, India

Suchit Tamboli
PhD DCH PGDAP PGDMLS
Director and Consultant
Department of Development and
Behavioral Pediatrics
Chiranjiv Clinic and Child
Development Research Institute
Ahmednagar, Gujarat, India

Sukanta Chatterjee MD FIAP
Retired Professor of Pediatrics
Government Medical College
Kolkata, West Bengal, India

Sunita Shanbhag
MBBS DPH MD (Community Medicine)
Professor
Department of Community
Medicine
Seth GS Medical College and KEM
Hospital
Mumbai, Maharashtra, India

Vibha Krishnamurthy MD
Medical Director
Ummeed Child Development
Center
Mumbai, Maharashtra, India

Preface to the Second Edition

COVID-19 has been an eye-opener to the mankind. People have become aware not only of the transmission, dynamics, and prevention of infectious diseases, but also of the mental health consequences of pandemic in particular and children in general. The pandemic has in fact brought out various complex issues regarding behavioral problems in children and adolescents. Parents have recognized many hitherto ignored behavioral issues, and many new challenges have also come to the surface. As a consequence, the pediatricians, psychiatrists, and behavioral therapists all have faced many questions, encountered many naive issues, and often discovered very receptive parents.

We have learnt that fostering children's peer social skills and behavior control may have a lifetime positive effect on children's developing behaviors, especially in dealing with crisis situations such as the COVID-19 pandemic. Parent distresses significantly predict behavior problems in children. More distressed parents reported more child behavior problems. Pre-pandemic peer social skills of children also significantly predicted behavior problems during the pandemic. More skilled children exhibited fewer behavior problems.

The pandemic has taught us vital lessons. We have learnt to think and retrospect. Let us channelize the acquired wisdom for the benefit of the children.

Various chapters in this second edition of *Behavioral Problems in Children and Adolescents* have been modified and updated keeping up with the current issues and understanding of the concept. New chapters have been added to fill-up the lacunae. I would like to express my sincere gratitude to all the contributors and the publisher.

Jaydeep Choudhury

Preface to the First Edition

In the early years of 20th century, medical fraternity recognized that children are not small adults, and they need to be understood and treated separately. The concept of child psychiatry developed in the 1920s and 1930s. It was recognized that children pass through intricate developmental phases as they traverse through childhood and adolescence on their inevitable journey to adulthood. The field of developmental pediatrics was gaining in importance. Gradually, the significance of mental health issues of children was recognized. Thus, the concept of developmental-behavioral pediatrics was evolving. The term "behavioral pediatrics" was first used in the early 1970s by Dr Robert J Haggerty and colleagues to study the behavioral concerns of children from a pediatrician's perspective and not only from a child psychiatrist's perspective. Dr Stanford B Friedman defined behavioral pediatrics as "an area within pediatrics which focuses on the psychological, social, and learning problems of children and adolescents".

There are two reasons why a primary care pediatrician should be oriented in problems and management of behavioral disorders in children and adolescents. The first is that they are the first contact physician, and they get to interact with the children and their families regularly. If they can detect the behavioral problems early, then it can be approached in the initial stage. The second reason is that on a broader perspective, there is some overlap between behavioral pediatrics and child psychiatry. The severe shortage of both child psychiatrists and behavioral pediatricians has encouraged primary care clinicians or pediatric practitioners to manage these various issues of behavioral pediatrics. Today, most of the parents are aware and well oriented about various developmental issues in children. They expect us to look at both the medical and behavioral health aspects that affect their children. There is no unequivocal line dividing the normal and abnormal behaviors in children and adolescents. It is often subjective, situational, and sometimes glaring.

Pervasiveness across situations and impairment are probably the two most important threshold criteria.

This book addresses general concepts and important topics of behavioral problems for children and adolescents.

Suggestions are welcome at: *drjaydeep_choudhury@yahoo.co.in.*

Jaydeep Choudhury

Acknowledgments

The editor wishes to thank all the contributors who have put in a lot of effort to chart the readers in this unexplored territory of behavioral pediatrics.

I express my sincere gratitude to Shri Jitendar P Vij (Group Chairman), Mr Ankit Vij (Managing Director), Mr MS Mani (Group President), Ms Chetna Malhotra (Senior Director—Professional Publishing, Marketing, and Business Development), Ms Pooja Bhandari (Director—Production), and the team of M/s Jaypee Brothers Medical Publishers (P) Ltd, New Delhi, India. I would also like to thank Ms Pallavi Mehrotra (Development Editor) and Mr Sabyasachi Hazra (Associate Director—Publishing and Digital Sales, Kolkata Branch), for their wholehearted effort and cooperation.

My family members have been extremely tolerant and cooperative during the hours that I have spent with the text and manuscript. I am grateful to them.

Contents

1. **Behavior Problems in Children: Looking Beyond the Surface** 1
   Jai Ranjan Ram
   • Why Pediatricians need to know about Behavioral Disorders? *1* • Behavioral Disorders: Cost to the Society *2* • How Common are Behavior Disorders? *3* • Understanding the Context: Why do Children Display Disruptive Behavior? *4*

2. **Intellectual Disability** 7
   Monidipa Banerjee
   • Definition and Disorder Characteristics *7* • Prevalence *8* Clinical Presentation *8* • Clinical Evaluation *10* • Important Points in Developmental History *12* • Management *22* • Long-term Outcome *23*

3. **Learning Disorders** 26
   Anjana Thadhani
   • Etiology *26* • Investigations *38* • Management *39* • Outcome of Specific Learning Disabilities *45*

4. **Developmental Coordination Disorder** 48
   Anjan Bhattacharya, Jewel Chakraborty
   • Definition *48* • Epidemiology *49* • Diagnosis *49* • Clinical Features *50* • Treatment *51*

5. **Stereotypic Movement Disorder** 60
   Jaydeep Choudhury
   • Epidemiology *60* • Diagnostic Criteria *61* • Clinical Features *61* • Course and Outcome *63* • Treatment *64*

6. **Communication Disorders** 65
   Vibha Krishnamurthy, Alafiya Nasrulla
   • Components of Language *65* • Normal Language Development *66* • Communication Disorders *67* • Assessment of the Child with Suspected Communication Disorder *68* • Common Communication Disorders *69*

- Link between Communication and Behavior Problems *71* • Role of the Team *72*

7. **Autism Spectrum Disorder** **77**
   Shabina Ahmed
   - History and Evolution *78* • Incidence and Epidemiology *79* • Clinical Features *79*
   - Diagnostic Criteria *81* • Etiology *85*
   - Clinical Features *88* • Laboratory Tests and Imaging *88*
   - Management *88*

8. **Attention-deficit/Hyperactivity Disorder** **98**
   Jai Ranjan Ram, Jaydeep Choudhury
   - History and Nomenclature *98* • Etiology *99*
   - Epidemiology *102* • Diagnosis *102*
   - Clinical Features *105* • Investigations *106*
   - Differential Diagnosis *107* • Treatment *109*

9. **Disruptive Behavior** **123**
   Jaydeep Choudhury
   - Oppositional Defiant Disorder *124* • Conduct Disorder *128* • Intermittent Explosive Disorder *133*

10. **Feeding and Eating Disorders in Infancy and Childhood** **135**
    Ketan Bharadva
    - Epidemiology *136* • Etiopathogenesis and Diagnosis *137* • Classical Eating Disorders *138*
    - Unclassified Eating Disturbances *142* • Management *147*

11. **Elimination Disorders (Urinary Incontinence and Encopresis)** **153**
    Nandita Chatterjee
    Urinary Incontinence 153
    - Daytime Incontinence *153*
    - Enuresis (Nocturnal Incontinence) *161*

    Encopresis 168
    - Incidence *168* • Classification *168* • Etiology *169*
    - Pathophysiology *169* • Toilet Training *170*
    - Toilet Refusal *170* • Toilet Training in Special Situation *171* • Clinical Features *172*

- Investigation *175* • Treatment *175*
- Outcome *178*

12. Tic Disorders 182
Jaydeb Ray, Jaydeep Choudhury
- Epidemiology *182* • Etiology *183*
- Clinical Features *183* • Diagnosis *188*
- Differential Diagnosis *188* • Treatment *188*
- Prognosis *191*

13. Sleep Problem 194
Jaydeep Choudhury
- Patterns of Normal Sleep *195* • Consequences of Poor Sleep *195* • Types of Sleep Problems *195*
- Evaluation *196* • Common Sleep Problems *196*
- General Management *201*

14. Mood Disorder 203
Saheli Misra
- Epidemiology *203* • Etiology *204* • Clinical Features *205*
- Diagnosis *206* • Differential Diagnosis *209*
- Treatment *210* • Prognosis and Outcome *212*

15. Anxiety Disorder 213
Ranjana Chatterjee, Mandira Roy
- Epidemiology *214* • Etiopathogenesis *214*
- Types of Anxiety Disorders *218* • Management *222*

16. Somatic Symptoms and Related Disorders 226
Mandira Roy
- What is Somatic Symptom Disorder? *226*
- Epidemiology *228* • Etiology *228*
- Clinical Features *232* • Diagnosis *234*
- Assessment *236* • Treatment *238*

17. Psychological Effects of Chronic Illness 242
Jai Ranjan Ram
- Epidemiology *242* • Factors Deciding Adaptation of Children to Chronic Illness *244*
- Children with Various Ailments *245*
- General Intervention Strategies *247*

18. Study Skills 249
Preeti M Galagali
- Definition *249* • Importance of Study Skills in an Indian Scenario *250* • Essentials for Learning *250*
- Early Foundations of Learning *252*
- Evidence-based Study Strategies *255*
- Classification of Study Skills *256*

19. School Problems 265
Ketan Bharadva
- School Refusal *265* • Bullying in School *270*

20. Fussy Child.. 276
Piyali Bhattacharya
- Common Childhood Illnesses which make a Child Fussy *277*
- Some Serious Conditions *279*

21. Behavioral Problems in Adolescents........................... 282
Suchit Tamboli

Eating Disorders *282*
- Risk Factors of Eating Disorders *282* • Barriers Influencing Eating Behaviors *283* • Anorexia Nervosa *283*
- Bulimia Nervosa *286* • Binge Eating Disorder *289*
- Eating Disorder not Otherwise Specified *290*
- Purging Disorder *291* • Night Eating Syndrome *291*
- Other Feeding or Eating Condition not Elsewhere Classified *291*
- Medical Complications of Eating Disorders *292*
- Management *295* • Prognosis *299*

Sexuality and Deviant Sexual Behavior *300*
- Sexualized Behavior *304* • Issues Bothering Girls *304*
- Issues Bothering Boys *304* • Gender Identity Disorder *305*
- Etiology of Deviant Sexual Behavior *306*
- Characteristics of Paraphilic Disorders *308*
- Management of Sexual Dysfunction *312*
- Treatment of Sexual Dysfunction *312*
- Distinguishing Sexual Exploitation *313*

Suicide *315*
- Assessment for Suicide Risk *316* • New Risk Syndromes Category *317* • Risk Factors for Suicide *319*

22. Adolescent Parenting 330
Sukanta Chatterjee
- Actions that should make Parents Cautious *330*
- Role of Parents *331* • Dealing with the Situation *332*
- Different Parenting Styles *332*

23. Digital Media and Children 336
Samir Hasan Dalwai
- Patterns of Media use in Children and Adolescents *336*
- Clinical Features *337* • Management *338*

24. Street Children 341
Sunita Shanbhag, Jaydeep Choudhury
- Categories *342* • Number *342* • Age *343*
- Location *343* • Gender *343* • Reasons why a Child Chooses Street to be his Home *344* • Physical Problems Faced by a Street Child *348* • Psychological Problems Faced by a Street Child *350* • Social Problems Faced by a Street Child *352* • Stigmatization *354*
- Immediate Measures *354* • Long-term Measures *355*

25. Substitute Care 357
Jaydeep Choudhury
- Reasons for Placement in Substitute Care *357* • Types of Substitute Care *358* • Challenges *358* • Common Behavioral Problems *359*

26. Substance-related and Addictive Disorders 363
Mandira Roy
- Epidemiology *363* • Etiopathogenesis *365*
- Clinical Features *366* • Stages of Adolescent Substance Abuse *366* • Screening and Assessment *367*
- Diagnosis *368*

27. Mental Health of Children during Pandemic 372
Jaydeep Choudhury
- Clinician's Approach *373* • Role of Parents *374*
- Management *375*

Index *377*

CHAPTER 1

Behavior Problems in Children: Looking Beyond the Surface

Jai Ranjan Ram

WHY PEDIATRICIANS NEED TO KNOW ABOUT BEHAVIORAL DISORDERS?

Pediatricians are most frequently the first port of call for parents when they realize that their child has behavior problems or developmental disorders. Most frequently, it is the pediatrician who suspects, picks it up, and expresses concerns about the child. The majority of the initial concerns, such as temper tantrums, feeding difficulties, and sleep problems, resolve with basic psychoeducation and a few simple tips on behavior management. Often, the reasons for behavior problems in young children are their underlying developmental disorders. A child may be more restless and inattentive compared to his peers, may have partial deafness, and hence does not look at his carers when called, leading to concerns from parents. In a multitude of situations like this, pediatricians are first consulted. Accredited Social Health Activist (ASHA) workers and Anganwadi workers very frequently refer children with developmental disorders and behavioral concerns in rural/urban settings, where medical resources are scarce.

For an office-based pediatrician, behavioral disorders contribute to 25–30% of some pediatricians' caseloads. Therefore, it is mandatory that pediatricians are updated with this subject.

If there was any doubt regarding the need to address behavior problems in children was a necessary skill for pediatricians, the COVID-19 pandemic ended that debate. Prolonged school closure, increased screen time, experience of bereavements, lack of outdoor activity, and financial hardships fractured the lives of many young people. Clinical experience confirmed spurts in behavior problems, self-harm, and even suicides.

Another important role for pediatricians is to identify and refer serious mental illnesses, a large majority of which starts by adolescence. Schizophrenia, recurrent depression, and bipolar mood disorders can have onset in adolescence and in very rare situations, prepubertal onset also. It is again within the remit of pediatricians to identify these symptoms and guide them for appropriate treatment pathways. Most families in India are reluctant to see a mental health professional for the fear of the child being labeled. Unless pediatricians dispel this fear, many families will not seek appropriate medical treatment for young people.

During my own work with parents, I have realized that many parents too suffer from mental illnesses, or they could be displaying broad phenotypes of conditions such as autism, which their child has. They very frequently test the patience of doctors, working in an overcrowded clinic. A father may forget to bring his daughter for scheduled vaccination. Could he be having ADHD (attention-deficit hyperactivity disorder)? The mother who is calling up the pediatrician repeatedly to cross-check the dose of the prescribed medicines. Could she be having OCD (obsessive-compulsive disorder)?

Knowledge about behavioral pediatrics actually enables the pediatricians to analyze and understand the child and the family's problems in a broader systematic perspective.

■ BEHAVIORAL DISORDERS: COST TO THE SOCIETY

There are huge societal costs if behavioral disorders are ignored or untreated. Severe behavior problems cause children, families, and schools considerable distress. The problems become more entrenched and become more difficult to treat as the disease trajectory progresses downward. There is an individual cost, in terms of social, educational, and occupational impairment, but there is also a more macroeconomic national cost. Drug addiction, violent crimes, and incarceration in prisons are often a sequela of unmet needs of children with behavioral problems. Ultimately, it is the taxpayers' money that gets diverted to law enforcement agencies and costs the nation harm.

■ HOW COMMON ARE BEHAVIOR DISORDERS?

A recent study published in *Lancet Psychiatry* found that disorders or developmental disorders that have the onset predominantly during childhood and adolescence, the crude prevalence for intellectual disability was 4.5%, conduct disorder had a prevalence of 0.8%, ADHD was 0.4%, and autism spectrum disorders (ASD) of 0.4%. The prevalence rates for both ADHD and ASD were lower if compared with international prevalence studies.

The National Mental Health Survey (2015–16) on prevalence of mental disorders in the age group 13–17 years was 7.3% and nearly equal in both genders. Nearly 9.8 million of young Indians aged 13–17 years are in need of active interventions. The prevalence of mental disorders was nearly twice (13.5%) as much in urban metros as compared to rural (6.9%) areas. The most common prevalent problems were depressive episode and recurrent depressive disorder (2.6%), agoraphobia (2.3%), intellectual disability (1.7%), ASD (1.6%), phobic anxiety disorder (1.3%), and psychotic disorder.

Roles of Pediatricians

As enumerated earlier, a key goal is early detection of behavioral disorders. The subsequent skill development need is developing a framework of understanding why the index child is displaying a behavioral disorder. This involves looking behind the surface, within the mind of the child. The severity of the presenting problems may be mild and often does not reach the category of a diagnosable disorder. All restless, inattentive behavior is not due to ADHD. It may be due to hunger or lack of stimulation in the child due to maternal depression.

Having a developmental perspective, which all pediatricians have, is a key asset. Separation anxiety in a toddler may be normal but may not be so in a 9-year-old child. Sexual play may be age appropriate in a 12-year-old child, but the same kind of play in a 6-year-old is not.

The key parameter is to distinguish whether the presenting problem/s which is used, is affecting the child's overall development. Is a child's restlessness making his behavior difficult to the extent that other children are avoiding him, his mother is feeling overwhelmed, and his learning is below par?

This child may be so restless that he is unable to sit at his desk in the class, may not be able to wait for his turn in joint play with other children, and always demands or needs attention when his mother is doing other household chores. A detailed evaluation will help the clinician to establish that the presenting problems are severe enough and reach the category of a disorder.

UNDERSTANDING THE CONTEXT: WHY DO CHILDREN DISPLAY DISRUPTIVE BEHAVIOR?

Children develop disruptive behavior because of complex interplay in their biological and psychosocial factors. For clinicians, it is important and vital to remember that the remedy for disruptive behavior will depend on how successfully we are able to piece together all the factors, which are contributing to the cause. A pediatrician usually knows the family best. He/she has a good insight into the dynamics of the family and the communication patterns. The analysis of the communication problems and conflicts within the family often helps to address the behavioral problems better.

A large number of children in India live in extremely vulnerable conditions. They are most at risk of developing behavioral disorders. The groups of children who are at more risk are:

- Those who have suffered abuse/neglect
- Homeless/street children
- Children in substitute care
- Young offenders
- Young people with physical disorders, especially neurological disorders
- Children of parents with mental illness, including substance misuse and personality disorders

For routine assessment, basic history taking and routine physical examination will suffice. The important issue for clinicians to remember is to view the child as a child in need, rather than labeling the child as "bad" child.

During an assessment, it is equally important to identify a disorder if present and also identify the environmental factors that are causing or maintaining the illness.

There are many important causal factors, which lead to disruptive behavior. Few of the important associations of disruptive behavior in children are the following:
- Attention-deficit hyperactivity disorder
- Autism spectrum disorders
- Undiagnosed mental illnesses such as anxiety disorders and mood disorders
- Tic disorders
- Academic difficulties
- Harsh and punitive parenting
- Overt parental conflict
- Abuse (sexual, emotional, and physical)
- Parental mental illness
- Excessive dependence on screen (mobiles/computers)

CONCLUSION

Meeting a child with disruptive behavior is actually a golden chance to change the child's life course for each of us. Skepticism has to give way to optimism, and children and young people have to be addressed respectfully to air their view. Harsh judgments need to be suspended and have no place in therapeutics. A young person displays disruptive behavior for many reasons. An assessment with a humane lens gives the young person an opportunity to change life's course. It is more pragmatic to view the young person as a child in need rather than just looking at the surface of external behavioral manifestations. Clinicians, especially pediatricians play a crucially important role in formulating opinion about a child presenting with behavior problems and even basic therapeutic intervention such as counseling the family to seek help can be life altering for the child and the family.

BIBLIOGRAPHY

1. Burke JD, Loeber R, Birhamer B. Oppositional defiant disorder and conduct disorder: a review of the past 10 years, part II. J Am Acad Child Adolesc Psychiatry. 2002;41:127593.

2. India State-Level Disease Burden Initiative Mental Disorders Collaborators. The burden of mental disorders across the states of India: the Global Burden of Disease Study 1990-2017. Lancet Psychiatry. 2020;7(2):148-61.
3. Rahman F, Adamson L, Spencer N, et al. Do community pediatricians contribute to a comprehensive CAMHS service? Arch Dis Child. 2006;91(Suppl. 1):A39.

CHAPTER 2

Intellectual Disability

Monidipa Banerjee

■ DEFINITION AND DISORDER CHARACTERISTICS
What is Intellectual Disability?
Intellectual disability (ID) is a condition that reflects impaired intellectual and adaptive abilities of varying severity, seen in a child or a young person before 18 years of age. In the fifth edition of the Diagnostic and Statistical Manual of Mental Disorders (DSM 5), the diagnosis of ID (intellectual developmental disorder) is revised from the DSM-IV diagnosis of "mental retardation." The term "mental retardation" has been considered derogatory over the last few decades. It was being used almost exclusively in scientific contexts. Alternative terms that were used included developmental delay, developmental disability, ID, learning disability, learning difficulties, etc. The DSM 5, which was published in May 2013, has brought a name change. *ID replaces "mental retardation"* used in previous editions of the manuals.

Early developmental impairment (EDI) is now replacing the term (*popularly known as global developmental delay or GDD* where developmental delay is noted across two or more domains). The term GDD has been noted to be confusing for parents as the word "delay" gives the impression of "catch up" at a later stage.

Early developmental impairment does not necessarily equate to ID in later life, although a strong correlation exists. Alternatively, not all children with EDI/GDD will meet the criteria for ID as they grow older.

A diagnosis of ID requires:
- Onset before 18 years of age
- Limitations in both adaptive and intellectual functioning

Disorder Characteristics

Intellectual disability involves impairments that affect functioning in three domains. In other words, it determines how well an individual copes with everyday tasks.

1. *Conceptual domain:* This domain includes skills in language, reading, writing, math, reasoning, knowledge, and memory.
2. *Social domain:* This domain refers to empathy, social judgment, interpersonal communication skills, the ability to make and retain friendships, and similar capacities.
3. *Practical domain:* This domain centers on self-management in areas such as personal care, job responsibilities, money management, recreation, and organizing school and work tasks.

An individual's symptoms must begin during the developmental period and are diagnosed based on the severity of deficits in adaptive functioning. Intellectual disability is further divided according to the level of disability as well as the level of support needed by an individual. Standardized tests used to measure intelligence quotient (IQ) are no longer used for the classification of ID. The DSM 5 classifies ID as mild, moderate, severe, or profound.

■ PREVALENCE

The prevalence of ID among the general population is approximately 1%. The prevalence of *EDI (popularly known as global developmental delay or GDD)* is said to be 1–3%. EDI, as we already know, does not necessarily equate to ID in later life, although a strong correlation exists.

■ CLINICAL PRESENTATION

How do Children with ID Present?

When considering ID in a child, we need to remember three important aspects:
1. Presenting symptoms
2. Associated conditions
3. Comorbid conditions.

Presenting Symptoms

Presenting symptoms vary according to the severity of affection.

Severe ID is picked up earlier than others and is usually diagnosed by 2 years of age. They usually come to attention because of GDD and associated conditions.

Mild-to-moderate ID may come to attention because of a *worried parent, family, or friend*. There may be parental concern over language delay [should be distinguished from autism spectrum disorder (ASD) with or without ID], immature self-help skills, or any other skills such as behavior or social, being delayed compared to siblings, particularly when compared to a younger sibling. *Routine surveillance* of childhood development is conducted in some countries, thereby picking up early delays. *School* may "red flag" some children, usually with mild ID, who may not have been detected until school age, till they exhibit learning difficulties. *Associated conditions*, with distinctive dysmorphic features, e.g., Down syndrome or the presence of known genetic disorders, in the family can help identify ID in infancy.

Associated Conditions

Numerous conditions are known to be associated with ID. Whenever children present with specific conditions/syndromes, they should be evaluated for ID so that they receive appropriate help. Common medical and/or physical associations with ID include the following:

- Cerebral palsy
- Congenital heart disease
- Gastrointestinal conditions such as constipation, gastroesophageal reflux disease (GERD), or early feeding difficulties
- Endocrine abnormalities (e.g., hypothyroidism, short or tall stature, cryptorchidism, ambiguous genitalia, and delayed puberty)
- Hearing loss
- Seizures and epilepsy syndromes
- Sleep disorders
- Vision impairment
- Presence of multiple congenital abnormalities
- Known syndromic and genetic conditions (Down, Turner, Prader-Willi, Angelman syndromes, etc.)

Comorbid Conditions

Comorbid conditions must be actively sought and managed appropriately:
- Neurodivergence, namely autism spectrum condition (ASC)—now replacing the term ASD and attention-deficit hyperactivity disorder (ADHD) are often present as comorbid conditions and may need specific management.
- Learning disabilities—when an individual has learning difficulties that are much more than what is expected for the child's intellectual level, and not explained by any other factor, the child is said to have a specific learning disorder in addition to ID.
- Feeding and related disorders—abnormal eating behaviors and major difficulty with feeding may be present.
- Constipation and incontinence leading to recurrent urinary tract infection (UTI) and other complications
- Sleep disorders, including sleep-disordered breathing
- Dental caries and other features of dental malocclusion
- Depression, low mood, and anxiety—depressive and anxiety disorders are frequent comorbid conditions.
- Movement disorders—stereotyped and complex motor mannerisms are often seen in severe ID.
- Self-injurious behaviors—these are often seen in individuals with ID, particularly where there are communication difficulties.

CLINICAL EVALUATION

How would you Diagnose Intellectual Disability?

Screening for ID—different countries have different policies for screening. Besides routine surveillance, developmental and behavioral screening should be performed if a concern is raised by either parent or a professional. The goal is early identification of developmental delay and providing early interventional support.

Evaluation for ID involves two parts:
1. Diagnosing ID
2. Finding an underlying cause for ID

Diagnosing ID

As with any condition, we must go through history, physical examination, and investigations to come to a diagnosis of ID and establish an underlying etiology. A detailed history and physical examination can identify an etiology in 17–34% of cases.

Often, one can begin with an open question like *"When did you first feel your child had a problem?"* It has been seen that parents felt something was wrong with their baby long before they voiced concerns.

History

Plenty of time is needed to elicit details of birth history (antenatal, perinatal), medical, developmental, and family history.

The following aspects should be looked at in particular:

- *Antenatal:* Any problems in pregnancy such as history of fever with rash, drugs taken during pregnancy, antenatal ultrasound (USG) findings
- *Perinatal:* Mode of delivery, resuscitation, neonatal problems
- *Medical history:* Major medical problems including history of seizures, meningitis, neurocutaneous markers, episodic decompensations, and previous hospitalizations
  A record of *all medications, treatments, and previous assessment reports* if any.
  Feeding problems including evidence of reflux, *bowel, and bladder* control including constipation and *sleeping habits* including features of obstructive sleep apnea
- *Developmental history* includes details of developmental milestones as well as any evidence for regression of milestones. Important points in developmental history are mentioned below.
- *Behavior concerns* in the child, preferably in more than one setting. Sometimes, disorder-specific questions may be needed to identify more frequent comorbidities such as ASD or ADHD.
- *Educational history* including any history of learning difficulties
- *Social history:* Look at *family dynamics*—Any situation that could lead to emotional deprivation of the child or other social concerns.

- *Family history*, preferably over three generations of neurodevelopmental or genetic disorders
  Consanguinity of marriage, miscarriages, stillbirths, neonatal deaths

IMPORTANT POINTS IN DEVELOPMENTAL HISTORY

When to Suspect?

The pediatrician is best placed to identify children who appear to have developmental delay, to address the concerns of parents or teachers, and to pursue the process of differential diagnosis and investigations as to an underlying cause.

The most important marker is a history of delay in reaching important milestones. For this, a thorough knowledge of normal developmental milestones is essential and does not stop with the child walking and talking. The following are the important milestones that must be assessed to determine ID:

- Commonly gross motor milestones delay present first, followed by delay in communication skills. With slow achievement of adaptive skills, obvious cognitive impairment often is not apparent until the child is older. Many cases of mild ID may not be identified until they enter formal education.
- In the first year of life, social smile and sitting are the milestones associated with the least individual variation. Social smiling with responsive vocalization (baby noises) not elicited by 8 weeks of age is a cause for concern. Visual and auditory impairment must be excluded, and unsuspected illness or seizure activity considered.
- Failure to demonstrate sitting (sitting upright on the hard floor for 5 minutes without any support) by 10 months very likely predicts later problems. Unfortunately, the milestones which are the easiest to observe (walking, talking) are not always the most meaningful clinically.
- Advanced motor development certainly does not mean higher intelligence. Manipulative development and the use of hands, especially the index finger approach and the pincer grasp, are much more important. If these appear at normal ages, ID is unlikely.

- There is a lot of individual variation in speech and language milestones. Normal children may say no words, particularly those with a family history, till they are 2 or 3 years old. However, it is important to note their understanding of spoken language. In young children, evaluation of receptive language offers the best prediction of mental age.
- Acquisition of self-help and social skills largely depends on the opportunity offered to the child. These skills can only be evaluated with knowledge of the cultural norms which apply to that family. However, given the same background, a child with ID will be slower than his normal sibling in the acquisition of these skills.
- The first true milestone of cognitive progress occurs around the age of 10 months, when normally developing infants acquire the concept of object permanence. Till then it is "out of sight, out of mind." Now they realize that objects continue to exist even when they cannot be seen. This can easily be checked in a clinical setting.
- Alternatively, a child may present with behavior problems or academic underachievement. Such a child may have normal developmental milestones. A careful history will elicit that the child is slow in the achievement of adaptive skills and is typically described by parents as "immature for his age."

Physical Examination

A thorough physical examination should include the following:
- *Anthropometry:* It is by far the most important aspect of physical examination. Head size (micro or macro) and stature (tall or short) are useful in the evaluation of syndromic cases. Any acceleration or deceleration of head circumference must be carefully monitored. It correlates well with changes in the infant's length and contemporaneous acceleration or deceleration of length may indicate growth spurt or severe malnutrition accordingly. One must bear in mind that normal growth of the brain is maintained preferentially in all but the most severe cases of systemic illnesses.

- *Face:* Who does your child look like? This helps establish the significance of dysmorphism. There is no facial appearance characteristic of all causes of mental retardation or ID. Diagnoses are based more on the basis of developmental delay rather than on appearance. The first mental retardation syndrome to be identified based on its characteristic physical appearance was Down syndrome, described by Langdon Down in 1866. Dysmorphic features that suggest syndromic etiology can guide in the choice of chromosomal or genetic tests.
- *Malformations:* Internal and external, particularly hands and feet, should be examined.
- *Skin, hair, nails, and teeth:* Important findings to look for include café-au-lait macules (think of neurofibromatosis), ash-leaf spots and adenoma sebaceum (consider tuberous sclerosis), facial hemangiomas (rule out Sturge-Weber syndrome), and bruises and unkempt skin as signs suggestive of neglect and abuse.
- *Bones* (scoliosis) and *joints* (laxity, contractures)
- *Chest and abdomen:* Presence of organomegaly and abnormal genitalia, cryptorchidism, etc.
- *Heart* for murmur heart rate and evidence of cardiac failure
- *Central nervous system (CNS):* Muscle tone is the most important aspect, abnormal movements (dystonia), reflexes (persistence of primitive reflexes), gait, and coordination. Complete neurologic and neurodevelopmental assessment is important.
- *Ophthalmologic and audiology review:* There is a need to check vision and structural abnormalities of the eye, as well as a hearing test for all children, as part of the physical examination. Children with ID often have accompanying sensory impairments.

Developmental Assessment

A complete developmental assessment of the child is needed and applies usually to children <5 years of age. A standard, available developmental tool must be used, which has been standardized for language and cultural differences. However, there is no substitute for a thorough practical knowledge of child development and each milestone should be interpreted in context. One must always remember to make appropriate corrections for early birth, up to the age of 2 years.

Speech delay is the most common presenting symptom leading to the eventual diagnosis of ID. In fact, it is the second most common cause of speech delay, after developmental expressive speech delay. Thus, these children need language assessment and the possibility of autism or language disorder needs to be ruled out.

Detailed observation of the child's behavior and social communication skills is very important and should form part of the developmental assessment. Parent/family behaviors in general and interactions particularly with the child may be observed. This often provides useful and invaluable information.

Definitive Assessment for Intellectual Disability

Significant limitations in individuals, as compared to that expected for age and sex, in intellectual and adaptive functioning give a diagnosis of ID. Onset should occur during the developmental period (<18 years of age). Thus, *the child is assessed in two domains, intellectual function and adaptive function.*

Earlier, mental retardation used to be diagnosed by a professional assessment of IQ. In DSM 5, ID is approximately 2 standard deviations or more below the population, which equals an IQ score of about 70 or below.

What has Changed in DSM 5?

The fifth edition of the Diagnostic and Statistical Manual of Mental Disorders emphasizes the need to use both clinical assessment and standardized testing of intelligence when diagnosing ID, with *the severity of impairment based on adaptive functioning rather than IQ test scores alone.* It is important to note that IQ or similar standardized test scores may still need to be included in an individual's assessment.

Adaptive function—adaptive impairment is essential for the diagnosis of ID.

Adaptive functioning refers to the skills needed to live independently. To assess adaptive behavior, professionals compare the functional abilities of a child to those of other children of similar age. Certain skills are important to adaptive behavior, such as *self-help skills* (such as getting dressed, using the bathroom, and feeding oneself), *communication skills* (such as understanding what is said and being able to answer in context), and *social skills* (with peers, family members, spouses, adults, and others).

The adaptive functioning should impact at least *one* of the three domains and be present across settings, such as home and school.

1. *Conceptual domain*—some examples include concepts of money and time, reasoning, memory, and handling of novel situations.
2. *Social domain*—some examples include social communication, empathy, age-appropriate social responsibility, self-respect, and the ability to follow rules.
3. *Practical domain*—examples include activities of personal care, such as preparing food and feeding, dressing, undressing, washing, brushing, toileting, and self-hygiene. Other examples include following a routine, understanding the concept of time, using telephone, managing money, independent traveling, and issues related to health and safety.

Two standard deviations below the mean on a standardized test assessing adaptive functioning indicate significant impairment. The assessment of intelligence across three domains (conceptual, social, and practical) will ensure that clinicians base their diagnosis on the impact of the deficit in general mental abilities on functioning needed for everyday life. Thus, a child with ID or intellectual developmental disorder may have some or all the following features:

- May be late in sitting, crawling, walking, and talking (developmental delay)
- Have trouble speaking (speech delay, shy of strangers)
- Find it hard to remember things
- Have trouble understanding social rules
- Have trouble discerning cause and effect, and this may lead to behavior problems.
- Have trouble solving problems
- Have trouble thinking logically
- Lack of sense of danger

Intellectual function includes academic learning, reasoning, problem-solving, abstract thinking, and decision-making. Assessment of intellectual function is one of the components of the diagnosis of ID. An IQ score that is 2 standard deviations or more below the mean (usually <70) indicates significant intellectual impairment. Standardized intelligence tests are used. Wechsler scale is commonly used. There are several more but need to be standardized for language and cultural variations.

Classification of severity—the severity of ID is dependent on the level of impairment as well as the level of support needed and is classified as mild, moderate, severe, and profound.

Finding a Cause for Intellectual Disability

Why should we find an Underlying Cause for Intellectual Disability?

Despite elaborate investigations, a cause may not be found in a certain proportion of cases. Finding a cause can provide more information to the family about the condition and its prognosis. It helps explain comorbidities and plan future needs as well as future pregnancies. Any specific available treatment can be discussed. It helps with genetic counseling for the immediate and extended family. It also helps parents accept the child's limitations and stop blaming themselves or their own parenting skills. It helps the family to have closure, get on with their lives while helping the child to achieve his or her full potential.

How do we Investigate a Child with Intellectual Disability?

The list of investigations is endless. On one hand, we must *rule out any treatable cause and establish a diagnosis* in view of future genetic counseling. On the other hand, we need to respect the views and wishes of the family, keeping in mind the financial implications, and not let our scientific curiosity take priority.

History and examination are the main ways in which a diagnosis is made. Investigations are most useful in confirming or clarifying a diagnosis. After a clinical evaluation, we can either have a clinical diagnosis or it can be ID of unknown etiology.

In the absence of major clues to the underlying cause, some baseline blood tests may be considered. These are in no way comprehensive or mandatory and are tailored as per individual needs and circumstances.

Some of the *first-line investigations to be considered* are as follows:
- *Hematological:* Blood count and peripheral smear examination, ferritin
- *Biochemistry:* Electrolytes, kidney function, bone profile, liver function, creatine kinase (in boys with language delay), thyroid function test, uric acid (raised in Lesch–Nyhan syndrome), biotinidase, lead levels
- *Audiometry:* To rule out hearing deficits

Other investigations are based on clinical suspicion of either of the following:
- Environmental causes
- Targeted specific disorders
- Metabolic disorders
- Neurologic causes
- Genetic causes.

Environmental Causes

Some cases are due to environmental causes which often have *a definitive history*. These may be classified as *prenatal, perinatal, and postnatal*.

Antenatal maternal illnesses like uncontrolled diabetes, nutritional deficiencies (folic acid), congenital infections [cytomegalovirus (CMV), rubella, varicella, herpes, etc.], antenatal exposure to teratogenic drugs (valproic acid), toxins, alcohol, substance abuse, etc., are risk factors. The timing (as the first trimester is most vulnerable) and extent of exposure decide the outcome.

Perinatal birth asphyxia, prematurity and its related complications including intraventricular hemorrhage, and postnatal infections including necrotizing enterocolitis (NEC), meningoencephalitis, etc., are other possible factors.

Testing for Specific Disorders

Children with characteristic features that suggest a particular syndrome should undergo specific chromosomal or genetic testing to diagnose that condition. *Examples include Down syndrome, fragile X syndrome, Rett syndrome, and Prader–Willi syndrome*, to name a few.

Metabolic Disorders

Metabolic disorders comprise an important group which are associated with ID. Most affected children have other manifestations of metabolic disease. Features suggestive of metabolic disorders in individuals with ID include:
- Consanguineous marriage
- Unexplained infant death in the immediate family
- Failure to thrive
- Hypotonia
- Recurrent unexplained illness (especially anorexia and vomiting)
- Episodic illness
- Any loss of acquired skills
- Coarse facial features
- Organomegaly
- Ocular abnormalities
- Macro- or microcephaly
- Seizure
- Evidence of encephalopathy

Initially, screening tests are performed based on clinical suspicion. These include blood for serum ammonia, pH, lactate, electrolytes, liver function tests, kidney function tests, plasma amino acids, very long chain fatty acids, and carnitine. Urine is checked for organic acids. Further, metabolic testing is performed depending on initial reports and is preferably guided by a specialist. *Hypothyroidism should be ruled out in countries where new-born screening program is not routinely performed.*

Neurological Causes

Intellectual disability can be present in children with neurological conditions such as epilepsy or brain malformations.

Clues to *structural brain malformation* may be derived from abnormal skull, focal deficit, loss of skills, micro- or macrocephaly, seizures, and visual abnormality.

If there is *progressive loss of skills*, we must be alert toward conditions such as hydrocephalus, poorly controlled epilepsy, metabolic disorder/neurodegenerative disorder, Rett syndrome, and other MECP2 deletions, duplications, mutations, and variations. Infection, particularly in an immunocompromised host (e.g., HIV/AIDS) may be a precipitating factor. Vascular problem, e.g., repeated minor strokes may be the cause. If *epilepsy is suspected*, it needs to be investigated carefully. Electroencephalography (EEG) is not a test for diagnosing epilepsies but may provide helpful information to confirm specific epilepsy types and helps in deciding management. In the presence of specific loss of language skills, EEG should be considered (Landau–Kleffner syndrome). Muscular hypotonia, weakness, or suspicion of neuromuscular disorder warrants further evaluation. Indicators of neuromuscular disorders are reduced fetal movements, early feeding difficulties, floppy infant, late motor milestones (not walking by 18 months), positive Gowers sign, not jumping by 3 years, or unable to hop by 5 years.

Muscular dystrophy—proximal muscle weakness in the presence of developmental delay often indicates muscular dystrophy. An elevated creatine kinase leads to specific genetic testing to confirm a specific diagnosis. In the presence of extrapyramidal signs, be alert to Wilson's disease and familial disorders related to chorea and athetosis.

Neuroimaging—magnetic resonance imaging (MRI) is the preferred imaging modality. Common findings include CNS malformations, white matter abnormalities, and cerebral atrophy. Some of the indications for MRI of the brain include the following (consider computerized tomography if calcification is suspected):

- Microcephaly (head circumference < 0.4th percentile)
- Macrocephaly (head circumference > 99th percentile)
- Changing head circumference, e.g., crossed >2 percentile lines
- Neurocutaneous stigmata
- Cerebral palsy including hemiplegia
- Focal onset epilepsy
- Myoclonic seizures in infancy
- Unexplained seizures
- Focal neurological signs
- Ataxia
- Evidence of loss of skills
- Severe visual impairment

Genetic Evaluation

Testing for specific disorders—a genetic evaluation is offered whenever there is a known genetic condition in the family and the child is symptomatic or sometimes even screened soon after birth, depending on the condition.

When to go for genetic testing in the absence of history of specific disorders?
A genetic disorder is suspected in a child with ID in the presence of:
- Consanguineous marriage
- Family history of unexplained infant deaths
- History of multiple miscarriages
- Congenital anomalies affecting various organs of the body (e.g., hearing loss, visual problems, congenital heart defects, or urogenital anomalies)
- Syndromic features
- Failure to thrive
- Abnormal tone (e.g., hypotonia, hypertonia, dystonia)

Karyotype is now done for confirmation of suspected specific chromosomal disorders such as Trisomy's, etc., or where microarray is not available. Chromosomal microarray (CMA) also looks at the chromosomal level, but can see in much more details, called copy number variations (CNV) or microdeletions and duplications. It has a much higher detection rate, compared to regular karyotyping, picking up microdeletions and microduplications. Some copy number changes may be reported as of uncertain significance and cannot be fully interpreted without investigation of parental samples. These will be requested in the report and only a targeted analysis of parental samples will be carried out with respect to the copy number change observed in the original test of the proband. When CMA fails to find any abnormality, whole exome sequencing (WES) can be considered. CMA testing has replaced karyotype analysis for patients who fulfill some of the following criteria:
- Developmental delay
- Learning disability
- Facial dysmorphism or congenital abnormalities
- Hypotonic infant

- Congenital heart disease
- Behavioral problems/autistic spectrum

Microarray will not exclude:
- Balanced rearrangements
- Point mutations
- Fragile X syndrome
- Single-gene disorders
- Some cases of Prader–Willi or Angelman syndrome
- Some cases of mosaicism (low level)

Always consult a clinical geneticist where possible, and counsel families adequately about the implications of the tests in detail.

MANAGEMENT

Currently, there is no "cure" for an established ID, though with appropriate support and teaching, most individuals can learn to do many things.

The medical contribution to the management of ID includes:
- Early identification
- Diagnosis of preventable and treatable causes such as phenylketonuria and hypothyroidism
- Ensuring access to genetic and metabolic tests and genetic counseling, wherever applicable
- Maintenance of the health of the child with reference to nutrition, vision, hearing, seizure control, gastroesophageal reflux, constipation, behavior issues, and mental health
- Detection of comorbidities or associated impairments
- Providing information to the family

Apart from medical management, these children need the help of a multidisciplinary team depending on their needs. These include the physiotherapist, occupational therapist, speech therapist, psychologist, and special educator. The parents need to be trained to be the key worker of the child.

Learning in the early years is most effective on a one-to-one basis. This is usually provided by the parent at home and the special educator at school. The slow learner may find it difficult to benefit from a classroom-like situation and hence needs to be integrated carefully. Most will need special educational support throughout their learning years.

LONG-TERM OUTCOME

Parents are usually anxious to know the future of their child. Will he walk? Will he talk? Will he study in a normal school? Will he ever be independent? The outcome obviously depends on the level of disability and the appropriate training opportunities available to the child.

Those with mild ID are educable and usually face academic underachievement in late school years. Adaptive behaviors, however, can be learned over a longer period. They can perform many simple but useful tasks without supervision. Independence is the realistic goal, but many need continued support and guidance regarding complicated decisions and in emergency situations.

People with moderate ID seem mildly delayed in the preschool years. They will acquire vocational and social skills, but academically may not progress beyond 6-7 years level. They will continue to need supervision for many daily routines in their adult life.

Children with severe ID are slow in acquiring speech and basic self-help skills. They need close supervision even for simple and repetitive tasks. If speech is not present by 10-12 years, it is unlikely to develop. They are trainable to some extent but need specialized care throughout their lives.

Those with profound ID face significant developmental delay in the early years. Seizures and medical complications are common. They may or may not walk, and speech may never develop. Multiple intensive supports are required to maintain an acceptable quality of life.

Expectation of life appears to be closely related to the severity of cognitive impairment. Uncontrolled seizure disorders are associated with shortened life. Some of the specific syndromes bring special risks, such as increased risk of death from heart disease or leukemia in Down syndrome. Immobility is also associated with shortened life. The child unable to roll or show purposeful hand use is at a much increased risk of early death. Children without complications, however, have a life expectancy equivalent to that of the surrounding population if equal healthcare facilities and nutrition are made available.

> **GUIDELINES FOR PARENTS**
> - Parents are the key workers for the management of these children.
> - With appropriate support and teaching, most individuals with ID can learn to do many things including activities of daily living.
> - Early identification and diagnosis of preventable and treatable causes are important aspects of management.
> - Maintenance of the health of the child, particularly nutrition, vision, hearing, seizure control, vomiting, bowel habit, and mental health, is important.
> - Many children with ID are educable to a certain extent and over time they develop adaptive behavior.

■ SUMMARY POINTS

- *ID* is defined as limitations in both intelligence and adaptive skills, affecting at least one of three adaptive domains (conceptual, social, and practical), with varying severity. The degree of impairment in adaptive functioning determines the severity of ID. Severity is directly proportional to the level of support needed and not just the level of IQ.
- The term ID replaces the older term of "mental retardation."
- *EDI* (popularly known as global developmental delay or GDD) is a term used where developmental delay is noted across two or more domains in children under 5 years of age. EDI does not necessarily equate to ID in later life, although a strong correlation exists.
- Children with *severe ID are diagnosed earlier* compared to children with mild ID.
- *Clinical and standardized assessments* are needed to diagnose ID.
- It is important to find an *underlying cause of ID*, for prognostic purposes as well as counseling for any future pregnancies. But this should always be done after proper consultation with the family, keeping their wishes and expectations in mind.
- *Early identification* and diagnosis of preventable and treatable causes are important aspects of management. With *appropriate support and teaching*, most individuals can learn to live meaningful lives and contribute to society in general.

BIBLIOGRAPHY

1. American Association of Intellectual and Developmental Disabilities (AAIDD), Definition of Intellectual Disability. [online] Available from http://aaidd.org/intellectual-disability/definition. [Last accessed August, 2023].
2. American Psychiatric Association. Diagnostic and Statistical Manual of Mental Disorders, 5th edition. Arlington: American Psychiatric Association; 2013.
3. Fox AM. An Introduction to Neurodevelopmental Disorders in Children, 2nd edition. National Trust for the Welfare of Persons with Autism, Cerebral Palsy, Mental Retardation, & Multiple Disabilities; 2005.
4. Horridge KA. Assessment and investigation of the child with disordered development. Arch Dis Child Educ Pract Ed. 2011;96:9-20.
5. Illingworth RS. Basic Developmental Screening: 0-4 Years, 5th edition. Hoboken, NJ: Wiley-Blackwell; 1990.
6. Leonard H, Wen X. The epidemiology of mental retardation: challenges and opportunities in the new millennium. Ment Retard Dev Disabil Res Rev. 2002;8(3):117-34.
7. Miller DT, Adam MP, Aradhya S, Biesecker LG, Brothman AR, Carter NP, et al. Consensus statement: chromosomal microarray is a first-tier clinical diagnostic test for individuals with developmental disabilities or congenital anomalies. Am J Hum Genet. 2010;86(5):749-64.
8. Moeschler JB, Shevell M, American Academy of Pediatrics Committee on Genetics. Clinical genetic evaluation of the child with mental retardation or developmental delays. Pediatrics. 2006;117(6):2304-16.
9. Shevell M, Ashwal S, Donley D, Flint J, Gingold M, Hirtz D, et al. Practice parameter: evaluation of the child with global developmental delay: report of the Quality Standards Subcommittee of the American Academy of Neurology and The Practice Committee of the Child Neurology Society. Neurology. 2003;60(3):367-80.
10. Shevell MI, Majnemer A, Rosenbaum P, Abrahamowicz M. Etiologic yield of subspecialists' evaluation of young children with global developmental delay. J Pediatr. 2000;136(5):593-8.
11. Szymanski L, King BH. Practice parameters for the assessment and treatment of children, adolescents, and adults with mental retardation and comorbid mental disorders. American Academy of Child and Adolescent Psychiatry Working Group on Quality Issues. J Am Acad Child Adolesc Psychiatry. 1999;38:5S-31S.

CHAPTER 3

Learning Disorders

Anjana Thadhani

■ INTRODUCTION

Learning is the process of acquiring and retaining knowledge and is closely related to development. It is a complex process that requires an efficient coordination of various areas of the central nervous system. In a regular classroom, about 20% of children struggle to cope up with the academic concepts as per the grade level. There are many reasons for children to perform poorly at school. It is very important to objectively look at these numerous causes as most of them would present early as childhood developmental disabilities and would later definitely interfere with the learning process.

■ ETIOLOGY

The causes for academic backwardness in children are multidimensional and could be attributed to both intrinsic and extrinsic causes. The intrinsic causes being chronic medical problems, sensory deficits, neurological disorders, epilepsy, psychiatric disorders, poor cognitive ability, specific learning disability (SpLD), attention-deficit hyperactivity disorder (ADHD), and behavioral problems. Poor sociocultural home environment, acute stress, abuse, domestic violence, multiple changes in school, and teaching methodology could significantly contribute as extrinsic factors related to learning difficulties.

Medical Disorders

Several chronic medical and neurologic conditions in children are associated with poor learning. Learning problems are commonly seen with conditions associated with any injury to the developing brain due to any hypoxic or metabolic insult. Prenatal and perinatal causes are of paramount importance and a detailed history is essential. Meningitis, epilepsy, and head injury are the conditions that affect cognition and learning in later years.

Epilepsy

Epileptic children have a higher chance of learning disorders. The neuropsychological approach to learning disabilities in epilepsy concentrates on analyzing the differential effects of epileptic factors on cognitive function. The impact of seizure activity, localization of epileptogenic foci, and antiepileptic treatment on cognitive functioning has been evaluated and seems to influence the learning outcomes. Studies showed a significant lower school achievement scores for the patients with idiopathic generalized epilepsy compared to the patients with localization-related epilepsy. Besides epilepsy, the long-term effects of antiepileptic medications such as phenytoin and phenobarbitone on cognitive function are well documented. It has been concluded that recent-onset epilepsy with higher seizure frequency or uncontrolled epilepsy has more learning problems. Therefore, it is essential to sensitize parents about these learning difficulties and the importance of starting early intervention.

Neurological Conditions

Neurological conditions are generally thought to be related to mental retardation but they may also have normal intelligence with learning disabilities. However, the risk of cognitive and learning deficits is estimated to be as high as three to five times in various studies.

Some neurological conditions such as neurofibromatosis, craniosynostosis, and Tourette syndrome (TS) are also associated with learning and behavioral disorders. More than 50% of children with neurofibromatosis type 1 have learning problems and a higher incidence of SpLD.

Fetal Alcohol Syndrome

Fetal alcohol syndrome presents with learning difficulties, poor fine motor coordination with hyperactivity. Early recognition of minor physical anomalies could result in prompt evaluation and treatment of these children.

Tourette Syndrome

Tourette syndrome is a neurological disorder characterized by repetitive, stereotyped, involuntary movements and vocalizations called tics. Poor school performance and severe behavioral concerns are usually seen in children with tic disorder. In a study, using a 1.5 standard deviation discrepancy, 51% met the criteria for learning disability in at least one academic area and 21% had a two standard deviation discrepancy. Specific cognitive deficits in TS consist of visuomotor integration problems, impaired fine motor skill, and executive dysfunction.

Others

Common conditions associated with academic and behavioral issues along with variations in head size including syndromes such as Sotos syndrome, mucopolysaccharidoses, and secondary microcephaly are seen to have developmental disabilities with associated motor, visual, and cognitive impairments.

Children with fragile X syndrome have demonstrated learning difficulties that included hyperactivity, visuomotor incoordination, language deficits, and academic delays in mathematics in various studies. Girls with Turner syndrome also differed from their respective comparison groups on math-related abilities, including visual-spatial, working memory and reading skills, and the associations between math and those related skills. Together, these findings support the notion that difficulty with math and related skills among girls with fragile X or Turner syndrome continues into late elementary school and that the profile of math and related skill difficulty distinguishes the two syndrome groups from each other. Children with Prader–Willi syndrome have moderate-to-severe learning difficulties, stubbornness, and verbal perseverance.

Chronic medical conditions: Other common chronic medical conditions associated with poor learning are poorly controlled asthma, thalassemia, chronic renal failure (CRF), cardiac conditions, etc. These children require repeated hospitalizations or daycare visits with frequent absenteeism, medical complications, drug-related side effects, and other psychological implications. All these problems could lead to poor academic achievement in children, but they can cope up well with parental and school support.

Attention-deficit/Hyperactivity Disorder

Another common disorder associated with poor learning is ADHD, which is seen in about 3–7% of schoolgoing children. The diagnostic criteria for this disorder are now applicable from 4 to 18 years as per the latest American Academy of Pediatrics (AAP) recommendations. The children are classified into inattentive type or hyperactive-impulsive type based on the cluster of the symptoms or a mixed type, which has a combination of these symptoms. ADHD has a very strong association with specific learning disability, which is as high as 20%. Most of these children with hyperactivity require help or medication during the initial years but usually settle by early adulthood. Diet modification in the form of reduction in chocolates and junk food helps. Medications are safe, effective, and easily available. Psychological testing and educational intervention are almost always required.

Psychiatric Disorders

Psychiatric and behavioral conditions also have a high incidence in childhood and affect school performance. Childhood depression and generalized anxiety disorder may be difficult to identify in children. These psychiatric disorders are pretty common in children. In addition to dysphoria, these children frequently have lower self-esteem, a reduced capacity for fun, massive guilt, social withdrawal, impaired school work, excessive fatigue, psychomotor retardation, and morbid or suicidal ideation. Some studies have mentioned that lateralized cerebral dysfunction in children is associated with specific clusters of cognitive deficits that impair learning. Right hemisphere learning disabilities may be etiologically related to childhood endogenous depressive illness, while left hemisphere learning disabilities may be reversibly worsened by such depression. It is suggested that diagnostic evaluation of learning disability should routinely include a search for childhood depressive illness.

Autism Spectrum Disorder

Another condition which is related to both learning and behavioral problems is autism spectrum disorder. The incidence is reported to be as high as 1-2% of schoolgoing children. Autism is a neurodevelopmental condition, which mainly affects areas of social interaction and communication. These children represent a spectrum of symptoms from avoidance of social situations and isolation to severe aggression with an inability to learn or function appropriately. The soft subtle signs of autism such as poor eye contact, speech delay, and difficulty in play and interaction with other children may present early. Inability to focus and hyperactivity with unpredictable aggression is noted in schoolgoing children. These children also may have some repetitive motor movements and behaviors such as hand flapping and rocking.

Specific Learning Disabilities

Specific learning disabilities are one of the most common neurodevelopmental disorders in children. Formal classroom learning involves processing information related to language and mathematical concepts, correlating it, storing it in memory, and retrieving it later for recall. These disorders manifest as deficits in one or more of the following areas such as attention, reasoning, processing, memory, communication, reading, writing, spelling, calculation, coordination, social competence, and emotional maturity.

Definition

National Joint Committee for Learning Disabilities (NJCLD) in the year 1988 defined SpLD as a generic term that refers to a heterogeneous group of neurobehavioral disorders manifested by significant unexpected, specific, and persistent difficulties in the acquisition and use of efficient reading (dyslexia), writing (dysgraphia), or mathematical (dyscalculia) abilities despite conventional instruction, intact senses, normal intelligence, proper motivation, and adequate sociocultural opportunity.

Types

Specific learning disabilities are classified as follows:

- *Dyslexia:* The word dyslexia is used as a synonym for learning disability but it actually presents as difficulty in reading, spelling errors, comprehension difficulties, fluency, and vocabulary.
- *Dysgraphia:* This type of disability signifies difficulty in written expression and poor handwriting.
- *Dyscalculia:* This type of SpLD refers to a disorder affecting mathematical reasoning, concepts, math fluency, and calculations.

Epidemiology

Among the three subtypes of SpLD, dyslexia (or specific reading disability) is the most common, accounting for 80% of all those identified as learning disabled. Earlier studies indicate a male preponderance, but recent data indicate that both boys and girls are equally affected. This pattern could be attributed to the gender bias in referrals and availing special needs services. Studies have shown that SpLD affects between 5 and 15% of schoolgoing children. The incidence of dyslexia in primary school children in India has been reported to be 2–18%, dysgraphia 14%, and dyscalculia 5.5%. Dyslexic children avail about 40% of utilized special needs services.

Pathophysiology

Etiology of SpLD is multifactorial and its association with many risk factors such as prematurity, birth complication, and epilepsy is well documented. Various theories have been postulated related to the deficits in children with learning disability and debated with scientific evidence over decades.

Neurobiological Basis

Neuroimaging has been considered a common investigation modality for clinical diagnosis and in research studies. Various studies have documented structural changes such as atypical hemispheric asymmetry, agenesis of the angular gyrus in the dominant hemisphere, minor migration cell defects, and tiny scars located selectively in the perisylvian areas of the left hemisphere in dyslexics. However, no specific structural lesion is detected in all children with SpLD and hence not advisable.

Positron emission tomography (PET) studies have demonstrated failure of activation of the left parietal and left middle temporal regions in response to an aurally presented rhyming task in dyslexic adults. Dyslexic readers also have reduced blood flow in the temporal cortex and left inferior parietal cortex, especially seen in pronunciation and decision-making tasks. An interesting study showed adequate activation of left temporo-parieto-occipital cortical regions during reading after educational intervention in a dyslexic child.

Genetic Basis

Academic history of parents, siblings, and close relatives should be documented as a part of history taking. A strong positive family history of academic concerns is seen in children presenting with academic difficulties. Four major genes related to cell migration, adhesion, and axonal guidance have been studied in dyslexic adults. Replicated linkage studies of dyslexia implicate loci on chromosomes 1, 2, 3, 6, 15, and 18 for the transmission of phonologic awareness deficits and subsequent reading problems. The gene *DCDC2A* may be related to cortical neuronal migration, which is also related to dyslexics.

A strong positive family history was noted in a significant number of children in the learning disability clinic when asked their history of failures, spelling errors, and difficulty in math. It is important to note that the parents were not diagnosed with SpLD using standardized psychoeducational tests.

Phonologic Basis

Children with dyslexia have difficulty with auditory processing, phonological awareness, auditory discrimination, and letter-sound association. The functional unit of phonology is "phoneme," which is the smallest segment of speech; for example, the word "boot" consists of three phonemes: /b/ /oo/ /t/. According to the "phonologic-deficit hypothesis," children with dyslexia have difficulty in decoding words into phonemes and also blending phonemes into meaningful actual words while reading tasks. Speech sound disorder (SSD) is also seen in dyslexic children, which causes developmentally inappropriate errors in speech production and reduces speech intelligibility.

Clinical Presentation

Children with SpLD present with poor school performance with below average grades in school. They may be referred from school or reported by parents. These children may present with learning difficulties from preprimary to secondary level depending on the severity, comorbidities, and awareness among parents or teachers.

Early red flag signs are difficulty in learning alphabets, numbers, days of the week, months, colors, or shapes. The child may have difficulty in rhyming, recalling, and sequencing stories or poems. The child may have trouble in pronouncing difficult words. The child may show confusion in space concepts, left versus right, over versus under, before versus after. These children may have problems in fine motor skills, abnormal pencil grip, delayed speech, and poor phonological awareness.

Children at primary and secondary levels present with:
- Difficulty in reading, slow, laborious, may skip words or lines
- Difficulty in blending and decoding words, confusion in homophones
- Spelling mistakes such as omissions, additions, substitutions, and transposition
- Written expression with poor sentence formation and punctuation errors
- Poor handwriting with refusal to write
- Poor academic fluency
- Calculation errors and difficulty in math reasoning, mental math, algebra, geometry, and word problems
- Poor recall and memory

Some children may have behavioral problems or symptoms of inattention and hyperactivity if ADHD is present. They may have difficulty with peer group and interpersonal relations. Some children exhibit severe aggression or withdrawn behavior.

Handwriting samples in children with dysgraphia are shown in **Figure 1**.

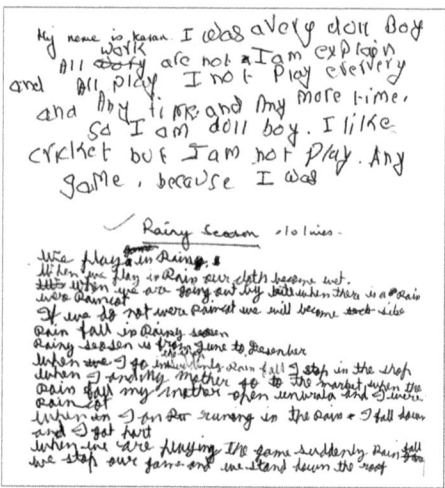

Fig. 1: Handwriting samples in children with dysgraphia.

Evaluation Procedure

A detailed multidisciplinary team is required for complete evaluation and intervention of a child presenting with poor school performance. The team should include pediatrician, developmental pediatrician, pediatric neurologist, child psychiatrist, ophthalmologist, psychologist, occupational therapist, special educator, and speech therapist.

This in-depth evaluation process includes:
- Medical and development history with clinical examination
- Academic history
- Vision and hearing evaluation
- Intelligence testing
- Educational testing
- Psychiatric or behavioral evaluation if needed
- Occupational therapist evaluation
- Speech evaluation if needed

Medical History

A prestructured case proforma helps to document all the relevant details and is critical to screen children with poor school performance in a busy clinic. Medical history related to head injury, trauma, headache, epilepsy, medications, chronic condition such as CRF, thalassemia, surgery, genetic conditions, or any other medical condition should be documented and evaluated for possible etiology.

Birth History

Birth history include antenatal history with detailed information during pregnancy regarding trauma, fall, pregnancy-induced hypertension, gestational diabetes mellitus, antepartum hemorrhage, nutritional deficiencies, febrile illness, and medications. Natal history related to prematurity, low birth weight (LBW), perinatal asphyxia, neonatal intensive care unit (NICU) stay, neonatal convulsion, jaundice, and ventilatory support should be asked specifically as many of these conditions are related to childhood disability. Many studies have proposed above factors as the cause of learning disabilities. Lilenfield and Pasamanick (1960) suggested that prolonged labor, malpresentation, and cord around the neck with hypoxic–ischemic injury to the brain could be responsible for learning disability in children. Davie et al. (1972) and Dunn et al. (1971) reported that appropriate for gestational age (AGA) children performed better academically than small for gestational age (SGA) babies. Prematurity and LBW are considered as important contributing factors for the development of learning disability and good antenatal care can reduce the disability burden.

Development History

Taking a descriptive development history with proper recording of milestones in all the domains is important in the evaluation of a child with poor school performance. Children with gross motor delays may present with generalized hypotonia, poor motor planning, dyspraxia, coordination, and clumsiness. Fine motor skills may be affected in some children with poor or awkward grip, confusion with laterality, delayed handedness, and hand manipulation function.

Speech and language development would present as a delay in the acquisition of meaningful words or phrases. Language processing skills include assimilation of words, phonological awareness, naming objects, comprehension, abstraction, analysis, memory, and recall.

In some children, persistent articulation errors may lead to faulty phonological association and spelling errors.

School History

The details of academic difficulties since primary level should be taken from the parents. Screening checklist could be used with specific questions such as spelling errors, reading difficulty, written expression, handwriting, calculation errors, mirror images, and recall. Any change of school, educational board, and change of curriculum should be asked. The teacher's feedback regarding the attentiveness and classroom participation of the child could give us insights into the child's problem. It is helpful to review the report card of previous 3 years.

Family History

Every child with poor school performance should be reviewed with regard to positive family history of academic difficulties in parents, siblings, or other close family members. A history of academic problems such as school dropout, failures, spelling errors, poor handwriting, and calculation errors is commonly reported by parents. Educational qualifications of the parents should be specifically asked in all cases. The positive family history of academic difficulty is around 40% in parents and siblings. "At risk" siblings should be started on preventive early intervention from the primary school level.

Social History

Detailed family history and socioeconomic status of parents should be recorded. Any acute stress in the family such as death, medical illness, separation, abuse, or domestic violence can lead to poor academic performance. In case of a change of school, adjustment issues should be taken into consideration.

Physical Examination

As learning disability may be present in few genetic conditions, dysmorphic features such as epicanthal folds, slanting palpebral fissures, microcephaly, and polydactyly may be present. Neurocutaneous syndromes such as neurofibromatosis and tuberous sclerosis are associated with learning disability, and hence markers such as hypopigmented macules (ash leaf macules), periungual fibromas or shagreen patches, and multiple café-au-lait spots should be looked for. However, most of the children with SpLD would not have any typical or consistent findings on physical examination.

Neurological Examination

The neurologic examination is generally normal in children with learning difficulties. Soft neurological signs may be seen in children, which suggest a neurologic deficit or immaturity of the central nervous system (CNS). These include repetitive finger tapping, dysdiadochokinesis, finger agnosia, and left–right (L–R) confusion. However, these signs are commonly seen till 7 years of age. Classic neurologic examination with asymmetry of reflexes, asymmetric gait, or an awkward posture may be observed in some children with LD secondary to epilepsy and neurologic deficits.

Cognitive Assessment

Intelligence or cognitive function should be done for every child with academic concerns to understand his ability or potential to learn. SpLD creates a discrepancy between the potential of a child and the academic performance; hence, both need to be tested using standardized structured tests. The Wechsler Intelligence Scale for Children (WISC-R) Indian adaptation is the commonly used test and consists of six verbal subtests and six performance subtests. The verbal and performance scores give a full-scale/global IQ.

The WISC-IV is another test commonly used by many psychologists but has not been standardized in the Indian population yet. Children with SpLD would have an average or above average IQ score (85 and above), while children having IQ score between dull-normal and borderline range (84–70) are categorized as slow learner. The WISC test is used for children between 6 and 16 years of age. Kamat Binet Test of Intelligence is also used for children above 4 years of age. For children above 16 years, the Wechsler Adult Intelligence Scale is administered.

Educational Assessment

Many standardized educational assessment tests are available. The informal or curriculum-based tests assess the performance of children related to grade level concepts and have tasks related to reading, written expression, spelling, comprehension, calculation, and math reasoning. Some educational tests are able to give information about the achieved grade level of the child in areas such as academic fluency, comprehension, reading, vocabulary, letter-word identification, phonology, handwriting, capitalization, punctuation, spelling, calculation, and mathematical concepts. These test results help in diagnosis as well as planning the individual education plan. Handwriting evaluation on various parameters such as letter formation, writing pressure, size, spacing, slant or alignment, rate, and legibility is also conducted.

These educational evaluations are conducted by a special educator trained in testing and commonly used tests are Diagnostic Test of Learning Disability, Curriculum-based Test, Woodcock-Johnson Psychoeducational Test of Achievement, standard and extended battery, Wide Range Achievement Test—Revised, etc.

■ INVESTIGATIONS

Sensory deficits need to be ruled out at the beginning of the evaluation of a child with academic concerns. Ophthalmological checkup with vision acuity by an ophthalmologist is a must. Hearing evaluation with an audiogram rules out any academic problems related to the inability to hear properly. It is also helpful in children with speech delay and articulation errors. Neuroimaging is not required unless there are any signs or symptoms of any underlying neurological condition. Many studies have documented few changes in computed tomography (CT) or magnetic resonance imaging (MRI) scan but they do not show any consistent structural abnormality seen in a large percentage of children diagnosed with learning disability. Functional studies are reserved for research purposes only. Electroencephalogram (EEG) studies need to be done in children with associated epilepsy.

The approach to a child with poor school performance is shown in **Flowchart 1**.

Flowchart 1: Approach to a child with poor school performance.

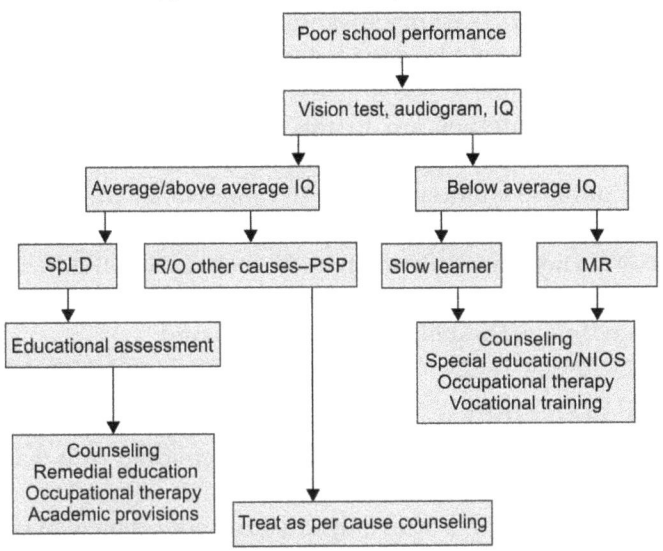

(MR: mental retardation; NIOS: National Institute of Open Schooling; PSP: progressive supranuclear palsy; R/O: rule out; SpLD: specific learning disability)

MANAGEMENT

Children with SpLD need a multidisciplinary team for both evaluation and subsequent management. Every pediatrician should be aware of the role of these rehabilitative professionals, so he can orchestrate the entire process right from screening to certification.

After the evaluation as discussed in the previous section, most parents depend on the clinician to interpret the psychoeducational and other evaluation reports and provide them guidance on future course of action. Most of the parents show difficulty in acceptance of the diagnosis and show extreme anxiety. They need a lot of answers ranging from etiology to long-term prognosis and would expect handholding from the pediatrician.

A clinician needs to give a clear message about SpLD, which would be helpful for the parents:
- Learning disability is a life-long condition and usually manifests in the school and college years.

- No medical treatment is available.
- Children with learning disability should study in regular schools and should be provided intervention and provisions as applicable.
- Long-term intervention in the form of special education, counseling, and therapies is extremely helpful.
- Most of these children do well in professional and vocational fields.
- SpLD is a benchmark disability and is included in rPWD Act 2016.
- These children should undergo government certification and obtain Unique Disability Identity (UDID) card.

Special Education

The only definitive treatment modality for children with learning disability is providing them with special education. Early intervention in the form of an individualized education plan should be implemented by qualified special educators as early as possible. It is important to provide intervention during the critical learning period, which is generally considered up to 8 years of age. Special educator is also involved in the educational assessment of the child. After the evaluation, an educator can enumerate the strengths and weaknesses of the child in various areas of learning. After applying a standardized test, the educator would know the learning gap, which would aid in writing the education plan. Long-term and short-term goals are defined by the educator and regular one-on-one sessions are started. This information is important for pediatricians as they may have to motivate the parents to continue the remedial education. It may take 2–3 years to bridge the gap.

Occupational Therapist

Children with SpLD may have difficulties in fine motor coordination, L–R orientation, and spatial relations. These would lead to deficits in motor planning and execution in organizing tasks and written expression. Younger children have visual and auditory perceptual difficulties, which affect learning and early concept formation. A thorough evaluation of gross and fine motor areas, pencil grip along with sensory and perception is desirable. Some children may need regular therapy to solve these issues. Occupational therapy also helps in inattention and sensory integration.

Role of Psychiatrist

Mental health issues in children with SpLD could be due to comorbid conditions such as ADHD, generalized anxiety disorder, performance anxiety, depression, and school phobia. Some children with learning disability may present with secondary behavior problems related to poor self-esteem, peer relations, aggression, severe anxiety, or withdrawal behavior. It is advisable to refer them to a psychiatrist for confirmation of diagnosis and treatment. Evaluation and management of ADHD can be done by the pediatrician.

Role of School and Classroom Teacher

Awareness among teachers and principals with regard to SpLD has been constantly increasing. The concept of inclusive education with mainstreaming of children with disabilities has been emphasized at policy level. Regular seminars and discussions are held in schools and other forums. It is important that the parents are aware of the support provided by the school before taking a decision to put the child in a particular school. The school should be willing to provide support in the form of a counselor, resource room facility, provisions during examination, and daily classroom modifications to augment their learning experience. Another issue is the acceptance of these children by peers and teachers with active support by school counselors and principals.

Resource Room at School

An inclusive school should have a resource room facility with counselor, occupational therapist, and special educator. The role of the counselor is to screen children with academic difficulties and follow their progress. They need to communicate their concerns with parents and support them through assessment and certification process. The counselor also conducts regular awareness programs for teachers and parents. Special educators start working with children by providing goal-oriented "Individualized Education Program." The children could attend the resource room facility depending on the class timetable. Counselor can also take individual counseling sessions for students in case of severe emotional problems and stress during examination.

Provisions at School and Educational Board

Most of the children struggle in regular schools and may drop out of the regular school as they are unable to cope in secondary and higher education As SpLD causes deficits in processing, comprehension, abstraction, reasoning, and calculation, these children perform poorly in timed tasks, and hence a provision of extra time is provided. Extra time is usually 25% of the allotted time for examination or task. Children with dysgraphia present with poor handwriting and written expression with better oral output, and hence a reader and writer facility is helpful. In a study conducted at LD clinic at LTMGH Mumbai, mean total marks had shown an increase of 22% from 41% marks before the provisions were given to 63% after availing provisions as applicable. This a significant change, especially during board examinations, as these marks help them seek better future prospects.

Provisions enable children with SpLD to continue education in regular mainstream schools with support from primary to higher education. The provisions vary as per the diagnosis, and it is important for the medical authorities to ensure a proper diagnosis and certification before offering any provisions. These children are given provisions from class standard I to class standard XII and are carried forward to university examinations and professional courses. The provisions offered are as per the latest circular from various educational boards and government departments.

Classroom Modifications

Simple interventions in the classroom help these children learn better in a regular classroom and can be easily implemented by the regular teacher:
- Preferential seating in the classroom in the first row, closer to the teacher, and away from distractions such as door or window.

This would enable the teacher to give individual attention and instructions if needed and minimize distractions for the child.
- "Buddy" system—assigning another student to help the child with SpLD with routine classroom work. This usually helps and works wonders with the child with disabilities but may require patience and some trial and error to get the correct and most helpful buddy.
- Individual attention and instruction from the teacher at the end of the lesson would be extremely helpful. The teacher could provide a brief summary or share a daily teacher schedule to prepare the child in advance.
- Multisensory teaching would be helpful as these children are better visual learners. Most of the classrooms use audiovisual aids, which aid in learning.
- The school should provide provisions during school examination as per the diagnosis. This includes giving extra time during examination, spelling concession, and use of a reader/writer and calculator.

Role of Government

Inclusion with mainstreaming of children with learning disabilities has been the focus at the policy level. The Right of Children to Free and Compulsory Education 2009 (RTE Act) makes education free and compulsory to all children, including those with disabilities in the 6-14 years age group. NEP 2016 and rPWD Act 2017 has increased the focus on providing support, rights, and provisions to children with 21 disabilities along with the formation of a central registry through a mandatory UDID card for taking any form of support. These initiatives will help us review the burden of disability and the need for additional support services.

Provisions

Prior to 2016, few state governments (Maharashtra, Karnataka, Tamil Nadu, Kerala, Goa, and Gujarat) and the National Educational Boards such as the Indian Certificate of Secondary Education (ICSE) and the Central Board of Secondary Education (CBSE) examinations formally granted children with SpLD the benefit of availing the necessary provisions. With the rPWD Act, the awareness and certification process has gained momentum across the country and all children with learning disability can avail the provisions and other benefits as prescribed under the Act.

Centers for Certification and Diagnosis of Specific Learning Disabilities

Infrastructure has to be upgraded at every district hospital to set up learning disability clinics for the assessment and certification of children. At present, many children with SpLD studying in non-English (vernacular) medium schools, especially in rural areas, are going undetected for nonavailability of standardized psychological and educational tests and also poor awareness among teachers and parents.

Courses in Special Education

It is very difficult to get teachers and other professionals for intervention as very few courses are available and the focus of such courses is mainly for mental retardation and other sensory disabilities. It is imperative that new courses should be introduced and advertised by the government-run institutions and universities. The universities should start the undergraduate degree course, B.Ed. (Special Education) and M.Ed. (Special Education) with curriculum specific to learning disabilities.

Counseling of Parents

- Counseling of the parents to understand various aspects of learning disability is very crucial.
- While interacting with parents whose child has been newly diagnosed with SpLD, the parents have many key issues, such as mainstreaming, which educational board gives support, prognosis, and future prospects; these need to be carefully explained to the parents.
- Pediatrician or the counselor could tell the parents that SpLD is a common disorder seen in many children. Parents should understand that their child has average or above average intelligence and learning disability is an information processing disorder. These children usually do well with timely intervention and support.

- Most parents are keen to know the cause for this disability, the multifactorial causation along with a strong genetic basis can be explained. Often during counseling, one of the parents may admit having a similar problem during his/her childhood. This understanding helps in reducing the stress on the child.
- Parents are keen to find a cure or medicine to help their child. Parents must be told that the child would gradually show improvement through special education, counseling, and occupational therapy. These interventions need to continue on a long-term basis to see a significant change in academics and behavior.
- During counseling, parents should be provided a list of provisions provided by the school and the educational board. The purpose of these provisions is to enable the child to achieve academic performance corresponding to his intellectual ability and continue education in a regular mainstream school.
- Parents should encourage their child to avail specific provisions provided by the educational and other authorities. These provisions are necessary as even after remedial education and other early interventions, subtle deficiencies in reading, writing, comprehension, reasoning, and mathematical abilities may persist and hence the need for this support.
- After appropriate understanding of the problem and intervention, the parents need to identify areas where they can help.

OUTCOME OF SPECIFIC LEARNING DISABILITIES

The outcome in a child with SpLD depends on the severity of the disability, the age or class standard when remedial education is started, the length and continuity of remedial education, the presence or absence of associated emotional problems, and parental and school support. With appropriate remedial education and provisions, most children with SpLD can be expected to achieve academic competence and complete their education in a regular mainstream school. However, some children are still unable to cope up and need to continue their education in special schools. Children with SpLD invariably fail to achieve school grades at a level that is commensurate with their intelligence. Their "academic problems" also have an adverse impact on their quality of life, namely self-image, peer and family relationships, and social interactions.

It is important to diagnose SpLD early as is the case for all other types of childhood disabilities for better long-term learning outcomes.

GUIDELINES FOR PARENTS

- *Keep things in perspective:* It is important for parents to support their child and to help them keep their self-esteem intact. Try not to be intimidated by the news that your child has a learning disability, please understand that all people learn differently. Challenges can be overcome. What is really important is providing your child with emotional, educational, and moral support.
- *Handling difficult behavior:* It is very essential parents understand the emotional trauma the child undergoes constantly due to academic failures. This leads to difficult behavior such as aggression, anxiety, and social isolation. The parents have to reach out to children and understand their emotional needs as well. If needed, the parents should take guidance from a counselor.
- *Show support and stand by your child:* One of the most important things to remember in rearing a child with LD is that you do not have to do it alone. Talk to your child's counselors, therapists, and teachers, and let the interventions be well coordinated with periodic reviews and group meetings among therapists.
- *Do your own research and become your own expert:* Learn about new developments in learning disabilities, different programs, and educational techniques that could make an impact with your child. You may instinctively look to others for solutions—schools, teachers, therapists, or doctors—but you need to take charge when it comes to finding the tools your child needs to continue learning.
- *Be an advocate for your child:* You may have to speak up time and again to get special help for your child. Embrace your role as a proactive parent and work on your communication skills. It may be frustrating at times, but your calm, reasonable, and firm voice may make the difference in achieving what you want for your child.
- *Take care of yourself:* Eat right, exercise, and find ways to reduce stress, whether it means taking a nightly bath or practicing morning meditation. If you do get really stressed, acknowledge it and get help.
- *Remember that your influence on your child outweighs all others:* Your child will follow your lead. If you approach the learning challenges with optimism, hard work, and a sense of humor, your child is likely to embrace your perspective or at least see the challenges as a detour rather than a roadblock.

BIBLIOGRAPHY

1. Aldenkamp AP, Alpherts WCJ, Dekker MJA, Overweg J. Neuropsychological aspects of learning disabilities in epilepsy. Epilepsia. 1990;31:S9-20.
2. Brumback RA, Staton RD. Learning disability and childhood depression. Am J Orthopsychiatr. 1983;53:269-81.
3. Hammill DD. On defining learning disabilities: an emerging consensus. J Learn Disabil. 1990;23:74-84.
4. Hyman SL, Arthur Shores E, North KN. Learning disabilities in children with neurofibromatosis type 1: subtypes, cognitive profile, and attention-deficit-hyperactivity disorder. Dev Med Child Neurol. 2006;48(12):973-7.
5. Identification of specific learning disabilities. US Department of Education, Office of Special Education Programs, 2006.
6. Karande S, Kulkarni M. Poor school performance. Indian J Pediatr. 2005;72(11):961-7.
7. Karande S, Sholapurwala R (Ed). Management of specific learning disabilities. Childhood Disability: A Pediatrician's Perspective—Textbook on Childhood Disabilities. Mumbai: Indian Academy of Pediatrics.
8. Kulkarni M, Thadhani A. Specific learning disability: clinical features and diagnosis. Childhood Disability: A Pediatrician's Perspective—Textbook on Childhood Disabilities. Mumbai: Indian Academy of Pediatrics.
9. Lyon GR, Shaywitz SE, Shaywitz BA. Specific language and learning disabilities. In: Kliegman (RM), Marcdante M, Behrman RE, Jenson HB (Eds). Nelson Textbook of Pediatrics, 18th edition. Philadelphia, PA: Elsevier; 2008. pp. 150-2.
10. Rowland LP, Pedley TA. Birth injuries and developmental abnormalities. In: Rowland LP (Ed). Merritt's Neurology. Philadelphia, PA: Lippincott Williams & Wilkins; 2000. pp. 572-3.
11. Shapiro BK, Gallico RP. Learning disabilities: the child with developmental disabilities. Pediatr Clin North Am. 1993;40(3):491-5.
12. Shaywitz BA, Shaywitz SE. Dyslexia. In: Swaiman KF (Ed). Pediatric Neurology: Principles and Practice, 3rd edition. St. Louis, MO: C.V. Mosby; 1999. pp. 857-94.
13. The Diagnostic and Statistical Manual of Mental Disorders, 4th edition, Text Revision (DSM-IV-TR) and DSM 5. Washington DC: American Psychiatric Association; 1994.
14. World Health Organization. The International Classification of Diseases, Volume 10: Classification of Mental and Behavioral Disorders. Geneva: World Health Organization; 1993.

CHAPTER 4

Developmental Coordination Disorder

Anjan Bhattacharya, Jewel Chakraborty

■ INTRODUCTION

Some children fail to perform the usual fine and gross motor tasks of daily living; they are casually branded as "clumsy," "lazy," "odd," or even "silly." These children are often victims of bullying and insults of all sorts. Even their parents, teachers, and near and dear can abuse them without realizing that these terms are detrimental. Many of them suffer from the malady of developmental coordination disorder (DCD). Developmental coordination difficulties are thought to affect between 5 and 10% of school-aged children. In the UK, these difficulties are often referred to as dyspraxia.

■ DEFINITION

Developmental coordination disorder is diagnosed when children do not develop normal motor coordination (coordination of movements involving the voluntary muscles) in keeping with their general developmental level.

Developmental coordination disorder is a common disorder affecting fine or gross motor coordination in children. DCD is distinct from other motor disorders such as cerebral palsy and occurs across the range of intellectual abilities. These may change over time depending on environmental demands and life experience. Children suffering from DCD often struggle with various physical activities and sports. Due to their limitations, they may appear somewhat awkward and clumsy. Their progression is slow when compared to other children. Children having dyspraxia or DCD encounter difficulty learning new movements. They also have limitations in transferring learned skills in different situations.

Developmental Coordination Disorder

EPIDEMIOLOGY

The exact causes of DCD in children are not known. It is thought to be caused by a disruption in the way messages from the brain are transmitted to the body. DCD is characterized by difficulty in planning smooth, coordinated movements. This leads to clumsiness and lack of coordination. Often, it can lead to problems with language, perception, and thought. DCD is a universal problem. Current estimates quote that as many as 6% of children between the ages of 5 and 11 years have DCD. Males and females are equally affected. But it is often seen that males are more commonly detected. It is also known to run in families.

In typically developing populations, the most frequently reported prevalence of DCD is 5–6%, and in preterm populations, the reported prevalence has varied between <10 and >50% depending on the definition of DCD, the sample size, and the sample composition. Prevalence rates are mostly based on cohorts born in the 1980s and 1990s and may not reflect outcomes after the advent of active perinatal care of the most immature children. In addition, there are very few recent studies that have reported associations between DCD and other comorbidities in children born extremely preterm.

DIAGNOSIS

The following are the diagnostic criteria as per the Diagnostic and Statistical Manual of Mental Disorders, Fifth Edition (DSM 5):

- The accusation and execution of coordinated motor skills are substantially below than expected given the individual's chronological age and opportunity for skill learning and use. Difficulties are manifested as clumsiness (e.g., dropping or bumping into objects) as well as slowness and inaccuracy of performance of motor skills (e.g., catching an object, using scissors and cutlery, handwriting, riding a bike, or participating in sports).
- The motor skill deficit in criterion A significantly and persistently interferes with activities of daily living appropriate to chronological age (e.g., self-care and self-maintenance) and impacts academic/school productivity, prevocational and vocational activities, leisure, and play.

- The onset of symptoms is in the early developmental period.
- The motor skill deficits are not better explained by intellectual disability (intellectual developmental disorder) or visual impairment and are not attributable to a neurological condition affecting movements (e.g., cerebral palsy, muscular dystrophy, degenerative disorder).

CLINICAL FEATURES

There are great variations in symptoms and signs. So the presentations vary widely. In some, this manifests as an inability to catch a ball or fashion a lace, while in others, DCD may present as an inability to draw objects or properly form printed letters.

There are six general groups of symptoms as follows:
1. General unsteadiness and slight shaking
2. Low muscular tone at rest (basal tone)
3. Consistently high muscle tone than normal
4. Inability to put subunits of the whole movement together (jerkiness)
5. Inability to produce written symbols
6. Nonsmooth movement associated with comorbidities

Comorbidities

Co-occurrence of various disease entities is well recognized for DCD:
- *Speech difficulties:* Dysarthria or subtler varieties and speech, language, and communication needs (SLCN)
- *Specific learning disabilities:* Dyslexia, dysgraphia, or dyscalculia
- *Attention and motor planning disorders:* Attention-deficit hyperactivity disorder (ADHD)/attention-deficit disorder (ADD)/hyperactivity disorder (HD) or deficits in attention, motor control, and perception (DAMP)
- *Eye–hand coordination disorders:* Visuospatial difficulties or orthoptic/optometric difficulties
- *Neurological diseases:* Epilepsy, cerebral palsy, or kernicterus
- *Genetic diseases:* Dysmorphisms, syndromes, or chromosomal abnormalities
- *Health conditions:* Obesity or atopy
- *Other:* Medication effects or nervous tics.

Secondary Morbidities or Impact

Although some children with milder variety can grow out of their DCD, about 9 out of 10 children are known to suffer throughout their life from the disease and/or its impact on their life, some of which are as follows:

- *Mental health problems:*
  - Low self-esteem
  - Chronic anguish
  - Depression
  - Miscellaneous, e.g., phobias, suicidal tendencies
- *Educational impact:*
  - Writing, reading, or spelling difficulties
  - Backbencher position
  - Bullying
  - Truancy, delinquency, school failure
  - Miscellaneous
- *Employment impairment:*
  - Avoid professions involving fine precision or visual discrimination, e.g., driving heavy vehicles or airplanes, fine machinery.
  - Occupational hazards, e.g., accident proneness
  - Miscellaneous
- *Social impairment:*
  - Stigmatization
  - Poor peer group acceptance
  - Behavioral problems, e.g., antisocial, substance abuse, criminality
  - Miscellaneous, e.g., leisure and recreational activities.

TREATMENT

As common to all developmental disorders, the management of the condition depends on the precise developmental diagnostic workup.

Screening

The Developmental Coordination Disorder Questionnaire (DCDQ) is a brief parent questionnaire designed to screen for coordination disorders in children aged 5-15 years. It was originally developed in the late 90s at the Alberta Children's Hospital, Calgary, Alberta, Canada. Through further study with a population-based sample of children, a revision has been developed, the DCDQ'07. It can be considered a valid clinical screening tool for children who have coordination challenges.

Role of Sensory Integration and Praxis Tests in Diagnosis of Developmental Dyspraxia

The condition *developmental dyspraxia* was first described by *A Jean Ayres*. He pioneered the theory of sensory integration (SI). Ayres interpreted that children with developmental dyspraxia often face challenges coping with various life situations, which may include normal childhood activities such as play, educational learning, and daily social behavior. The limitations of this disorder have a deep impact on these children and their daily life activities.

Developmental dyspraxia was first identified with a measuring instrument developed by Ayres in 1972 as the *Southern California Sensory Integration Test (SCSIT)* and then the *Sensory Integration and Praxis Tests (SIPT)* in 1989. Through the development of SCSIT and SIPT, initially Ayres and later Mulligan were able to correlate poor discrimination of tactile, vestibular, and proprioceptive input with dyspraxia. This confirmed association between developmental dyspraxia and sensory discrimination contributed to the development of management protocols for developmental dyspraxia.

Sensory integration is one of the key factors to approach developmental dyspraxia. To understand developmental dyspraxia, the three processes of praxis have to be approached from an SI perspective. Ideation, motor planning, and motor execution are processes which are usually implicated when praxis is deficient. Ayres and Mulligan identified the four types of dyspraxia: *Visiodyspraxia, somatodyspraxia, bilateral integration and sequencing deficits,* and *dyspraxia on verbal command.*

The SIPT measures visual, tactile, and kinesthetic perception as well as motor performance. It is composed of the following 17 tests. A prototype case with a low average score is represented in **Figure 1**.

1. Space visualizations
2. Figure-ground perception

Developmental Coordination Disorder

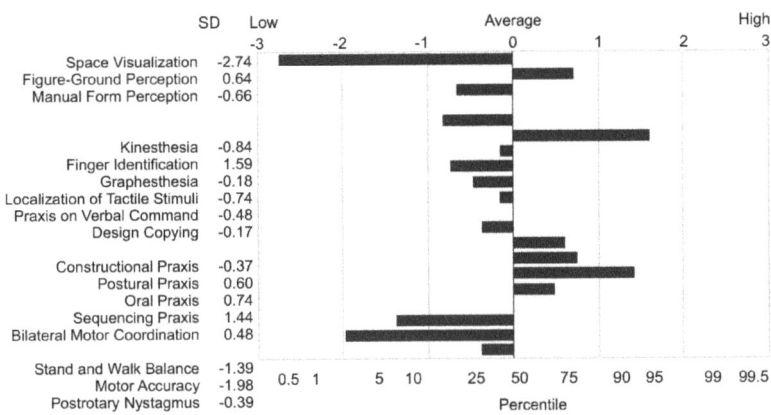

Fig. 1: Bar graph score shows the child has *low average scores* in the area of Figure-ground perception, Manual form perception, Kinesthesia, Graphesthesia, Localization of tactile stimuli, Praxis on verbal command, Design copying, Constructional praxis, Oral praxis, Bilateral motor coordination, Postrotary nystagmus, and Postural praxis.

3. Standing/walking balance
4. Design copying
5. Postural praxis
6. Bilateral motor coordination
7. Praxis on verbal command
8. Constructional praxis
9. Postrotary nystagmus
10. Motor accuracy
11. Sequencing praxis
12. Oral praxis
13. Manual form perception
14. Kinesthesia
15. Finger identification
16. Graphesthesia
17. Localization of tactile stimuli

The assessment is scored and interpreted through computerized scoring. The subject's raw scores are entered into the SIPT scoring program, which are converted to standard deviation (SD) scores. SIPT test results are expressed in SD scores. Scores between –1.0 and +1.0 SD are considered average, score of –2 to –1.0 suggests mild difficulties, score of −2.5 to −2 indicates definite dysfunction, and score of −3 to −2.5 indicates severe dysfunction. A score of +1.0 to +2.0 indicates above-average functioning and a score of +2.0 to +3.0 indicates advanced functioning. The computer-generated report describes each test and also the obtained standard score. It has a summary bar graph that depicts the major results and lists various scores such as the Standard Error of Measurement (SEM), SD scores, measurements of lateral function, and also an audit of test data. It also shows a summary graph comparing the child's SD scores to that of the significant cluster group mean scores.

The child has *definite dysfunction* in the areas of standing/walking balance and motor accuracy and *severe dysfunction* in the area of space visualization.

Six prototypic groups have been identified to describe the child's condition including dysfunctional, average, and superior patterns of SI. These six groups are as follows:
1. Low average bilateral integration and sequencing
2. Low average SI and praxis
3. Dyspraxia on verbal command
4. Generalized SI dysfunction
5. Visuo-and somatodyspraxia
6. High average SI and praxis

D-squared value of the SIPT scores indicates similarity to these six prototypic groups. A small D-squared value indicates a close fit and a large D-squared value indicates a poor fit with these six prototypic groups.

D-squared value of the below-mentioned scores in **Figure 2** indicates that the child has *low average bilateral integration and sequencing dysfunction.*

Precise tools like SIPT thus help pinpoint the functional barrier, which helps clinicians to target management precisely and accurately. Wherever properly *trained* professionals are employed to identify and treat these conditions, the results are rewarding to a surprising extent.

International Classification of Functioning (ICF) is another tool from the World Health Organization (WHO) that helps planning holistically in managing the child's all necessary aspects of management. A competent coordinating professional, like

Developmental Coordination Disorder

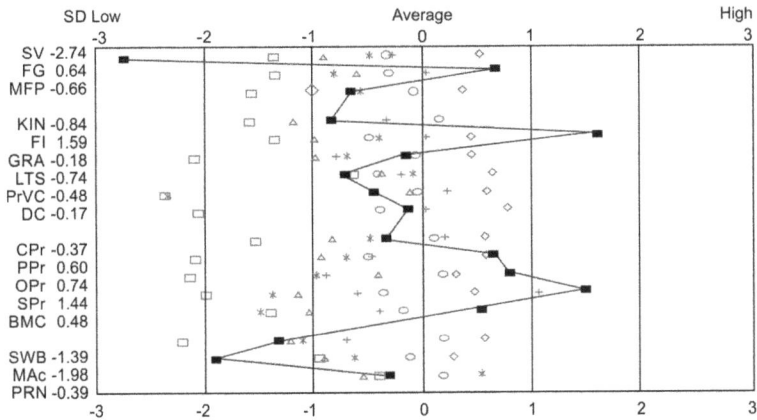

Fig. 2: D-squared value compared to diagnostic prototypes. (BMC: bilateral motor coordination; CPr: constructional praxis; DC: design copying; FG: figure-ground perception; FI: finger identification; GRA: graphethesia; KIN: kinesthesia; LTS: localized tactile stimuli; MAc: motor accuracy; MFP: manual form perception; OPr: oral praxis; PPr: postural praxis; PRN: postrotary nystagmus; PrVC: praxis verbal command; SPr: sequencing praxis; SWB: stand and walk balance)

a developmental pediatrician of quality, can ensure complex multidisciplinary care coordination in a simple and deliverable manner compared to incompetent handling, which is both cost-intensive and suboptimally effective.

Management

Primary care: Doctors, child health doctors, school nurses, school-based school health professionals such as special educational need coordinator (SENCO), teachers, social workers, and parents have a statutory (legal) obligation to refer the child "at risk" to school health team or community child health clinic.

Secondary care: Screening and referral to Child Development Centre (CDC), if concern persists with local advice and support until definitive management is instituted.

Tertiary care: Every borough (equivalent to Zilla or Talukas in the Indian system) in the UK has a Child Development Centre or equivalent to rule out other developmental disorders and institute early intervention (EI) to remediate if a definitive diagnosis is made.

Components of Management

Management involves EI involving a multidisciplinary team (MDT). The management modalities involve the following:

Therapeutic management: Remediation

School-based management: School health team

Resourced information and advice: Health education and information

Medical management: Primarily regular health promotional and preventative work and secondarily medication for comorbidities, advice and training for disability limitation, care coordination, transitional care modules, etc.

It is important to encourage children with DCD to actively participate in and get involved in physical activities. Swimming is a simple activity which is particularly good for children with DCD. It is basically repetitive sequential movements. Most importantly, it is not complicated and unpredictable as any team and ball games. Sometimes, it is difficult to learn the early skills but children should be encouraged to persevere as he or she will eventually become quite proficient. Swimming can also aid in the development of balance, physical strength, body flexibility, endurance, and coordination along with the enhancement of self-esteem and social skills. These children need constant encouragement and individual-focused attention to prevent them from quickly becoming dissatisfied and disillusioned.

GUIDELINES FOR PARENTS

- Reward the efforts.
- Participation and imbibing fun should be encouraged in all activities rather than competition.
- To start with, skills in smaller, more manageable parts should be taught.
- Give clear, concise instructions and repeat these for the child if necessary.
- It may be helpful to use pictures to illustrate the required action if the child has real difficulty focusing on verbal instructions.
- Swimming is particularly beneficial for children with DCD as it is made up of repetitive sequences of movements and it is not as complicated and unpredictable as team and ball games.

BIBLIOGRAPHY

1. Alloway TP, Archibald L. Working memory and learning in children with developmental coordination disorder and specific language impairment. J Learn Disabil. 2008;41(3):251-62.
2. Alloway TP. Working memory, reading, and mathematical skills in children with developmental coordination disorder. J Exp Child Psychol. 2007;96(1):20-36.
3. Ayres AJ. Interpretation of the SIPT scores. In: Ayres AJ (Ed). Sensory Integration and Praxis Tests Manual. Updated Edition. Los Angeles: Western Psychological Services; 2004. pp. 131-52.
4. Ayres AJ. Sensory Integration and the Child. 25th Anniversary Edition, revised and updated by Pediatric Therapy Network. Los Angeles: Western Psychological Services; 2005.
5. Barnhardt C, Borsting E, Deland P, Pham N, Vu T. Relationship between visual-motor integration and spatial organization of written language and math. Optom Vis Sci. 2005;82:138-43.
6. Barnhart RC, Davenport MJ, Epps SB, Nordiquist VM. Developmental coordination disorder. Phys Ther. 2003;83(8):722-31.
7. Beery KE. The Beery-Buktenica Developmental Test of Visual-Motor Integration: VMI with Supplemental Developmental Tests of Visual Perception and Motor Coordination: Administration, Scoring and Teaching Manual. Parsippany, NJ: Modern Curriculum Press; 1997.
8. Bolk J, Farooqi A, Hafström M, Åden U, Serenius F. Developmental coordination disorder and its association with developmental comorbidities at 6.5 years in apparently healthy children born extremely preterm. JAMA Pediatr. 2018;172(8):765-74.
9. Broeck JV, Ramokolo V, Dierkes J. Good clinical practice. In: Epidemiology: Principles and Practical Guidelines. Berlin: Springer; 2013. pp. 401-14.
10. Bundy AC, Murray EA. Sensory integration: a Jean Ayres' theory revisited. In: Bundy AC, Lane SJ, Murray EA (Eds). Sensory Integration Theory and Practice, 2nd edition. Philadelphia: FA Davis Company; 2002. pp. 3-33.
11. Butterfield SA, Loovis EM. Influence of age, sex, balance, and sport participation on development of throwing by children in grades K-8. Percept Mot Skills. 1993;76:459-64.
12. Cairney J, Hay JA, Faught BE, Hawes R. Developmental coordination disorder and overweight and obesity in children aged 9-14 y. Int J Obes (Lond). 2005;29:369-72.
13. Crawford SG, Brenda NW, Dewey D. Identifying developmental coordination disorder: consistency between tests. Phys Occup Ther Pediatr. 2001;20:29-50.

14. Dewey D, Cantell M, Crawford SG. Motor and gestural performance in children with autism spectrum disorders, developmental coordination disorder, and/or attention deficit hyperactivity disorder. J Int Neuropsychol Soc. 2007;13(2):246-56.
15. Dewey D, Kaplan BJ, Crawford SG, Wilson BN. Developmental coordination disorder: associated problems in attention, learning, and psychosocial adjustment. Hum Mov Sci. 2002;21(5-6):905-18.
16. Dewey D, Wilson BN. Developmental coordination disorder: what is it? Phys Occup Ther Pediatr. 2001;20(2-3):5-27.
17. Diagnostic and Statistical Manual of Mental Disorders, 5th edition. Washington DC: American Psychiatric Association; 2013.
18. Gains R, Missiuna C. Early identification: are speech/language-impaired toddlers at increased risk for Developmental Coordination Disorder? Child Care Health Dev. 2007;33(3):325-32.
19. Gibbs J, Appleton J, Appleton R. Dyspraxia or developmental coordination disorder? Unravelling the enigma. Arch Dis Child. 2007;92:534-9.
20. Gillberg G, Kadesjö B. Why bother about clumsiness? The implications of having developmental coordination disorder (DCD). Neural Plast. 2003;10(1-2):59-68.
21. Green D, Bishop T, Wilson B, Crawford S, Hooper R, Kaplan B, et al. Is questionnaire-based screening part of the solution to waiting lists for children with developmental coordination disorder? Br J Occup Ther. 2005;68(1):2-10.
22. Hurst CMF, Van de Weyer S, Smith C, Adler PM. Improvements in performance following optometric vision therapy in a child with dyspraxia. Ophthalmic Physiol Opt. 2006;26(2):199-210.
23. Jellinek MS, Murphy JM, Little M, Maria EP, Comer DM, Kelleher KJ. Use of the Pediatric Symptom Checklist to screen for psychosocial problems in pediatric primary care: a national feasibility study. Arch Pediatr Adolesc Med. 1999;153(3):254-60.
24. Kadesjo B, Gillberg C. Tourette's disorder: epidemiology and comorbidity in primary school children. J Am Acad Child Adolesc Psychiatry. 2009;39(5):548-55.
25. Lingam R, Hunt L, Golding J, Jongmans M, Emond A. Prevalence of developmental coordination disorder using the DSM-IV at 7 years of age: a UK population-based study. Am J Pediatr. 2009;123(4):e693-700.
26. Pal DK, Li W, Clarke T, Lieberman P, Strug LJ. Pleiotropic effects of the 11p13 locus on developmental verbal dyspraxia and EEG centrotemporal sharp waves. Genes Brain Behav. 2010;9(8):1004-12.
27. Peters JM, Barnett AL, Henderson SE. Clumsiness, dyspraxia and developmental co-ordination disorder: how do health and educational

professionals in the UK define the terms? Child Care Health Dev. 2001;27(5):399-412.
28. Rasmussen P, Gillberg C. Natural outcome of ADHD with developmental coordination disorder at age 22 years: a controlled, longitudinal, community-based study. J Am Acad Child Adolesc Psychiatry. 2009;39(11):1424-31.
29. Richardson AJ, Montgomery P. The Oxford–Durham Study: a randomized, controlled trial of dietary supplementation with fatty acids in children with developmental coordination disorder. Pediatrics. 2005;115(5):1360-6.
30. Scabar A, Devescovi R, Blason L, Bravar L, Carrozzi M. Comorbidity of DCD and SLI: significance of epileptiform activity during sleep. Child Care Health Dev. 2006;32(6):733-9.
31. Stevenson J. Recent research on food additives: implications for CAMH. Child Adolesc Ment Health. 2010;15(3):130-3.
32. Visser J. Developmental coordination disorder: a review of research on subtypes and comorbidities. Hum Mov Sci. 2003;22:479-93.

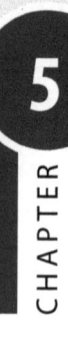

Stereotypic Movement Disorder

Jaydeep Choudhury

■ INTRODUCTION

Stereotypic movements are purposeless, repetitive, mostly rhythmic movements that can be voluntarily suppressed. Stereotypic movement is a nonfunctional motor behavior that seems to be compulsive. Some movements such as head banging, body rocking, or hand flapping are self-soothing or self-stimulating. To some extent, it occurs in normal children. But, it occurs with increased frequency in children with autism and mental retardation. Certain habits such as nail biting, thumb sucking, and nose picking are not included in stereotypic movement disorders as they rarely cause impairment. Stereotypic movements such as head banging, face slapping, hand biting, and eye poking can cause significant self-harm.

■ EPIDEMIOLOGY

About 7% of normal children have transient stereotypic movements. The prevalence is up to 20% in children <6 years. Nail biting is a common problem and affects almost 50% school-age children. Thumb sucking and rocking are normal in young children, but they are maladaptive in older children and adolescents. These types of isolated disorders do not constitute a stereotypic movement disorder. The causes of pathological stereotypic movement disorder are as below:
- Mental retardation
- Autism spectrum disorder
- Rett syndrome
- Williams syndrome
- Tardive dyskinesia
- Akathisia
- Neuroacanthocytosis

- Schizophrenia
- Catatonia
- Obsessive-compulsive disorder
- Tourette syndrome
- Restless legs syndrome
- Epileptic automatism
- Psychogenic

Stereotypic behavior is more common in boys. It is common among children with mental retardation; about 10–20% children are affected. The incidence of self-injurious behavior in children and adolescents with mental retardation is 2–3%. Self-injurious behaviors are also seen in Lesch–Nyhan syndrome and some patients with Tourette's disorder. Stereotypic behaviors are common in children with sensory impairments such as deafness and blindness. Genetic disorders such as Lesch–Nyhan syndrome, Rett syndrome, fragile X syndrome, Cornelia de Lange syndrome, and Smith–Magenis syndrome have stereotypic movement disorders.

DIAGNOSTIC CRITERIA

- Repetitive, seemingly driven and apparently purposeless motor behavior (e.g., hand shaking or waving, body rocking, head banging, self-biting, and hitting own body)
- Repetitive motor behavior interferes with social, academic, or other activities and may result in self-injury.
- Onset is in the early developmental period.
- The repetitive motor behavior is not attributable to the psychological effects of a substance or neurological condition and is not better explained by another neurodevelopmental or mental disorder (e.g., trichotillomania or obsessive-compulsive disorder).

CLINICAL FEATURES

- Onset is usually before 3 years of age.
- Most children have almost daily occurrence, but typically, it does not occur during sleep.
- The typical duration of episodes lasts <10 seconds in about one-third of patients, and it may last >60 seconds in another third. So, the range is wide.

- The movement generally involves flapping, shaking, clenching–stiffening–posturing.
- Triggers include various conditions such as sudden excitement, boredom, being focused or engrossed in some activity, and sometimes anxiety or stress.
- Some children may have comorbid attention-deficit hyperactivity disorder (ADHD) or learning disability (LD).
- There may be a history of similar stereotypies in family members.

Rett syndrome: It is a typical example of such a disorder. It is characterized by marked stereotypies. This condition is also one of the most frequent causes of mental retardation in females. Most cases of Rett syndrome are caused by mutations in the gene for methyl-CpG-binding protein 2 (MeCP2).

The onset of typical clinical presentation is at 6–18 months of age in girls with previously normal growth and development. The affected patients gradually regress in their verbal and motor skills. They lose purposeful use of their hands, and they often have jerky ataxia and typical stereotyped movements of the hands. It may resemble handwashing and kneading movements. Some other symptoms include breath-holding spells, hyperventilation, loss of facial expression, poor eye contact, bruxism, dystonia, occasional seizures, and apparent insensitivity to pain. They may have a variety of self-injurious and aggressive behaviors.

Features to be specified:
- Child with self-injurious behavior (or even behavior that would result in an injury if preventive measures were not used)
- Child without self-injurious behavior
- If the child is associated with a known medical or genetic condition, neurodevelopmental disorder, or other factors, such as Lesch–Nyhan syndrome, intellectual disability, and intrauterine alcohol exposure.

Severity

Mild: When symptoms are easily suppressed by sensory stimulus or some distraction.

Moderate: If symptoms require explicit protective measures and behavioral modification.

Severe: Symptoms which require continuous monitoring and when protective measures are required to prevent serious physical injury.

Differential Diagnosis

Normal Development

To some extent, simple stereotypic movements are common in infancy and early childhood. Rocking movements may occur in transition from sleep to awake phase, and resolve with age. The disorders are suppressed by distraction and sensory stimulation.

Autism Spectrum Disorder

Characteristically, some stereotypic movements may be the presenting feature of autism spectrum disorder. The distinguishing feature is the lack of social communication in autism spectrum disorder.

Tic Disorder

Typically, stereotypic disorders are earlier in onset, at about 3 years of age than tic disorders which start usually at 5-7 years. The former is consistent in pattern and topography than tics, which are variable. Both are reduced by distraction.

Other Neurological Conditions

Mannerisms, habits, paroxysmal dyskinesia, and chorea may present like stereotypic disorders. Neurological examination helps to exclude these conditions.

COURSE AND OUTCOME

Most of the normal children who exhibit rhythmic activities that seem purposeful and comforting seem to disappear by 4 years age. Stereotypic behaviors when accompanied by intellectual inability or autism spectrum disorder tend to fluctuate in episodes and severity. In some patients, stereotypic behaviors are prominent in early childhood and diminish as the child grows older. Children who have frequent, severe, self-injurious stereotypic behaviors have poor prognosis.

TREATMENT

Behavioral Modification

Habit reversal: The child is trained to replace the undesired repetitive behavior with a more acceptable behavior.

Differential reinforcement: Reducing unwanted behavior.

Drugs

Drugs are indicated only to minimize self-injury to children. Phenothiazines, dopamine antagonists, and opiate antagonists have been used.

GUIDELINES FOR PARENTS

- Stereotypic behaviors, to some extent, are normal behavior in children.
- Parents can try to distract the child to interrupt stereotypic behaviors.
- Scolding often complicates the situation and causes exacerbation when they are out of reach of their parents.
- Medical intervention should be sought when stereotypic behaviors lead to self-injury or it is accompanied by other conditions.

BIBLIOGRAPHY

1. Diagnostic and Statistical Manual of Mental Disorders, 5th edition. Washington DC: American Psychiatric Association; 2013.
2. Ghosh D, Rajan PV, Erenberg G. A comparative study of primary and secondary stereotypies. J Child Neurol. 2013;28:1562.
3. Sadock BJ, Sadock VA. Kaplan and Sadock's Concise Textbook of Child and Adolescent Psychiatry. Philadelphia: Lippincott Williams and Wilkins; 2009.
4. Sanger TD, Chen D, Fehlings DL, Hallett M, Lang AE, Mink JW, et al. Definition and classification of hyperkinetic movements in childhood. Mov Disord. 2010;25:1538.

Communication Disorders

Vibha Krishnamurthy, Alafiya Nasrulla

■ INTRODUCTION

Communication is a fundamental need for all human beings. Communication can be defined as the exchange of ideas verbally or nonverbally between people. Language can be defined as "a socially shared code or conventional system for representing concepts through the use of arbitrary symbols and rule-governed combinations of those symbols." When a child does not talk, or his language is delayed, it has far-reaching consequences on many aspects of his development, including school performance, social interactions, and emotional well-being. The parents of a language-delayed child will first turn to their pediatrician or primary healthcare provider for advice when they notice that their child's language is not like that of other children. It is therefore essential for every pediatrician to be aware of the course of normal language development and delays or deviations of the same.

■ COMPONENTS OF LANGUAGE

Language development can be broadly divided into two categories:
1. *Expressive language:* This is the means by which an individual relays or expresses thoughts or information to others.
2. *Receptive language:* It is the means by which an individual receives and understands messages from others.

Furthermore, primary components of language consist of the following:
- *Phonology:* It is the sound production of speech.
- *Morphology:* The structure of words
- *Syntax:* The grammar

- *Semantics:* The meaning of language
- *Pragmatics:* The appropriate usage of language, including the social context

NORMAL LANGUAGE DEVELOPMENT

Prelinguistic Period

When we think of the beginning of language development in a child, we usually think of the child's first words such as "mama" or "dada." However, language begins long before that, in early infancy. At the earliest, the infant's crying and response to sound are forms of communication. At 2–3 months, smiling and cooing appear. At 4–6 months, the infant laughs, blows raspberries. At 6–8 months, babbling begins and there is clear turn taking during interactions with adults. At 10–15 months, infants start to indicate desires as well as share with adults, using a combination of gestures and sounds.

Language Development in Toddler and Preschool Years

As in other streams of development, language development follows a predictable sequence. **Table 1** provides a broad outline of language development in the toddler and preschool child.

TABLE 1: Language development in toddler and preschool child.

Age	Comprehension	Expression
1–1.6 years	• Comprehends simple commands with cues • Can bring simple objects from another room • Indicates body parts on self	• Has a vocabulary of at least 10 words by 1.6 years • Names objects
1.6–2 years	• Points to pictures when named • Follows a two-step command by 2 years	• Two-word sentences • Uses one pronoun, e.g., my shoes
2–2.11 years	• Understands spatial concepts • Understands several pronouns	• Can express negation using negative forms • Combines 3–4 words in spontaneous speech

Contd...

Contd...

Age	Comprehension	Expression
	• Recognizes actions in picture • Understands use of object • Understands descriptive concepts	• Uses plurals • Answers what, where, and yes/no questions • Uses verb+ ing
3–3.11 years	• Understands spatial concepts, e.g., in, on, under • Understands negatives • Identifies colors • Compares objects • Makes inferences	• Describes how an object is used • Talks about remote events • Answers "when" questions
4–4.11 years	• Understands complex instructions • Understands descriptive concepts • Understands time concepts • Understands quantity concepts	• Describes a procedure • Names members of category • Defines words • Names categories • Responds to why questions by giving a reason

■ COMMUNICATION DISORDERS

The American Speech-Language-Hearing Association (ASHA) defines communication disorders as "disorders of speech (articulation, voice, resonance, and fluency), orofacial, myofunctional patterns, language, swallowing, cognitive communication, hearing, and balance." Communication impairments can either be congenital or acquired. Acquired communication impairments can be a result of accidents, traumas, illnesses, or environmental factors. Socioenvironmental factors include impoverished families in which shelter, food, hygiene, and medical care are affected.

Several research studies have identified that children raised in lower socioeconomic families have lower level of cognitive functioning, verbal ability, and academic achievement compared to economically advantaged families. Additionally, some studies in the United States found that factors such as lower maternal education, lower maternal age, and poor parent-child relationship predicted poorer language and academic achievement in children. Therefore, careful assessment of the child's environmental factors is also warranted as it can have far reaching effects on a child's language development and learning patterns.

ASSESSMENT OF THE CHILD WITH SUSPECTED COMMUNICATION DISORDER

History

A careful history with details of pregnancy and birth to look for risk factors for developmental delay as well as other conditions such as hearing loss is important. Details of all streams of development should be obtained to ascertain whether this is an isolated delay or a global developmental delay. Other information includes details of how the delay impacts the child's performance in school and interaction with peers. A family history of language delays, hearing loss, and learning disabilities should be obtained. As discussed above, history of the cause and background of socioenvironmental factors that may be affecting the child's communication should also be obtained.

Examination

Apart from a routine physical examination, this should include a search for dysmorphic features, detailed examination of the oromotor structures, and a thorough neurological examination. Every child with a communication disorder or language delays should have a formal audiology assessment.

Developmental screening for language skills should be done using a standardized tool. Below the age of 3 years, the ELMS (Early Language Milestone Scale) or the CLAMS (Clinical Linguistic and Auditory Milestone Scale) part of the Capute scales may be used. A scale developed in India is the 3D-LAT (three-dimensional language acquisition test). A developmental quotient (DQ) may be calculated for language skills by the formula: Language age/chronological age × 100. A DQ <70 is considered a delay and referral for further assessment and follow-up must be made. Formal language development of the older child may be beyond the scope of the routine pediatric visit. The following chart may be used as a guide for referral to a good speech and language pathologist.

Red Flags in a Preschooler

- Unintelligible >10% of the time
- Significant discrepancy between nonverbal tasks (e.g., puzzles) and communication
- Does not ask questions/dislikes or frustrated by questions
- Dislikes listening to stories
- Does not understand or like rhymes
- Frequently says "what" despite normal hearing
- Rarely talks spontaneously during play
- Cannot relate an event/story
- Substitutes semantically related words, for example, "*chair*" for "*sofa*" or "*knife*" for "*scissor*".

Possible Causes of Communication Impairments

The following are the differential diagnoses of communication impairments:
- Hearing deficit
- Global developmental delays/mental retardation
- Autism
- Selective mutism
- Developmental articulation disorder (e.g., cerebral palsy)
- Developmental language disorder (specific language impairment)
- Impoverished environment.

COMMON COMMUNICATION DISORDERS

Autism Spectrum Disorder

Autism spectrum disorder (ASD) is a developmental disorder characterized by core deficits in communication (receptive and expressive), social reciprocity, and play skills. In the early years, lack of reciprocity is seen in the form of children showing lack in joint attention and referencing. For example, the child might show no interest in looking at a book or toy together with a parent or in showing his parent a toy he likes. When the parent is looking at a toy with the child, the child may be more interested in examining the toy rather than sharing that interest with the parent. Since it is a spectrum disorder, symptoms can vary greatly from one child to another. Therefore, language characteristics in children with autism may also vary greatly. Some children on the spectrum may be verbal or nonverbal, in which case speech therapy can aid in teaching functional augmentative or alternate means of communication using graphic symbols, pictures, manual signs, or voice output communication aids. Verbal individuals with ASD may appear to have a good command of the language system, but in some instances, their language may reflect repetitions of dialogue heard elsewhere (echolalia) and/or vocabulary may not be as expansive as utterances suggest. Additionally, they may have difficulty understanding figurative language (idioms, metaphors, etc.), drawing inferences from conversations, understanding humor, and expanding meaning of specific words based on their context.

Although prevalence data of autism in India has not yet been established, the data released by the Centers for Disease Control in April 2012 places prevalence of autism in the United States at approximately 1 in 88 children. The pediatrician's role is crucial in recognizing the symptoms and diagnosing autism with appropriate diagnostic tools. Early identification and intervention are strongly recommended for children with ASD. Children should be referred to a speech-language pathologist and occupational therapist to teach functional communication and self-help skills to the child. A special educator and counselor referral can be made based on the needs of the child and family. When such specialized professionals are not available, as is often the case in India, it is important to use available resources such as local teachers and experienced parents. Empowering parents and helping them teach their child functional skills in various areas of development are crucial to the progress of the child.

Dysfluency or Stammering

This is a difficulty with the rate and rhythm of speech. Stammering or stuttering often begins in the preschool years and usually between 2 and 4 years of age. Three quarters of all those who begin to stutter will recover by late childhood, leaving about 1% of the population with a long-term problem. The physician's role is crucial in counseling the family and making an appropriate referral when stuttering appears to be severe or persists beyond the normal developmental speech dysfluency. Therapy ranges from parental counseling alone for very young children, to direct instruction for older children.

Disorders of Articulation and Phonology

In general, 75% of a child's speech should be intelligible to strangers by 3 years of age, and nearly 100% intelligible to strangers by 4 years of age. The acquisition of all speech sounds is expected to be complete by the 8th year of life, although there is considerable variability. Factors that can cause articulation disorders include hearing loss, structural disorders of the oral cavity (e.g., cleft palate), central nervous system disorders such as cerebral palsy and oromotor dyspraxia. Treatment ranges depending on the severity of the speech disorder from traditional speech therapy to the use of augmentative communication, i.e., the use of sign language, a communication board, etc.

Developmental Language Delay

Clinically, this is a diagnosis of exclusion. This usually occurs in children with normal intelligence quotient (IQ) and hearing. In these children, the language stream of development is significantly delayed as compared to nonlanguage areas of development. The delay may be in expressive language alone, or in expressive and receptive language. It is important that the language delays of these children be addressed at an early age as they are at high risk for reading and writing failure later in school.

LINK BETWEEN COMMUNICATION AND BEHAVIOR PROBLEMS

Children with communication disorders often find it difficult to express themselves. Many times, their basic wants and needs are not met due to poor expressive and receptive communication. A recent study conducted at the University of Minnesota found that young children with language delays/disorders are at an increased risk for behavior problems. In addition, strong expressive language skills appear to reduce the risk of behavior problems as rated by teachers.

Behaviors that children demonstrate are most likely to communicate a need. Behavioral manifestations in children could be due to a variety of reasons. Therefore, a functional behavioral assessment by a therapist or a pediatrician can help in determining the cause of the behavior, and subsequent steps can be taken to replace inappropriate behaviors with appropriate ones. Functional behavioral analysis involves asking the following questions to understand the behavior:
- How often does the problem behavior occur?
- In what settings do the behaviors occur?
- What events precede the behavior and what are the immediate events that follow the behavior?
- What is the function of the behavior-attention-seeking, wants to express a need, sensory seeking?
- What appropriate behavior can you teach the child to replace the unwanted behavior?

It is important to remember that "positive, nonaversive approaches to address challenging behaviors are the most effective, evidence-based practice for individuals with disabilities."

ROLE OF THE TEAM

Many children with speech and language delays will require an assessment by a multidisciplinary team. This is crucial to work your way through the differential diagnosis as given below, and the approach outlined in **Table 1**. The team members should include a pediatrician, speech and language pathologist, clinical psychologist, and audiologist. Depending on the child, involvement of an occupational therapist, behavior therapist, or special educator may be required.

It is crucial for every pediatrician to be vigilant for parental concerns regarding their child's speech and language. Pediatricians need to be aware of normal speech and language milestones and be familiar with at least one tool for the screening of speech and language delays. Screening should be followed up by definitive diagnostic evaluation by a speech and language therapist or a multidisciplinary team whenever possible. An audiology assessment is an essential part of every work-up for a child with language delays. Speech and language therapy should be provided for the child with language delays whenever appropriate. Diagnostic approach to a child with speech and language delay is shown in **Flowchart 1**.

As mentioned earlier, a pediatrician can utilize screening tools such as the ELMS/CLAMS/3D-LAT to evaluate a speech and language delay in a child with a suspected communication disorder. If there is no delay, it is important to reassure, monitor progress, and reevaluate the child in 6 months. If there is a delay, an audiological assessment is warranted. Depending on the nature of the hearing loss (sensorineural or conductive), referrals should be made to a team

Flowchart 1: Diagnostic approach to a child with speech and language delay.

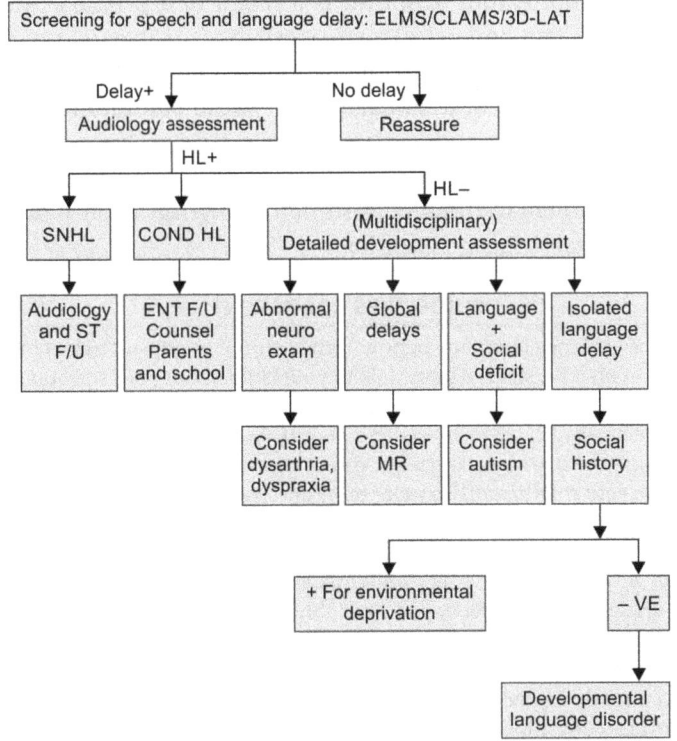

(CLAMS: Clinical Linguistic and Auditory Milestone Scale; COND HL: conductive hearing loss; ELMS: Early Language Milestone Scale; ENT: ear, nose, and throat; F/U: follow up; HL: hearing loss; MR: mental retardation; SNHL: sensory neural hearing loss; ST: speech therapy; 3D-LAT: three-dimensional language acquisition test)

consisting of an ENT (ear, nose, and throat) specialist, audiologist, and speech therapist. If an audiological assessment is negative for a hearing loss, a complete developmental assessment should be initiated. Ideally this should be an assessment by a multidisciplinary team. This could consist of a pediatrician, pediatric neurologist, speech and language pathologist, and clinical psychologist, depending on the presentation of the child's cognitive-linguistic abilities and overall developmental concerns. The evaluation should determine the pattern of development and look at whether there is delay, dissociation, or deviation across various streams of development. Based on the evaluation, it can be determined if the child's communication disorder is a result of a primarily motor disorder (e.g., cerebral palsy), or suggestive of involvement of more than one stream of development, for example, global developmental delays or deficits in both language and social communication, as in autism. If an isolated language delay is present, a careful social history should be obtained to determine if a deprivation in the socioenvironmental structure exists or the language delay is due to a developmental language disorder.

GUIDELINES FOR PARENTS

- *Start early:* Since language begins from birth, it is important to talk to your child even if he/she is a baby. Talk to your child about your surroundings. Label objects/situations in the surrounding. Be animated when talking to your baby so they are looking at you. As your child is growing, talk through the day regarding what you or your child is doing.
- *Follow your child's lead:* Use motivators and your child's interest to interact with him/her. Involve yourself in your child's play so that you can increase your child's engagement with you. Make learning fun and interactive—take turns with your child while playing, sing nursery rhymes, action songs, and story books he/she likes. When speaking or playing with your child, bend down and be at their eye level so you have their attention.
- *Model and expand language:* Adjust your language to your child's level and provide models of language. For example, if your child is using one word to communicate, model a two-word response. Avoid asking too many questions to your child, comment on their play instead. Use visual cues such as gestures and pictures while speaking and giving directions to your child. Remember the three S—Simplify your language, Speak slowly, Stress important words.

Contd...

Contd...

- *Waiting is important:* Create opportunities for your child to communicate by waiting for him/her to initiate or respond during play activities that your child enjoys. Takes Two to Talk® Hanen program outlines the OWL model → Observe, Wait, and Listen. Observe what your child is doing. Wait for your child's initiation or response. Listen to what your child is saying as it boosts their self-confidence and self-esteem.
- *Read to your child:* When your baby is 3–4 months old, start looking at picture books together. By the time your child is 8–9 months old, set aside a short time every day to read aloud. Read story books to your child to improve his/her listening skills. Make reading fun and interactive by being animated, modulating your voice, and showing pictures in the book.
- Give a lot of praise to your child to encourage and motivate language development further.

■ BIBLIOGRAPHY

1. American Speech-Language Hearing Association (ASHA). (2006). Guidelines for speech-language pathologists in diagnosis, assessment, and treatment of autism spectrum disorders across the life span. [online] Available from chrome-extension://efaidnbmnnnibpcajpcglclefindmkaj/https://faculty.washington.edu/jct6/ASHAGuideLinesAutismAssessmentScreening.pdf [Last accessed August, 2023].
2. Bradley RH, Whiteside-Mansell L. Children in poverty. In: Ammerman RT, Hersen M (Eds). Handbook of Prevention and Treatment with Children and Adolescents: Intervention in the Real World Context. New York, NY: John Wiley and Sons; 1997. pp. 13-58.
3. Caputo AJ, Palmer FB, Shapiro BK, Wachtel RC, Schmidt S, Ross A. Clinical linguistic and auditory milestone scale: prediction of cognition in infancy. Dev Med Child Neurol. 1986;28:76271.
4. Centers for Disease Control and Prevention. (2012). Data and statistics on autism spectrum disorder. [online] Available from http://www.cdc.gov/ncbddd/autism/data.html. [Last accessed August, 2023].
5. Coplan J. Early Language Milestone Scale. Tulsa, OK: Modern Education Corp.; 1983.
6. Dollaghan CA, Campbell TF, Paradise JL, Feldman HM, Janosky JE, Pitcairn DN, et al. Maternal education and measures of early speech and language. J Speech Lang Hear Res. 1999;42(6):1432-43.
7. Duncan GJ, Brooks-Gunn J, Klebanov PK. Economic deprivation and early childhood development. Child Dev. 1994;65(2 Spec No):296318.

8. Frank D, Zuckerman B. Infancy and toddler years. In: Levine M, Carey W, Crocker A (Eds). Developmental-Behavioral Pediatrics, 2nd edition. Philadelphia: WB Saunders Co.; 1992. pp. 2738.
9. Guitar B, Conture E. The Child Who Stutters: To the Family Physician. Publication No. 24. Memphis: Stuttering Foundation of America; 1992. pp. 34.
10. Ingersoll B, Dvostcsak A. Teaching Social Communication to Children with Autism: A Manual for Parents. New York: Guilford Press; 2010.
11. Manolson A. It Takes Two to Talk. Toronto: The Hanen Center; 1992.
12. Owens RE. Language Development: An Introduction, 6th edition. Boston: Allyn and Bacon; 2005.
13. Panoscha R. The child who does not speak. In: Capute A, Accardo P (Eds). Developmental Disabilities in Infancy and Childhood, Vol II, 2nd edition. Baltimore: Paul H. Brookes Publishing Co.; 1996. pp. 337-45.
14. Preferred Practice Patterns for the Profession of Speech-Language Pathology. Rockville: American Speech-Language-Hearing Association (ASHA); 1997. p. I64iii.
15. Shonkoff J. Preschool. In: Levine M, Carey W, Crocker A (Eds). Developmental-Behavioral Pediatrics, 2nd edition. Philadelphia: WB Saunders Co.; 1992.
16. Vaidyanathan R. 3-Dimensional Language Acquisition Test. T.N.B.Y.L. Nair Hospital.
17. Van Ijzendoorn MH, Dijkstra J, Bus AG. Attachment, intelligence, and language: a meta-analysis. Social Dev. 1995;4:11528.
18. Vicker B. Social Communication and Language Characteristics Associated with High Functioning, Verbal Children and Adults with Autism Spectrum Disorder. Bloomington: Indiana Resource Center for Autism; 2009.
19. Wadsworth J, Taylor B, Osborn A, Butler N. Teenage mothering: child development at five years. J Child Psychol Psychiatry. 1984;25:30513.
20. Zimmerman IL, Steiner VG, Pond RE. Preschool Language Scale-3. San Antonio: The Psychological Corporation; 1992.

CHAPTER 7

Autism Spectrum Disorder

Shabina Ahmed

INTRODUCTION

Autism spectrum disorder (ASD) is an early onset neurodevelopmental disorder of the central nervous system which has a tremendous impact on the normal functioning of the brain, challenging child development, particularly of social, emotional, and communication competence, and all their activities are directed by their own self needs. Phenotypically, they appear disobedient, arrogant, and selfish; prefer to stay alone absorbed in their own world with minimal contact with people; and communicate with parents when they want something by pulling their hands and directing it to the item with minimal use of communicative language. They have limited ability to respond to the surrounding environment on command.

They are characterized by a set of behaviors:
- Impairment of social interactions
- Disordered verbal and nonverbal communication
- Limited ability to participate in imaginative play
- Preference for routine and insistence on sameness
- Repetitive and stereotyped mannerisms in some cases.

Symptoms of this condition are evident either from birth or may begin to appear after a period of normal development, but definitely by the time the child is 2½ years old.

Emergence of behavioral symptoms of ASD may follow various patterns:
- *Early onset:* Where symptoms become apparent shortly after birth (Kanner)
- *Plateau:* Where after a period of more or less typical development, the rate of acquisition of skills slows down and the child's development stagnates

- *Regression:* Where the child loses previously acquired skills of social and communication by 2 years of age
- *Delays plus loss:* Where there is a delay in acquisition of development followed by loss of acquired social communicative skills in the second year of life.

■ HISTORY AND EVOLUTION

Autism is not a modern predicament although its vast recognition emerged in recent times. In 1911, the word "autism" was coined by Eugen Blueler, a psychiatrist, the term coming from the Greek word "auto" meaning "self," and he considered it to be another manifestation of schizophrenia.

In 1938, Leo Kanner, an Austrian–American psychiatrist termed it "early infantile autism" and in 1943, autism was claimed to be an inborn developmental problem affecting the social and emotional perspective of the child. Another pioneer in autism research was Hans Asperger, a scientist and a pediatrician, who defined a specific type of high-functioning autism children and labeled it as Asperger's syndrome in 1944. The American Psychiatric Association in 1994 classified autism as a pervasive development disorder in the Diagnostic Statistical Manual-4 for children with the onset of distortions of multiple psychological functions involving social behavior and language. Pervasive developmental disorder (PDD) is the umbrella term that encompasses various conditions, which include autistic disorder, Asperger's disorder, childhood disintegrative disorder, Rett's disorder, and pervasive developmental disorder-not specified (PDD-NOS).

Pervasive developmental disorder-not specified is a group of disorders which has an unusual presentation of autism at a later age of onset and the symptoms fall below the threshold for clinical impairment. The term PDD is somewhat misleading as the deficits shown are not fully pervasive and there is great variability in their presentation; hence, in 1960, Lorna Wing gave the term Autism Spectrum Disorder. In 2013, autism has been addressed in the Diagnostic and Statistical Manual of Mental Disorders, Fifth Edition (DSM 5) as a specific identity of ASD and that all other conditions mentioned earlier under PDD are only different presentations of the disorder. Rett's syndrome will become its own entity and not a part of the autism spectrum. These changes have been necessitated by the need to define the diagnosis in terms of severity, and it has been endorsed as a sensitive tool across age and all abilities.

INCIDENCE AND EPIDEMIOLOGY

There has been a dramatic increase in the prevalence of autism over the last few years. The US Center for Disease Control and Prevention (CDC, 2009) placed autism prevalence at 1:110 children. But recently, CDC has reported an increase in the prevalence to 1:88 children. Similar increases in autism have been observed worldwide (MMWR Surveillance Summaries). In another study in Korea, in association with the Yale Child Study Centre, Klinger et al., in 2011, found a prevalence rate of 1:38 among regular school children, who remained undiagnosed.

There are no studies on the incidence of autism in India; extrapolating from international data, the number of individuals with autism in India could be estimated to be approximately 2 million. Action for Autism (New Delhi) has cited the prevalence as 1:250.

However, the ratio of males to females diagnosed with autism has remained unchanged over the years at approximately 4:1.

CLINICAL FEATURES

The most important information one can gather to assist in formulating a diagnosis of autism relates to the child's development. The areas most impacted by the disorder are communication, socialization, and the demonstration of restrictive and repetitive behavior. Although there are no absolute makers, uneven skill development is the hallmark of autism. Certain behaviors and features tend to be more commonly encountered in children with autism, and the presence of one or more of these features should alert the treating doctor.

Socialization

These children prefer to be alone. They remain unaware of another person's existence.

- Do not respond to their name. They on many occasions appear deaf
- Tend to avoid gaze or sometimes show unusual eye contact
- Do not reach out spontaneously in anticipation of being picked up
- Do not seek comfort from others even when hurt or ill
- Do not reciprocate by smiling in response to parent's face or smile
- Have difficulty in interacting and playing with other children
- Do not finger point to ask for an object
- Do not try to attract attention of others to his/her own activity
- Do not look at an object across the room when an adult points at it
- Do not look at things adults like looking at
- Have difficulty taking usual turns in turn-taking games and activities
- Do not imitate adult actions
- Do not have pretend play, or have unusual or repetitive play, or have limited pretend play
- Do not cuddle, and stiffen when hugged or cuddled
- Like sameness in everyday routines. They may protest and resist changes in routine or surrounding.

Emotions

- Show apparent insensitivity to pain
- Show extreme distress for no obvious or apparent reason
- Appear unaware and insensitive to distress in others
- Have extreme unusual fears or have poor awareness of danger or do not show fear.

Communication

- Display good rote memory for nursery rhymes and some commercial jingles, which are often heard
- Often utter irrelevant talk
- Show delay or lack of language development or loss of early acquired language

- Rarely use gestures to communicate
- Lead adult by the arm to have needs met or use adult hand as an object
- Pronoun reversal
- Echo words or phrases (echolalia)
- Have difficulty initiating and sustaining conversation
- Do not address mother by her name in some cases.

Repetitive Action

- Display repetitive actions and asks repetitive questions
- Display unusual behavior or body movements such as spinning, hand flapping, head banging or rocking
- Enjoy revolving, rotating, or spinning objects or serially lining up objects, twirling twigs, or flapping paper
- Often occupied or even obsessed with parts of objects such as knobs, switches, and wheels.

There is great phenotypic heterogeneity; no two children of autism are the same, but social dysfunction has been the hallmark and unifying feature of autism since its initial description. It particularly affects both simple social behavior, for example, shared gaze, and complex social behaviors such as triadic attention sharing. In addition to the above, some children present with increased sensitivity to sound, touch, or light.

Thus, the basic problems in autism are as follows:
- Limited capacity for emotional involvement with others
- Limited capacity for understanding the mental state
- Limited capacity for abstraction and symbolism
- Altered capacity for sensory input modulation.

■ DIAGNOSTIC CRITERIA

To diagnose autism, we need to compare the individual's behavior with the criteria laid out in DSM 5 and the International Classification of Diseases, Tenth Revision (ICD-10). It may be pertinent to mention here that DSM 5 has been published in May 2013, and ICD-10 is under revision.

There is no medical or biological marker for ASD. There is an ongoing research to identify the problem by biological markers for evidence-based practice.

To be called autistic, a child must exhibit a given number of qualitatively impaired behaviors in each of the three categories mentioned in DSM 5.

The key features of DSM 5 are that they must show qualitative defects in all three domains of social and communication and two areas of restricted, repetitive pattern of behavior. These features must be present in early childhood and the symptoms limit everyday functioning. The latest development in the diagnostic process is a shift from categorical to dimensional and the new criteria try to fit in the medical conditions as specifiers and modifiers. For example, genetic disorders such as Rett's syndrome and fragile X syndrome as specifiers, and modifiers include, for example, seizures and intellectual disability. The cases are further defined according to the severity levels. It is based on the amount of support needed. They are labeled as follows: Level 1, level 2, or level 3.

Social deficits in ASD tend to precede impairment in other domains emerging within the first year of life.

The children of autism can be divided into three groups.

1. *Classical autism:* The symptomatology and behavioral characteristics conform to the abovementioned areas. There is good physical growth and the child is reared in a good home setting and parenting style.
2. *Double syndrome:* The child presents with features of autism with associated syndromic features as in Angelman's syndrome, Down syndrome, William's syndrome, and fragile X syndrome, to name a few.
3. *Transient autism:* There is a group of children who achieve motor development normally but have some features of atypical social, behavioral, or language aberrations, which start becoming evident around 18 months of age, the age when joint attention is the most prominent infant behavior. If intervention is started at this point, some children gradually show recovery and start reciprocal communication and gradually get imbibed into the social system.

Diagnostic Criteria According to DSM 5
Criterion A
Persistent deficits in social communication and social interaction across contexts, not accounted for by general developmental delays and manifested by all three of the following:
1. Deficits in social-emotional reciprocity, ranging from abnormal social approach and failure of normal back-and-forth conversation through reduced sharing of interests, emotions, and affect and response to total lack of initiation of social interaction
2. Deficits in nonverbal communication behaviors used for social interaction, ranging from poorly integrated verbal and nonverbal communication, through abnormalities in eye contact and body language, or developmental deficits in understanding and use of facial expressions or gestures.
3. Inability in developing and sustaining relationships, appropriate to developmental level of the child (beyond those with caregivers). It may range from difficulties adapting behavior to suit different social contexts through difficulties in performing imaginative play and in making friends to an apparent lack of interest in people.

Criterion B
Restricted, repetitive patterns of behavior, interest, or activities as manifested by at least two of the following:
- Stereotyped or repetitive speech, motor movements, or use of objects (such as simple motor stereotypies, echolalia, repetitive use of objects, or idiosyncratic phrases)
- Excessive adherence to routines, ritualized patterns of behavior of verbal or nonverbal communication, or excessive resistance to change (such as motoric rituals, insistence on the same route or food, repetitive questioning, or extreme distress at small changes)
- Highly restricted, fixated interests that are abnormal in intensity or focus (such as a strong attachment to or preoccupation with unusual objects, excessively circumscribed or perseverative interests)
- Hyper- or hyporeactivity to sensory input or unusual interest in sensory aspects of the environment, such as apparent

indifference to pain, heat, cold, adverse response to specific sounds or textures, excessive smelling or touching of objects, fascination with lights or spinning objects.

Criterion C
Symptoms must be present in early childhood (but may not become fully manifest until social demands exceed limited capacities).

Criterion D
Symptoms together limit and impair everyday functioning.

ASD DSM 5 Diagnosis: Specifiers and Modifiers
With the new criteria, if the child meets the criteria for ASD, he or she will receive a diagnosis with the etiology as a specifier, e.g., ASD with Rett's syndrome, ASD with fragile X. One can also receive a diagnosis with a modifier indicating another important factor, e.g., ASD with tonic-clonic seizure, ASD with intellectual disabilities.

Early history is also specified. This includes age and pattern of onset of loss of skills, e.g., ASD with onset before 20 months and loss of words, ASD with onset before 32 months and loss of social skills, ASD with no clear onset and no loss, or ASD-Asperger's type.

The levels of severity of ASD are shown in **Table 1**.

TABLE 1: Levels of severity of autism spectrum disorder (ASD).

Severity level for ASD	Social communication	Restrictive interests and repetitive
Level 1: Without support	Some significant deficits in social communication	Significant interference in at least one context
Level 2: Requires substantial support	Marked deficits with limited initiations and reduced or atypical responses	Obvious to the casual observer and occur across contexts
Level 3: Requires very substantial support	Minimal	Marked interference in daily life

Along with DSM 5, certain other diagnostic assessment tools need to be used. The gold standards for diagnostic assessment tools are parent-based ADI-R (Autism Diagnostic Interview-Revised), observation-based ADOS-2 (Autism Diagnostic Observation Schedule 2), and CARS-2 (Childhood Autism Rating Scale, Second Edition).

Further, a child's current developmental functioning, with a focus on speech and language communication, and cognitive and sensory evaluation, must be ascertained by appropriate professionals experienced in assessing ASD.

ETIOLOGY
Neurobiological Basis

Development disorders, such as autism, have generally presented formidable problems for scientific investigations. We do not yet have a specific cause for autism, but now there is agreement that a degree of brain dysfunction, however subtle, underlies the condition rather than a reaction to adverse environmental influence, given that all children of autism have some degree of social dysfunction. Neuropathology in the brain systems concerned with social information processing is the key focus in autism research. These deficits in the brain systems exert secondary peripheral impacts on the development of the child, and many of them have associated seizures and abnormal electroencephalogram (EEG) without seizures.

There are several hypothesized anatomic and neurophysiologic explanations for autism. The brainstem hypothesis of autism proposes that the etiology is related to the compromised brainstem and diencephalic structures. Courchesne's findings appear to implicate neurophysiologic abnormalities in the parietal and frontal association cortex. The different patterns or behavioral symptomatology in autism may result from neuropathology in restricted and different parts of the medial temporal lobe.

The recent understanding in ASD is the perception of biological motion. It has been observed that children with ASD display reduced sensitivity to human motion, which is linked to the superior temporal sulcus, and face perception to the fusiform gyrus.

Neurochemical Research

Research on autism has been performed for more than 30 years. Strong cases can be made for the possible involvement of the monoamine, dopamine, norepinephrine, serotonin, and neuropeptides such as opioids in autism, especially beta-endorphins and adrenocorticotropic hormone (ACTH).

Another line of peptide research has investigated patterns of urinary peptide excretions. Although several reports of marked differences in excretion patterns between autistic and control groups have appeared, the nonquantitative and subjective nature of the work has hindered replications and interpretation.

Genetic Factors

Hereditary factors in the etiology of idiopathic autism are well established, but particular genetic mechanisms have not been identified.

There is a higher genetic liability to autism in siblings of autistic probands than expected from the population prevalence. The condition runs with 2–3% of siblings affected. It appears likely that both parents and siblings have a higher liability for social cognitive deficits that are milder but conceptually similar to those found in autism. Concordance for autism is much higher in monozygotic than in dizygotic twins. Studies of extended families also support a strong genetic component to etiology as reported by Jorde et al. in 1990. A small number of cases have been described with chromosomal defects, especially the fragile X syndrome.

Etiology of diseases of epigenetic origin involves genes and the environment. Fifteen genes might be involved in ASD; the strongest evidence points to areas on chromosome 2, which has the homeobox or *HOX* genes that control growth and development very early in life. Chromosome 7 houses the *AUTS1* gene, related to speech and language disorders. The *MET* gene signals neocortical and cerebellar growth and maturation, immune function, and gastrointestinal repair.

In a minority of cases, the condition arises on the basis of a well-identified entity. This may be infective (congenital rubella), metabolic (phenylketonuria), genetic/developmental (tuberous sclerosis, Rett's syndrome), toxic (fetal alcohol syndrome), or of unproven etiology (e.g., infantile spasms).

Immune System Role in the Biology of Autism

The most recent research concerning the potential role of immune system dysfunction in autism has revealed a finding of autoantibodies targeting brain protein in children and their mothers, and this poses great potential as a biomarker for disease risk and may provide an avenue of therapeutics.

Emerging evidence over the last decade has clearly identified a range of medical and biological irregularities such as oxidative stress, neuroinflammations, mitochondrial dysfunction, abnormalities in glutathione, and a critical antioxidant and detoxifier. There is presently a growing sense of whole-body involvement, where the brain is affected in parallel to other systems. These suggest that environmental factors have a role in the inception and lifelong modulation of autism.

Associated Medical Conditions

Mental retardation: It is the most common comorbid condition with 75% of individuals of autism having mental retardation. The level of intelligence ultimately determines the adaptability and functionality of the child.

Seizures: Approximately one-third of the children of autism have seizure disorders. Seizures are more likely to emerge during infancy and adolescence. In fact, the discovery of a high incidence of seizures with autism revealed that it is a biological disorder rather than an emotional or a psychological one.

Savant skills: Some of the children have extraordinary skills, particularly in rote skills, mathematical calculation, and unusual talent in music or art.

Sensitivities and perceptual problems: They have certain sensory sensibilities and have difficulty filtering and processing sensory information in hearing, vision, touch, and smell.

CLINICAL FEATURES

Physical and neurological examination of children of autism generally is normal. However, checking specifically for signs and symptoms of medical conditions known to be associated with autism is important; for example, small or large head circumference, neurocutaneous signs of tuberous sclerosis, and facial features typical of fragile X syndrome can provide valuable clues.

LABORATORY TESTS AND IMAGING

Laboratory tests and brain imaging studies remain controversial. Some experts advocate EEG and brain magnetic resonance imaging for most children, while others tailor it to specific findings. But close attention to possible genetic or metabolic indications should guide clinicians' actions.

MANAGEMENT

There are no etiologically based treatments available to cure autism. Multidisciplinary team and parent partnership are essential in managing autism. This should begin with an explanation to the parents about the nature of the diagnosis, its probable cause and the way of helping the child, with its likely outcome, and that early intensive intervention can modify functionality.

Presently, the need of the hour is that pediatricians must take responsibility of early diagnosis of autism and involve the parents in providing comprehensive care of the child. Pediatricians need to create the optimum support system for parents by placing the issue in its proper perspective, avoiding delay in referrals, and initiating early intervention in centers that have the necessary resources that cater to this special population. It is necessary to reassure the parents that their parenting has not been the cause of this condition. Neither drugs nor psychotherapy has a place in the management. The main goals of management are as follows:

- Fostering of normal development
- Reduction of rigidity and stereotype that often dominate the life for the child and family
- Removal of maladaptive behavior
- Alleviation of family distress.

These goals are most likely to be met by a combination of counseling, behavior modification, and special schooling, encouraging normal development by parental participation in providing intense and stimulating experience for early vocalization and socialization.

Over the years, there have been treatments developed for children with autism evolving from different philosophies.

Behavioral intervention: Applied behavior analysis, discrete trial training, pivotal response training.

Developmental intervention: Greenspan Model, Denver Model, Early Start Denver Model, Cognitive Behavioral Model (TEEACH).

Augmentative or alternative communication system: For those nonverbal or limited-verbal language individuals.

Parent-mediated intervention: Longitudinal research has shown that responsive parental behaviors reliably predict subsequent language growth in children. Hence, there is now stress on a family centered approach for early interventional programs.
- Parents need to increase their fund of knowledge.
- They should accommodate different learning styles.
- They must use natural environments for teaching.
- Parents must play an active role in problem-solving.
- They should use functional words in communication.
- Parents must be able to synchronize with the child and recognize "ups and downs" of their child's social engagement.
- They should develop special playtime routine to develop eye contact, joint attention, and communicative gestures.

The models have to be carefully selected to suit the child, based on individual needs, strength, and family needs. Comprehensive treatments generally refer to those that address core deficits of autism disorder, across different contexts, such as communication, play, and aberrant behavior. Those with sensory problems, such as hyperacusis, and motor coordination problems, benefit from sensory integration and occupational therapy.

Delivery of intervention needs to be given in a special school with favorable teacher–pupil ratio in a highly structured and predictable.

However, many interventions claimed to cure or treat autism have not been scientifically established. There is a need for reliable methods for evaluating the effectiveness of an intervention.

Pharmacotherapeutics

No pharmacological strategy is available to treat the "core" features of autism. We are therefore forced to adopt a behavioral, dynamic, and psychopharmacotherapeutical approach when making a therapeutic decision using a dimensional approach to symptoms, rather than a categorical approach, because symptomatic improvement is the goal. It is useful to assess and classify the symptoms as follows:
- *Medication responsive:* Symptoms that may be medication responsive (hyperactive, obsession, rituals, and attention deficit)
- *Responsive to behavioral intervention:* Symptoms that may be responsive to behavioral intervention but may require medication (aggression, anxiety, depression, impulsivity, and sleep difficulties)
- *Nonresponsive to medication:* Symptoms which need specific skill remediation and are usually nonresponsive to medication (deficits in academic, social, or sport domains).

The dosage and range of psychotropic medication used in children and adolescents with autism are shown in **Table 2**.

Dietary Intervention

People with autism are more susceptible to allergies and food sensitivities than the average person. Hence, gluten- and casein-free diets seem to help some individuals.

Vitamins

Vitamin B_6 and magnesium continue to be suggested and there is some rationale since B_6 is related to neurotransmitter formation. Vitamin B_6, along with zinc and magnesium, are cofactors in the serotonin and other amino acid pathways. Clinical effects are sustained longer if magnesium is administered with the vitamin.

TABLE 2: Dosage and range of psychotropic medication used in children and adolescents with autism.

Symptom	Drug	Dosage
Inattention, hyperactivity, impulsivity, and behavioral symptoms of attention deficit hyperactivity disorder (ADHD)	Methylphenidate Dextroamphetamine Pemoline Imipramine Desipramine Clonidine	5–60 mg/day 2.5–40 mg/day 37.5–112.5 mg/day 10–20 mg/day In <6 years olds 10–75 mg/day In >6 years olds 50–150 mg/day 0.05–0.4 mg/day
Obsessions, compulsions, depression, chronic aggressive outbursts	Clomipramine Fluoxetine Fluvoxamine Sertraline Paroxetine Citalopram Venlafaxine	10–200 mg/day 10–60 mg/day 50–300 mg/day 25–150 mg/day 10–60 mg/day 20–30 mg/day 37.5–150 mg/day
Delusions, hallucinations, psychotic	Haloperidol Clozapine Pimozide Olanzapine Risperidone Quetiapine	0.5–8 mg/day (prepubertal) 1–16 mg/day (postpubertal) 50–600 mg/day 1–12 mg/day 2.5–20 mg/day 0.25–6 mg/day 25–250 mg/day
Epilepsy, symptoms, and prophylaxis of bipolar illness	Carbamazepine Sodium valproate Clonazepam	5–10 mg/L (serum level) 50–100 mg/L (serum level) 0.5–4 mg/day
Anxiety with hyperactivity, aggression, self-injurious behavior	Buspirone Naltrexone	10–45 mg/day 12.5–50 mg/day

Alerting Signs

Early suspicion and detection of children with ASD and referral for appropriate interventions can influence the long-term outcome. Hence, clinicians and health professionals must be familiar with the alerting signs. Parents often observe deviance in their children's development, and their observations could provide important information for early detection.

Recognition of early autism also depends upon the awareness of pediatricians and physicians, and other professionals whom the parents solicit help. It is important to put the child through common questionnaires and testing if there is suspicion of autism.

Early Alerting Signs

- 6 months—no big smile or other warm, joyful expressions
- 9 months—no back-and-forth sharing of sounds, smiles, or other facial expression
- 12 months—no back-and-forth gestures such as pointing, showing, reaching, or waving
- 16 months—no words
- 24 months—no two-word meaningful phrases
- At any age—any loss of speech or babbling or social skills.

The American Academy of Pediatrics (AAP) recommends that all children be screened for possible ASD at 18 months and 24–30 months of age in the context of routine developmental surveillance. Any child suspected to have deficits must go through a screening tool. The Modified Checklist for Autism in Toddlers (M-CHAT) is one of the several recommended tools. M-CHAT is shown in **Table 3**.

M-CHAT scoring instructions: A child fails the checklist when two or more critical items are failed or when any three items are failed. Yes/No answers convert to pass/fail responses. Below are listed the failed responses for each item on the M-CHAT. **Bold capitalized items are CRITICAL items.** Not all children who fail the checklist will meet the criteria for a diagnosis on the autism spectrum. However, children who fail the checklist should be evaluated in more depth by the physician or referred for a developmental evaluation with a specialist.

1. No	6. No	11. Yes	16. No	21. No
2. **NO**	7. **NO**	12. No	17. No	22. Yes
3. No	8. No	13. **NO**	18. Yes	23. No
4. No	9. **NO**	14. **NO**	19. No	
5. No	10. No	15. **NO**	20. Yes	

TABLE 3: M-CHAT table.

Parents to fill out the following about how the child usually is. If the behavior is rare, e.g., they have noticed it once or twice, consider that the child does not do it.

1.	Does your child enjoy being swung, bounced on your knees, etc.?	Yes	No
2.	Does your child take an interest in other children?	Yes	No
3.	Does your child like climbing on things, such as upstairs?	Yes	No
4.	Does your child enjoy playing peek-a-boo/hide-and-seek?	Yes	No
5.	Does your child ever pretend, for example, to talk on the phone or take care of dolls, or pretend other things?	Yes	No
6.	Does your child ever use his/her index finger to point, to ask for something?	Yes	No
7.	Does your child ever use his/her index finger to point, to indicate interest in something?	Yes	No
8.	Does your child look you in the eye for more than a second or two?	Yes	No
9.	Can your child play properly with small toys (e.g., cars or bricks) without just mouthing, fiddling, or dropping them?	Yes	No
10.	Does your child ever bring objects over to you (parent) to show you something?	Yes	No
11.	Does your child ever seem oversensitive to noise? (e.g., plugging ears)	Yes	No
12.	Does your child smile in response to your face or your smile?	Yes	No
13.	Does your child imitate you? (e.g., you make a face—will your child imitate it?)	Yes	No
14.	Does your child respond to his/her name when you call?	Yes	No
15.	If you point at a toy across the room, does your child look at it?	Yes	No
16.	Does your child walk?	Yes	No
17.	Does your child look at things you are looking at?	Yes	No
18.	Does your child try to attract your attention to his/her own activity?	Yes	No
19.	Have you ever wondered if your child is deaf?	Yes	No

Contd...

Contd...

20.	Does your child sometimes stare at nothing or wander with no purpose?	Yes	No
21.	Does your child look at faced with something unfamiliar?	Yes	No

(M-CHAT: Modified Checklist for Autism in Toddlers)

Source: Robins D, Fein D, Barton M, Green J. The Modified Checklist for Autism in Toddlers: an initial study investigating the early detection of autism and pervasive development disorder. J Autism Dev Disord. 2001;31(2):131-44.

Outcome

Autism is almost always a life-long condition. Approximately two-thirds of the diagnosed children remain dependent on adults throughout their lives and require continuing care at home. Only 10% achieve a significant degree of independence. 50% remain without spoken language, while 50% of individuals experience aggravation of their behavioral problems as they enter adolescence.

The best predictors of outcome for independent living are the measured intelligence of the child; those with a nonverbal IQ over 70 do well later on. Presence of socially useful language by 5 years of age and the early development of constructive play also show good progress in life.

GUIDELINES FOR PARENTS

- Everybody should learn about autism. The more one knows about ASDs, the better equipped one will be to make positive decisions for your child.
- Figure out what triggers your child's disruptive behaviors and what elicits a positive response.
- Practice acceptance. Enjoy your child's special quirks and celebrate small successes. Stop comparing your child to others. Feeling unconditionally loved and accepted will help your child more than anything else.
- Do not give up. It is impossible to predict the course of an ASD.
- Creating consistency in the child's environment is the most appropriate way to reinforce learning. Children with autism have a tough time adapting what they have learned in one setting to others, including the home. Explore the possibility of having therapy take place in more than one place in order to encourage your child to transfer what he or she has learned from one environment to another.

Contd...

Contd...

- Stick to a schedule. Children with autism tend to do best when they have a highly structured schedule or routine. Disruptions to the routine should be minimum. If there is an unavoidable schedule change, the child should be prepared well in advance.
- Good behavior should be rewarded. Positive reinforcement can be very effective in children with autism.
- Create a home safety zone. Certain modifications in the house may be necessary to make it safety proof, particularly if the child is prone to tantrums or other self-injurious behaviors.
- Look for nonverbal cues. Pay attention to the kinds of sounds they make, their facial expressions, and the gestures they use when they are tired, hungry, or want something.
- Figure out the need behind the tantrum. Throwing a tantrum is their way of communicating their frustration and getting your attention.
- Make time for fun. There are tremendous positive effects from your enjoyment of your child's company and from your child's enjoyment of spending quality unpressured time with you. Play is an essential part of learning and should not feel like compulsive work.
- Attention should be paid to the child's sensory sensitivities. Children with autism are usually hypersensitive to light, sound, touch, taste, and smell. Some children with autism are "undersensitive" to various sensory stimuli. Parents should understand what affects the child, thus they will be better at preventing situations that cause difficulties and creating good experiences.
- The child's treatment should be modified according to his or her individual needs.
- No matter what autism treatment plan is chosen, parents' involvement is vital to success. Parents can help the child get the most out of treatment by working hand in hand with the autism treatment team and following through with the therapy regularly at home.

BIBLIOGRAPHY

1. Ahmed S. Understanding of Autism, 2nd edition. Guwahati: EBH Publishers; 2008.
2. Autism and Developmental Disabilities Monitoring Network Surveillance Year 2008 Principal Investigators, Centers for Disease Control and Prevention. Prevalence of autism spectrum disorders—Autism and Developmental Disabilities Monitoring Network, 14 sites, United States, 2008. MMWR Surveill Summ. 2012;61(3):1-19.
3. Barua M. Action for Autism. [online] Available from: www.autism-india.org. [Last accessed August, 2023].

4. Cavine MD, Caney WB, Crocker AC. Developmental-Behavioral Pediatrics, 2nd edition. Philadelphia: W.B. Saunders; 1992. p. 593.
5. Coleman M. Clinical review: medical differential diagnosis and treatment of the autistic syndrome. Eur Child Adolesc Psychiatry. 1993;2(3):161-8.
6. Courchesne E. A neurophysiological view of autism. In: Schopler E, Mesibov G (Eds). Neurobiological Issue in Autism. New York: Plenum Press; 1987. pp. 258-324.
7. Diagnostic and Statistical Manual of Mental Disorders (DSM 5), 5th edition. Washington DC: American Psychiatric Association; 2013.
8. Diagnostic and Statistical Manual of Mental Disorders, 4th edition. Text Revision (DSM IV-TR). Washington DC: American Psychiatric Association; 2000.
9. Fox AM. An Introduction to Neurodevelopmental Disorders of Children. New Delhi: The National Trust; 2003.
10. Frequently Asked Questions. Ask IAP. Series-Basics and Beyond. IAP Action Plan. Mumbai: Indian Academy of Pediatrics; 2006. pp. 60-1.
11. Goines P, Van de Water J. The immune system's role in the biology of autism. Curr Opin Neurol. 2010;23:111-7.
12. Graham P, Turk J, Verhulst F. Child Psychiatry: A Developmental Approach. London: Oxford University Press; 1999.
13. Herbert MR. Contributions of the environment and environmentally vulnerable physiology to autism spectrum disorders. Curr Opin Neurol. 2010;23:103-10.
14. Jorde LB, Mason-Brothers A, Waldmann R, Ritvo ER, Freeman BJ, Pingree C, et al. The UCLA-University of Utah epidemiologic survey of autism: genealogical analysis of familial aggregation. Am J Med Genet. 1990;36:85-8.
15. Kanner C. Autistic disturbance of affective contact. Nervous Child. 1943;10:217-50.
16. Kent RG, Carrington S, Le Couteur A, Gould J, Wing L, Maljaars J, et al. Diagnosing autism spectrum disorder: who will get a DSM 5 diagnosis? J Child Psychol Psychiatry. 2013;54:1242-50.
17. Kim YS, Leventhal BL, Koh YJ, Fombonne E, Laska E, Lim EC, et al. Prevalence of autism spectrum disorders in a total population sample. Am J Psychiatry. 2011;168(9):904-12.
18. Landa RJ, Holman KC, Garrett-Mayer E. Social and communication development in toddlers with early and later diagnosis of autism spectrum disorders. Arch Gen Psychiatry. 2007;64:853-64.
19. Lelord G, Callaway E, Muh JP. Clinical and biological effects of high doses of vitamin B6 and magnesium on autistic children. Acta Vitaminol Enzymol. 1982;4(1-2):27-44.
20. Lord C, Rutter M, Le Couterer A. Autism Diagnostic Interview-Revised: a revised version of a diagnostic interview for caregivers of individuals

with possible pervasive developmental disorders. J Autism Dev Disord. 1994;24:659-85.
21. Luyster R, Richler J, Risi S, Hsu WL, Dawson G, Bernier R, et al. Early regression in social communication in autism spectrum disorders: a CPEA study. Dev Neuropsychol. 2005;27(3):311-36.
22. Mahoney WJ, Szatmam P, Maclean JE, Bryson SE, Bartolucci G, Walter SD, et al. Reliability and accuracy of differentiating pervasive developmental disorder subtypes. J Am Acad Child Adolesc Psychiatry. 1998;37:278-85.
23. McPartland JC, Coffmen M, Pelphrey KA. Recent advances in understanding the neural basis of autism. Curr Opin Paediatr. 2011;23:628-32.
24. Molloy CA, Murray DS, Akers R, Mitchell T, Manning-Courtney P. Use of the Autism Diagnostic Observation Schedule (ADOS) in a clinical setting. Autism. 2011;15(2):143-62.
25. Rimland B. Infantile Autism: The Syndrome and Its Implications for a Neural Theory of Behavior. New York: Appleton-Century-Crofts; 1962.
26. Robins D, Fein D, Barton M, Green J. The Modified Checklist for Autism in Toddlers: an initial study investigating the early detection of autism and pervasive developmental disorders. J Autism Dev Disord. 2001;31(2):131-44.
27. Siller M, Hutman T, Sigman M. A parent-mediated intervention to increase responsive parental behaviors and child communication in children with ASD: a randomized clinical trial. J Autism Dev Disord. 2013;42:540-55.
28. Suzanne L, Campbell D, Gengoux GW, Saulmier CA, Klin AJ, Chawarska K. Predicting developmental status from 12 to 24 months in infants at risk for autism spectrum disorder: a preliminary report. J Autism Dev Disord. 2012;42:2636-47.
29. Volkmar FR, Klin A, Siegel B, Szatmari P, Lord C, Campbell M, et al. Field trial for autistic disorder in DSM-IV. Am J Psychiatry. 1994;151:1361-7.
30. Wing L, Gould J. Severe impairments of social interaction and associated abnormalities in children: epidemiology and classification. J Autism Dev Disord. 1979;9:11-29.
31. World Health Organization. The ICD-10 Classification of Mental and Behavioral Disorder: Clinical Descriptions and Diagnostic Guidelines. Geneva: World Health Organization; 1992.
32. Zwaigenbaum L, Bryson S, Rogers T, Roberts W, Brian J, Szatmari P. Behavioral manifestations of autism in the first year of life. J Dev Neurosci. 2005;23:143-52.

CHAPTER 8

Attention-deficit/Hyperactivity Disorder

Jai Ranjan Ram, Jaydeep Choudhury

■ INTRODUCTION

The syndrome of restless, inattentive, and impulsive child behavior is known as attention-deficit/hyperactivity disorder (ADHD) in North America and hyperkinetic disorder (HD) in Europe. It is one of the most commonly diagnosed behavioral disorders of children, and it occurs in approximately 6–9% of school-aged children. It is more common in boys. As per the onset criteria of ADHD as laid down in the Diagnostic and Statistical Manual of Mental Disorders (DSM 5), the inattentive or hyperactive–impulsive symptoms are present prior to age 12 years.

Hyperactivity, a term commonly used to describe this behavior, is an ambiguous term and ideally should not be used by professionals. ADHD is the manifestation of a condition of the brain that makes it difficult for the children to control their behavior. It is caused by a complex interplay between genetic and environmental risk factors. These risk factors affect the structural and functional capacity of brain networks and lead to ADHD symptoms, neurocognitive deficits, and a wide range of functional impairment. Those with ADHD have trouble paying attention at home or in school. They are much more active and impulsive. These aspects of their behavior cause problems in learning, relationships, and day-to-day activity.

■ HISTORY AND NOMENCLATURE

About 2,500 years ago, Hippocrates described patients who had "quickened responses to sensory experience, but also less tenaciousness because the soul moves on quickly to the next impression." The evidence base for the diagnosis and management of ADHD has been evolving exponentially since the syndrome was first described by the German physician Melchior Adam Weikard in 1775. In 1937, the efficacy of amphetamine uses to reduce symptom severity was serendipitously discovered. In the 1940s, the brain was implicated as the source of ADHD-like symptoms, which were described as minimal brain damage in the wake of an encephalitis epidemic. In 1980, the third edition of the Diagnostic and Statistical Manual of Mental Disorders (DSM 3) created the first reliable operational diagnostic criteria for the disorder. These criteria initiated many programs of research that ultimately led the scientific community to view ADHD as a seriously impairing, often persistent neurobiological disorder of high prevalence. Differences in diagnostic criteria between Europe and North America were markedly obvious in the 1940s. Since then, various labels have been applied to the clinical condition. The use of different labels to describe children with ADHD had hampered the acceptance of this diagnosis as a legitimate condition. There is still enormous controversy and disquiet about whether the condition is overdiagnosed or underdiagnosed. The critics of the label ADHD have the view that it unnecessarily stigmatizes children and medicalizes their problems. The history of ADHD is presented in **Flowchart 1**.

In 1998, the National Institute of Mental Health, United States agreed that ADHD is a legitimate psychological condition even though its definition has not been fully penned down.

Diagnostically, there are three main groups of symptomatology—overactivity, impulsivity, and inattentiveness. For a diagnosis of HD under the International Classification of Diseases (ICD), the presence of all three is required. HD is viewed as a unitary condition. In the North American classificatory system DSM 5, there are three possible subtypes of ADHD, and the presence of one or two symptom clusters is enough to make a diagnosis. The three subtypes are hyperactive-impulsive, inattentive, and combined. It is the combined type that is most common and closest to HD.

ETIOLOGY

Attention-deficit/hyperactivity disorder is principally a behavioral diagnosis, and the disorder is heterogeneous. It does not have any

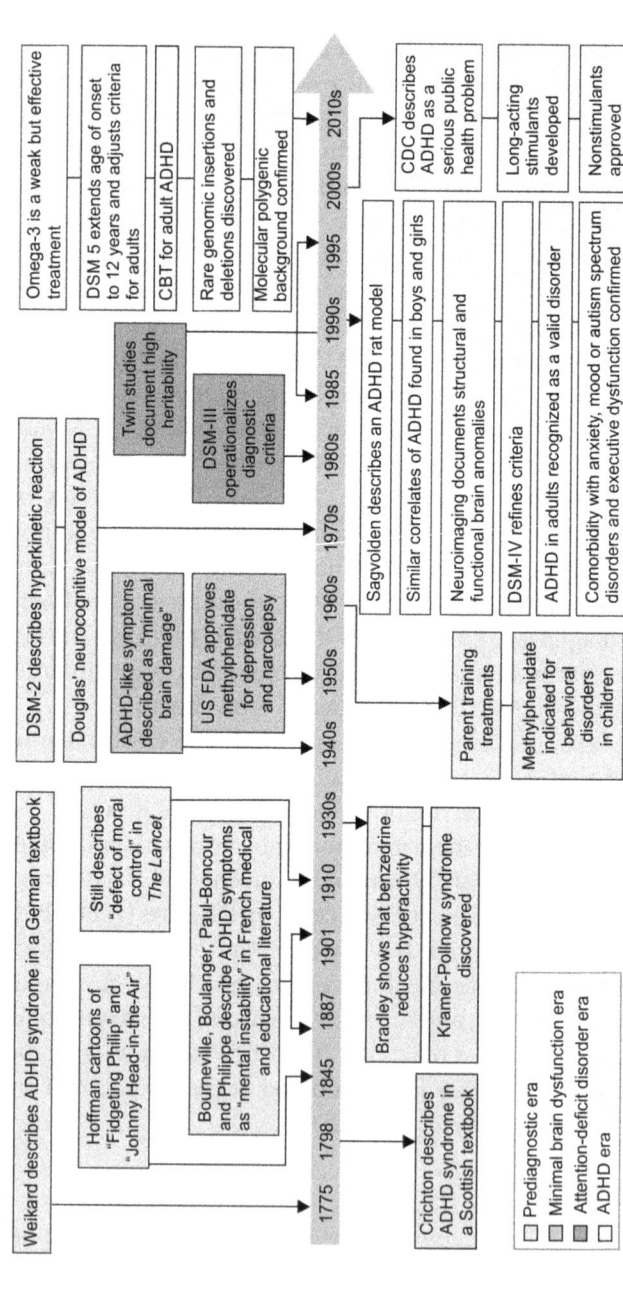

Flowchart 1: The history of attention-deficit/hyperactivity disorder (ADHD). ADHD "syndromes" have been described in the medical literature since the eighteenth century, but the growth of systematic research required the development of operational diagnostic criteria in the late twentieth century. This schematic outlines selected important developments in the history of ADHD research.

(CBT: cognitive-behavioral therapy; CDC: Centers for Disease Control and Prevention; DSM: Diagnostic and Statistical Manual of Mental Disorders; US FDA: United States Food and Drug Administration) single biological marker. Each of the various proposed etiologies leads to the same behavioral presentation.

Brain Dysfunction

The concept of minimal brain dysfunction (MBD) evolved in the 1960s. The impairments of perception, language, memory, attention, and motor activities were associated with functional problems in the central nervous system.

Anatomical Lesions

Various brain imaging studies, such as positron emission tomography (PET) and single photon emission computed tomography (SPECT), have demonstrated differences between children diagnosed with ADHD and controls. The differences are particularly in the anterior region and striatum.

Genetic and Biochemical

The first-degree relatives of children with ADHD have a five times greater risk for ADHD. Specific genes have not been found. Twin studies show that ADHD has a heritability of 70–80% in both children and adults, with little or no evidence that the effects of environmental risk factors shared by siblings substantially influence etiology. Environmental risk factors play their greatest part in the nonshared familial environment and/or act through interactions with genes and deoxyribonucleic acid (DNA) variants that regulate gene expression.

Environmental Risk Factors

The complexity of environmental risk factors makes it difficult to associate them with the cause of ADHD. Environmental associations might arise from multiple sources, such as from child or parental behaviors that shape the environment; sometimes, they might reflect unmeasured third variables. For example, children with ADHD might evoke "hostile" styles of parenting. Genes linked to ADHD might explain the association of certain parental variables, such as maternal smoking during pregnancy.

Some other environmental risk factors that have been associated with ADHD include prenatal and perinatal factors, such as maternal smoking and alcohol use, low birth weight, preterm birth, and exposure to certain environmental toxins, such as organophosphate pesticides, polychlorinated biphenyls, excessive zinc, and lead. Animal models have also contributed largely to the study of environmental risk factors. Similar to genetic risk factors, the effects of any particular environmental risk factor are small and could reflect either minor effects in many cases or major effects in a few cases. Furthermore, rather than being specific to ADHD, these environmental risk factors are associated with many other psychiatric disorders.

EPIDEMIOLOGY

The differences in diagnostic practice have had a profound impact on estimates of the prevalence of the disorder and its treatment. There have been concerns expressed in many quarters in North America and Europe regarding the overinclusiveness of the diagnosis and appropriateness of treating children with stimulant medication without exercising sufficient diagnostic rigor. The prevalence of ADHD is around 3–5%. It is more common in males, and the ratio of male to female ratio is 3:1 in community samples.

DIAGNOSIS

The diagnosis of ADHD is mainly clinical, based on the evaluation of the child, which includes interviews with parents about the child's development and behavior. Information from school, particularly from the teachers, is essential. The assessment is incomplete without input from the teachers. A direct examination of the child is also important. There are several semi-structured interviews that can be used and are better than questionnaires or diagnostic checklists as they elicit information from a range of situations.

The diagnostic criteria for ADHD in DSM 5 are similar to those in DSM-IV. Diagnosis by these criteria requires that the onset of symptoms must occur before the age of 12 years. The symptoms must be present for 6 months or longer. They should be pervasive across two or more major life settings (such as home and school).

Evidence will require information from more than one source, say from parents and teachers. Parental reports about classroom behavior are unlikely to be sufficient. The frequency and severity should be greater than those children at a compatible developmental level. The features should be clinically significant impairment in social, academic, or occupational functioning. Out of nine symptoms listed for each dimension, six are required to be present:

A. A persistent pattern of inattention and/or hyperactivity-impulsivity that interferes with functioning or development as characterized by 1 and/or 2.
   1. *Inattention:* Six or more of the following symptoms persisting for at least 6 months:
      i. Often fails to give close attention to details or makes careless errors in schoolwork, work, or other activities
      ii. Often fails to sustain attention in tasks or play activities
      iii. Often appears not to listen to what is being said to him
      iv. Often fails to follow through on instructions or to finish schoolwork, chores, or duties in the workplace (not because of oppositional behavior or failure to understand instruction)
      v. Often impaired in organizing tasks or activities.
      vi. Often avoids or strongly dislikes tasks such as homework that require sustained mental effort
      vii. Often loses things necessary for certain tasks or activities
      viii. Often easily distracted by external stimuli
      ix. Often forgetful in the course of daily activities
   2. *Hyperactivity-impulsivity:* Six or more of the following symptoms persisting for at least 6 months:

      Hyperactivity
      i. Often fidgets with hands or feet or squirms on seat
      ii. Often leaves seat in classroom or in other situations in which remaining seated is expected
      iii. Often runs about or climbs excessively in situations in which it is inappropriate (in adolescents, only subjective feelings of restlessness may remain)
      iv. Often has difficulty playing or engaging in leisure activities quietly

v. Often "on the go" or often acts as if "driven by a motor"
vi. Often talks excessively

Impulsivity
i. Often blurts out answers before questions have been completed
ii. Often has difficulty awaiting turn
iii. Often interrupts or intrudes on others

B. Several inattentive or hyperactive–impulsive symptoms were present prior to the age of 12 years.
C. Symptoms present in two or more settings (e.g., at home, school, or work; with friends or relatives; in other activities)
D. There is clear evidence that the symptoms interfere with or reduce the quality of social, academic, or academic functioning.

Specify Whether

Combined presentation: If both criterion A1 (inattention) and criterion A2 (hyperactive–impulsive) are met for the past 6 months. The majority of children and adolescents with ADHD have combined presentation.

Predominantly inattentive presentation: If criterion A1 (inattention) is met but criterion A2 (hyperactive–impulsive) is not met for the past 6 months.

Predominantly hyperactivity–impulsivity presentation: If criterion A2 (hyperactive–impulsive) is met but criterion A1 (inattention) is not met for the past 6 months.

Specify if

In partial remission: When full criteria were previously met, fewer than the full criteria have been met for the past 6 months, and the symptoms still result in impairment in social, academic, or occupational functioning.

Specify Current Severity

Mild: Symptoms result in minor impairment in social or occupational functioning.

Moderate: Symptoms or functional impairment between mild and severe are present.

Severe: Symptoms result in marked impairment in social or occupational functioning.

CLINICAL FEATURES

The cardinal features of ADHD are excessive and impairing levels of activity, inattention, and impulsiveness, which are a persistent pattern of behavior for the child. They are more pronounced in situations that require the child to be focused and restrained. The disorder is recognized purely by behavioral signs. Laboratory findings, such as continuous performance test, although illuminating, do not help the clinician.

Children with ADHD have great difficulty remaining seated when required to. They are more active than their peers in unstructured situations such as in the playground. They fail to pay attention to instructions, have difficulty in withholding a response until appropriate moment, have difficulty in waiting for their turn, and are easily distracted. One of the paradoxical features of ADHD that clinicians need to be aware of is that many children with ADHD can focus for long periods on screens, such as mobile phone games or computers/iPad on themes that are of interest to them.

Assessment

Diagnosis is based primarily on a clinical evaluation, which includes interviews with parents about the child's development and behavior. Information from the school is essential, and a direct examination of the child is important. There are several semi-structured interviews that can be used and are better than questionnaires or diagnostic checklists as they elicit information from a range of situations. A review on scales used for assessment of ADHD listed 11 scales, which are commonly used in North America and the United Kingdom. The scales which are used in some clinics in India are Conner's Rating Scales-Revised (CRS-R) version. The CRS-R includes items specific to DSM-IV-defined ADHD and its associated features, updating age and gender normative values.

Parent and teacher forms are available in full (80-item, 59-item) and abbreviated (27-item, 28-item) versions.

Another commercially available scale, which is occasionally used in India, is ACTeRS (Attention-deficit/Hyperactivity Disorder Comprehensive Teacher's Rating Scale) second edition (Ullman RK, et al., 2000) scale that has found some popularity in school settings. It was originally developed as a teacher rating scale derived in part from a scale used to study behavioral difficulties in children with lead exposure (Needleman HL, et al., 1979). Clinicians and parents of ADHD children provided input to the development of the scale. Its 11 items assessing inattention and hyperactivity are comparable to *DSM-IV* form includes an additional scale with descriptors of early childhood behaviors thought to be associated with the development of ADHD, such as difficult temperament.

However, both these and most other scales developed for use in the assessment of ADHD can only be bought and are not available for free use. This problem is circumvented by a scale developed by R Goodman and is known as strengths and difficulties questionnaires (SDQ). It is a 25-item scale with satisfactory psychometric properties and normative data. It covers five domains: Emotional symptoms (5 items), conduct problems (5 items), hyperactivity/inattention (5 items), peer relationship problems (5 items), and prosocial behavior (5 items). It is available over the internet at www.sdqinfo.com and has been used widely in research studies, especially in the United Kingdom and India. It is essential to assess the presence of learning disability, exclude hearing problems, and test for motor coordination. Stimulant medication can slow growth, and therefore it is important to record the baseline height and weight measurements.

■ INVESTIGATIONS

No specific physical investigations are needed or indicated to diagnose ADHD. Neuroimaging [computed tomography (CT) scan, magnetic resonance imaging (MRI), PET, and SPECT] and electroencephalography (EEG) should not be carried out without any specific clinical indication. In cases where lead toxicity is suspected, i.e., when history reveals exposure to lead plumbing or high lead levels in the environment, lead levels should be checked. The thyroid profile should be tested only when clinical features are suggestive of a thyroid disorder. EEG is only indicated if there is a suspicion of coexisting seizure disorder.

DIFFERENTIAL DIAGNOSIS

Attention-deficit/hyperactivity disorder can be conceptualized as a manifestation of one or more underlying pathological processes rather than simply a collection of symptoms, irrespective of etiology. ADHD should not be diagnosed if the symptoms are better accounted for by any other mental disorder. There are a number of other conditions/circumstances that can produce a reaction in a child that superficially mimics ADHD. Many of these conditions can also coexist with ADHD. These two separate issues, differential diagnosis and comorbidity, can cause difficulty for a professional who merely relies on the presence of behavioral items on a checklist to make a diagnosis of ADHD.

- *Normal variation:* There is no unequivocal dividing line between normal and abnormal levels of activity, impulsivity, and inattention. Pervasiveness across situations and impairment are therefore important threshold criteria. The impression and views of the teachers are important as they have experience with the normal range of behavior at a particular age.
- *Intellectual developmental disorder:* Children with moderate and severe mental retardation may have attention and activity levels that are appropriate for their developmental but not their chronological age. The fact that ADHD is more prevalent among children with borderline low levels of intelligence further complicates this.
- *Consequences of neglect, indulgence, or chaotic parenting:* This issue is often overlooked, but poor, chaotic parenting can result in a child who has not learned discipline and self-restraint. These children usually pester adults for the sake of attention-seeking and social involvement.
- *Restlessness, demanding behavior in the presence of maternal depression:* Mothers suffering from depression may be

unresponsive to the child's demands. Thus, children of mothers who are clinically depressed may be restless and demanding as a reaction to her unresponsiveness.
- *Sense organ deficits:* Fluctuating hearing loss in otitis media or fixed unilateral hearing losses due to various causes can elude clinical identification and present in children as apparently inattentive behavior.
- *Conduct disorder:* This may be a differential diagnosis as well as a comorbid condition. Restlessness and inattention are common among conduct-disordered children. A good developmental history will clarify which came first and a full assessment will sort out whether the inattentive restlessness is sufficiently severe to merit separate diagnosis.
- *Bipolar mood disorder:* It can also mimic ADHD. It can be both a differential diagnosis and a comorbidity. Eliciting a longitudinal history of symptom evolution, a family history of mood disorder, and the prominence of mood symptoms are factors that need to be clarified in detail.
- *Specific learning disorder:* Children with specific learning disorder may appear inattentive due to inability to learn, frustration, and lack of interest.
- *Autism spectrum disorder:* ADHD and autism spectrum disorder exhibit inattention, social dysfunction, and difficult-to-manage behavior.
- *Medications:* Anticonvulsants such as phenobarbitone, lamotrigine, clonazepam, and vigabatrin can cause irritability that mimics ADHD. Benzodiazepines and sedative antihistamines can have paradoxical excitatory effects. Even bronchodilators can cause hyperactivity in some individuals.

Comorbid Conditions

Comorbid problems are common in ADHD, and children with comorbidity are more likely to be brought for treatment in a clinical setting. Conduct disorders are prominently associated with ADHD, and it is often very difficult to distinguish from ADHD.
- *Learning disorders (LD):* Children with ADHD show an increased rate of specific learning disorder. It is estimated that one-third

of ADHD children have problems in reading, spelling, and mathematics unaccounted for by low intelligence.
- *Oppositional defiant disorders (ODD):* ODD and conduct disorders are characteristically associated with ADHD, so their differentiation is often impossible.
- Anxiety and mood disorders
- Language and communication disorders
- Tic disorders, such as Tourette syndrome
- Personality disorders
- *Emotional disorders*: It is also found in children with ADHD. As a matter of fact, clinical anxiety may represent a subgroup of ADHD. Follow-up of ADHD patients over a prolonged period suggests an increased risk of depression and substance abuse in late adolescence and adult life.

Other coexisting difficulties of these children are the following. These are not clinical conditions but are problems that have to be detected and managed accordingly.
- Difficulties in establishing relationships with peers and family members
- Poor self-esteem
- General academic underachievement
- Sleep–wake problems.

Longitudinal Course

It is important to remember that for many children, ADHD is a long-lasting impairing condition that affects not only their academic performance but also their overall development and achievements in life. **Flowchart 2** gives a snapshot of how the symptoms play out beyond childhood.

TREATMENT

The treatment of ADHD is by a multimodal approach. The key to successful management is making the parent and the child partners in treatment by providing them with age-appropriate information. Parents, schoolteachers, and clinicians must work together to help children and adolescents with ADHD achieve maximum potential.

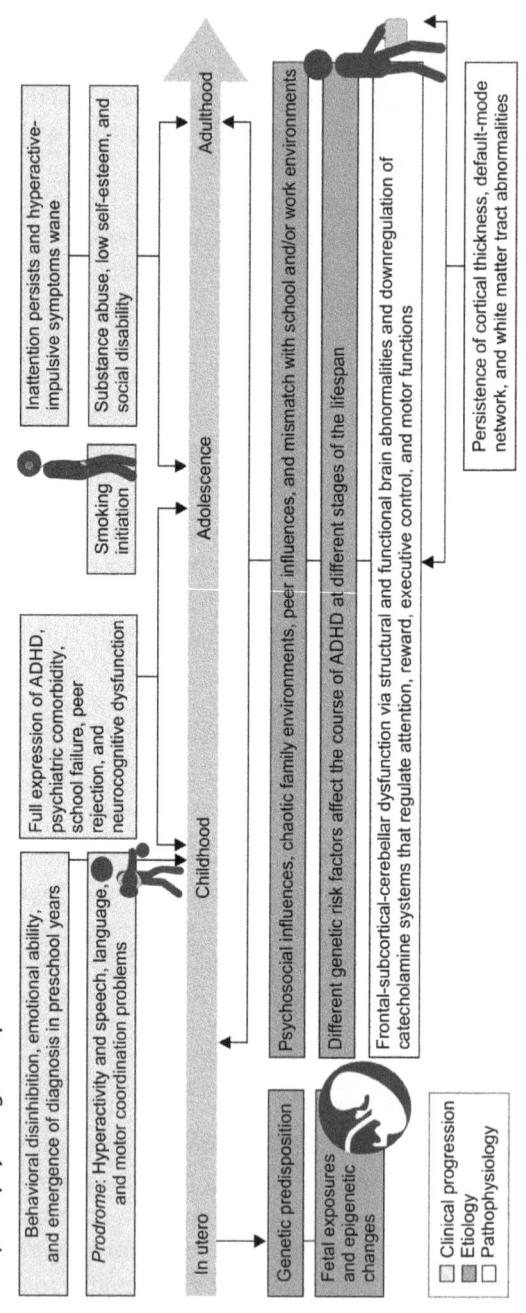

Flowchart 2: Developmental course of attention-deficit/hyperactivity disorder (ADHD) in persistent cases. Although no single sequence of events describes the pathway from in utero to adulthood, this figure describes key developmental events, with boxes spanning their approximate onset along with hypotheses about the timing of the biological underpinnings of etiological events and pathophysiological expression.

The overall plan for the management of children with ADHD is as follows:
- Education and information for parents and children
- Family intervention
- Behavioral management
- School interventions
- Individual cognitive approaches
- Medication.

The modality of treatment has to change, keeping in mind the age and context of the child and the family. The treatment approach for the child when he/she is 4 years old has to be different when the same child is 13 years old. The various tools in our treatment toolkit have to be modified and used in keeping with the evolving needs of the child.

Education and Family Interventions

It often helps to describe ADHD as essentially a limitation or handicap, a problem for the child to live with and for which treatment is available. The common goal of therapy is to help parents of children with ADHD recognize and believe that the child is not exhibiting the symptoms voluntarily. A child suffering from ADHD is capable of being responsible for meeting reasonable expectations. Parental training is an integral part of psychotherapy.

Parent management training centers on helping parents to manage their child. Strategies based on behavioral techniques are taught to the parents so that they are in control of the child's behavior. To build attention, parents can encourage the child to attempt short tasks with clear endpoint. Puzzles, drawing, and building small models can be used, and immediate praise for concentrating and finishing is crucial.

Behavioral Management

Behavior therapy represents a broad set of specific interventions that have a common goal of modifying the physical and social environment to alter or change behavior. The antecedents-behavior-consequences (A-B-C) analysis is used to target improved behavior.

Behavior therapy is usually implemented by training parents and teachers in specific techniques for improving behavior. There are three basic categories of behavioral training for children with ADHD:
1. Parent training in effective child behavior management methods
2. Classroom behavior modification techniques and academic interventions
3. Special educational placement.

Behavior modification is commonly used with younger children, but it can be used in adolescents and even adults. In children and adolescents, the two basic principles of behavior modification are as follows:
1. *Positive reinforcement:* Modeling behavior by encouraging good and acceptable behavior with healthy praise or rewards. The basis of this is positive reinforcement. It works best if the reward or praise of a particular action immediately follows the positive behavior.
2. *Negative reinforcement:* At the same time, the bad behavior has to be negatively reinforced. Rather than reprimanding the child, this can be achieved by allowing appropriate consequences to occur naturally following unacceptable behavior.

Repetitive application of the rewards and consequences gradually shapes behavior. Although behavior therapy shares a set of principles, it includes different techniques with many of the strategies often combined into a comprehensive program. The following are the seven steps of behavior modification program for the parents:
1. *Evaluation and repairing the relationship:* If one has developed patterns of becoming impatient, agitated, and angry each time the child misbehaves, or if one finds oneself shouting and punishing with much frequency, but without results, it is better to try first by taking some time to repair the relationship with the child.
2. *Choosing a behavior:* In order to help children with ADHD develop better habits and behaviors, one specific behavior has to be selected to work on at a time. Later, one or two more behaviors can be added. To start with, the behavior that has the most

demanding negative effect on the child's life and self-esteem has to be adapted.

3. *Choosing a reward:* Rewards should not be monetary but must be a token and tangible, interesting reward for an extended period of time of compliance.
4. *Choosing a consequence:* Consequences should be conveyed calmly each time. Using a time out often works well. During time out, there should not be any conversation of any kind. The child should not be able to participate in any "goings on" in their surroundings or in any discussion. The child should be gently removed from the environment and be left alone for a few minutes.
5. *Consistency:* Consistency is vital. If one is not consistent with resultant rewards, the child will not have the same motivation to act correctly.
6. *Variety:* One can add variety to the behavior program without altering the rules. By adding variety in behavior programs, the child will not become bored with the new way. Rules should remain the same, but changing the delivery pattern can help to keep it fresh.
7. *Continuing to another behavior:* When the child has mastered the initial behavior and is performing well, one has to proceed to something else.

Behavior Management Strategies for Preschoolers (5 years and below)

- Consistent routine, both for the days and for the structure of the activities, is important. The children should be conveyed when the routine is changing or something unusual will happen, be it a trivial one.
- Clear boundaries and expectations should be provided to the child. These guidelines and instructions are best given right before the activity or situation.
- An appropriate reward system for good behavior or for completing a certain number of positive behaviors, with a specific small reward such as a favorite activity, should be the norm. Food or candy as rewards should ideally be avoided.

- Engaging the child in constructive, interactive, and mind-building activities, such as reading books, participatory games, and puzzles by parent's participation.
- Using a timer for activities is a good way to build, maintain, and reinforce structure. For example, setting a reasonable time limit for a bath or playtime helps train the child to expect limitations, even on pleasurable activities.

Behavior Management Strategies for 6–12 years Children

- Clear instructions and explanations should be laid down for tasks throughout the day. A complex or lengthy task has to be broken down into smaller steps that are more manageable and achievable, keeping in mind that as the child learns to manage their behavior, the steps and tasks can gradually become more complex.
- Setting up of a clear pattern and system of rewards and rewarding for good behavior and tasks completed are required
- As the child gets older, they will be more concerned about how they appear to others and may overreact or be unduly ashamed when they are disciplined in the presence of others. Thus, it is important to have a plan for appropriate discipline for misbehaving that does not require carrying out in front of others.
- Regular communication with the child's schoolteachers so that behavior patterns can be dealt with properly before they become a major concern and before the teachers get overly frustrated with the situation is important.
- Children with ADHD need role models for behavior more than other children. The adults in their lives are very important role models.

Behavior Management Strategies for Teenagers

- As the child grows and steps into teenage, it is important to involve them in setting expectations, rewards, and consequences. Empowerment of the teenagers in this manner will improve their self-esteem and reinforce the concept that they are eventually the masters of their own behavior and can achieve positive results with good behavior.

- Teenagers are usually very sensitive to how they appear to others and may overreact or be unduly embarrassed when they are disciplined in front of others. As adolescents, they are going through a phase of hormonal changes and sexual development, and this brings up host of new issues. Teenage years can be tough enough even without ADHD, so parents have to be gentle and understanding.
- Regular communication with the child's teachers has to be continued as before.
- Having an understanding, predictable, and reasonable parent is always an advantage for children with ADHD.
- Children with ADHD need role models, and the adults in their lives, particularly parents, are very important.

Pharmacotherapy

The clinician should develop a comprehensive management plan focused on the target outcomes. The basic psychopharmacologic principles of management of ADHD that have to be remembered when providing children and adolescents with medications are as follows:

- Educate the patient, parents, and family about the purpose of these medications and clarify the goals of medications. The physician should clarify that medication use alone is not the remedy to all the problems. Medications are not curative.
- Any myths about the medicines should be corrected.
- A trial period of medication should be instituted first before embarking on medication management. The drugs should be started at a low dose and slowly increased till target symptoms are sufficiently improved.
- Other management strategies, such as behavior therapy, should be supported.
- The responsibility should be shared, clearly stating the issues the family, the school, and the physician must work on.

Assessment: Various methods can be used to assess medication efficacy, including interviews, report cards, and teacher and parent ratings. The goal of using medications is to use optimum dose with minimum adverse effects.

Stimulant medication: For most children, stimulant medication is highly effective in the management of the core symptoms of ADHD. In many cases, stimulant medication also improves the child's ability to follow rules and decreases emotional over-reactivity, thereby leading to improved relationships with peers and parents.

- Stimulants, in general, are not generally prescribed for children younger than 6 years. Methylphenidate is the only stimulant medication that is available in India now.

The potential benefits of stimulant medications are as follows:
- Enhanced concentration
- Reduced hyperarousal state
- Reduced impulsivity
- Reduced motor restlessness
- Improved school and homework performances
- Less aggressive and antisocial behavior

The common adverse effects of stimulants are headache, abdominal pain, jitteriness, anorexia, insomnia, social withdrawal, and weight loss due to poor appetite.

Methylphenidate: It is a well-known psychostimulant. It is safe, effective, and the most widely prescribed medication for ADHD. It is available as 10-mg scored tablets. The usual starting dose is 5 mg and is increased in 5-mg increments to a maximum of 60 mg/day. The half-life of methylphenidate is 2 hours. Most children will need three daily doses at 8 AM, 12 PM, and 4 PM. Slow-release preparations of methylphenidate allow for a single daily morning dose, and the effect lasts for the school day. However, it is not available in India at present.

Other Drugs

Clonidine: It is used as an alternative or adjunct to methylphenidate. Its sedative adverse effect counteracts insomniac effects of methylphenidate. It is useful for ADHD children with tics and whose problems tend more toward impulsivity and aggression. It does not improve attention dysfunction.

Tricyclic antidepressants: They are considered as the second-line therapy. They are particularly useful in children or adolescents with ADHD and depression.

Atomoxetine is a selective noradrenaline reuptake inhibitor, taken as once-daily dose in the morning. Some individuals may benefit by dividing the daily dose and taking it twice daily, once in the morning and second dose in the late afternoon or early evening.

It is effective in reducing both inattention and hyperactive/impulsive symptoms. The half-life of the drug is about 5 hours; it can be administered either once or twice daily. The adverse effects are relatively mild. As it is not a psychostimulant, it does not have any abuse potential. An advantage with atomoxetine is that it is freely available in the market, in contrast with the restrictions placed on methylphenidate.

The pharmacotherapy needs careful titration between the desired gains and the adverse effects. There is no concrete evidence on the effectiveness of "drug holidays"; hence, it is reasonable to treat each child on merit. The various medications used in the treatment of ADHD are shown in **Table 1**.

Duration of treatment: The duration of treatment depends on whether the symptoms remit in a particular child. Dose reduction may be attempted in early adolescence. It is best done during vacations in progressive decrements of 25% of the total daily dose. If dose reduction precipitates the emergence of ADHD symptoms, going back to the original dose is indicated.

Schooling Issues of Attention-deficit/Hyperactivity Disorder Children

Two important factors are to be considered before considering the placement of an ADHD child in school:
1. *Coexisting learning disability:* About one-third of ADHD children also have learning disability, and these children need special guidance and support.
2. *Successful medication:* In such situations, the teachers need to understand the effect and side effects of the medication.

The best type of classroom has defined rules and schedules. The activities should be stimulating. However, if the environment is too stimulating, then the child will not be able to concentrate. The desk should be closer to the teacher, not near the door, window, or the far end. The teacher should have correct information about ADHD. It is

TABLE 1: Various medications used in the treatment of attention-deficit/hyperactivity disorder (ADHD).

Medication	Daily dose (mg/kg)	Common side effects
• Stimulants		
– Methylphenidate	0.3–2.0 (2–4 divided doses)	Headache, abdominal pain, jitteriness, anorexia, insomnia
– Pemoline	0.5–3 (1–2 divided doses)	Possibly hepatotoxic
– Dextroamphetamine	1–1.5 (2–4 divided doses)	Evening anorexia, insomnia
• Antidepressants		
– Tricyclic	1–5	Cholestatic jaundice, tachycardia, delirium, neuropathy, tremor, lowered seizure threshold, weight gain, constipation, skin rash
– Bupropion	3–6 (2–4 divided doses)	Insomnia, irritability, seizure
• β-2 agonists		
– Clonidine	3–10 (2–4 divided doses)	Sedation, depression, dry mouth
• Noradrenaline reuptake inhibitors		
– Atomoxetine	0.5–1.4 (1–2 divided doses)	Decreased appetite, fatigue, sedation

preferable to divide works into "small chunks" with frequent breaks and teach concepts and not burden the memory with information. Communication between home and school is essential.

Safety Measures for Attention-deficit/Hyperactivity Disorder Children

A child with ADHD may not be aware of the dangers and is prone to get hurt. They should be closely supervised, especially in the following situations:
- Traffic
- Source of fire and firearms

- Swimming pool
- Sharp objects and potentially harmful instruments
- Poisonous chemicals and medicines.

Prognosis

The course of ADHD is variable. Remission is unlikely before the age of 12 years. When remission does occur, it is usually between the age of 12 and 20 years.

Attention-deficit/hyperactivity disorder continues into adulthood in most cases, but often they get better as they grow older. They learn to adjust to their problems. Hyperactivity usually stops in the late teenage years. Many of them continue to be easily distracted and have mood swings, hot tempers, and inability to complete tasks. Children with motivated, loving, supportive parents who work together with school staff, doctors, and mental health workers have the best chance of becoming well-adjusted adults.

Often, the symptoms continue into adolescence and adulthood. These patients are vulnerable to antisocial behavior, substance abuse, and mood disorders. Learning disorders often continue throughout life.

Role of the Pediatrician

The role of the pediatrician as the primary care clinician is pivotal in the successful management of ADHD children:
- Synthesize and interpret information about a child's behavior.
- Identify other medical or psychosocial problems that might be causing and/or exacerbating the child's symptoms.
- Refer to Special Educators or Clinical Psychologists for further evaluation where needed.
- Arrange other treatment (educational, psychosocial) as needed.
- Provide appropriate medical treatment, including prescribing atomoxetine.
- Monitor progress.
- Support parents in their role as advocates for the child.

It must be remembered that ADHD is a clinical diagnosis, and merely relying on a checklist is often inadequate.

> **GUIDELINES FOR PARENTS**
> - Children with ADHD may be difficult to parent. They may have trouble understanding directions.
> - Children with ADHD are usually in a constant state of activity. This can be a challenge to adults. The parents may need to change their home life a bit to help their child.
> - *Make a schedule:* Specific times for waking up, studying, playing, watching TV, eating, and going to bed
> - *Make simple house rules:* The virtue of obeying the rules and the consequences of not obeying them must be explained.
> - Reward good behavior. Focus on effort, not grades
> - Make sure the child is supervised all the time.
> - A child with ADHD may not be aware of dangers and is prone to getting hurt. They should be closely supervised, especially in the following situations—traffic, source of fire, swimming pool, sharp objects, potentially harmful instruments, poisonous chemicals, and medicines.

BIBLIOGRAPHY

1. Abikoff H, Klein RG. Attention-deficit hyperactivity and conduct disorder: comorbidity and implications for treatment. J Consult Clin Psychol. 1992;60:881-92.
2. American Academy of Pediatrics. Clinical practice guideline: treatment of the school-aged child with attention-deficit/hyperactivity disorder. Pediatrics. 2001;108:1049-92.
3. Balan A. Attention-deficit/hyperactivity disorder: identification and intervention. Indian J Pract Pediatr. 2007;9:6-12.
4. Barkley RA. Attention-Deficit Hyperactivity Disorder: A Handbook for Diagnosis and Treatment. New York: Guildford Press; 1990.
5. Barkley RA, McMurray MB, Edelbrock CS, Robbins K. Side effects of methylphenidate in children with attention deficit hyperactivity disorder: a placebo-controlled evaluation. Pediatrics. 1990;86:184-92.
6. Barkley RA, Peters H. The earliest reference to ADHD in the medical literature? Melchior Adam Weikard's description in 1775 of "attention deficit" (Mangel der Aufmerksamkeit, Attentio Volubilis). J. Atten Disorder. 2012;16:623-30.
7. Chatterjee A. Behavior modification. Indian J Growth Dev Behav Pediatr. 2006;2:15-9.
8. Diagnostic and Statistical Manual of Mental Disorders, 5th edition. Washington DC: American Psychiatric Association; 2013.
9. Faraone S, Asherson P, Banaschewski T, Biederman J, Buitelaar JK, Ramos-Quiroga JA, et al. Attention deficit/hyperactivity disorder. Nat Rev. 2015;1:1-23.

10. Gillberg C, Melander H, von Knorring AL, Janols LO, Thernlund G, Hägglöf B, et al. Long-term stimulant treatment of children with ADHD symptoms: a randomised, double-blind, placebo-controlled trial. Arch Gen Psychiatry. 1997;5:857-64.
11. Greydanus DE, Pratt HD, Sloane MA, Rappley MD. Attention-deficit/hyperactivity disorder in children and adolescents: interventions for a complex costly clinical conundrum. Pediatr Clin North Am. 2003;50:1049-92.
12. Guevara J, Lozano P, Wickizer T, Mell L, Gephart H. Psychotropic medication use in a population of children who have attention-deficit/hyperactivity disorder. Pediatrics. 2002;109:733-9.
13. Harold GT, Leve LD, Barrett D, Elam K, Neiderhiser JM, Natsuaki MN. Biological and rearing mother influences on child ADHD symptoms: revisiting the developmental interface between nature and nurture. J. Child Psychol Psychiatry. 2013;54:1038-46.
14. Hill P, Cameron M. Recognising hyperactivity: a guide for the cautious clinician. Child Psychol Psychiatry Rev. 1999;4:50-60.
15. Ivanov I, Newcorn J. Attention-deficit hyperactivity disorders. In: Sexon SB (Ed). Child and Adolescent Psychiatry, 2nd edition. Massachusetts: Blackwell Publishing; 2005. pp. 91-104.
16. Larsson H, Chang Z, D'Onofrio BM, Lichtenstein P. The heritability of clinically diagnosed attention deficit hyperactivity disorder across the lifespan. Psychol Med. 2014;44:2223-9.
17. Overmayer S, Taylor E. Principles of treatment for hyperkinetic disorder. J Child Psychol Psychiatry. 1999;40:1147-57.
18. Pisterman S, McGrath P, Firestone P, Goodman JT, Webster I, Mallory R. Outcome of parent-mediated treatment of preschoolers with attention deficit disorder with hyperactivity. J Consult Clin Psychol. 1989;57:628-35.
19. Prendergast M, Taylor E, Rapoport JL, Bartko J, Donnelly M, Zametkin A, et al. The diagnosis of childhood hyperactivity. A US-UK cross national study. J Child Psychol Psychiatry. 1988;29:289-300.
20. Reiff MI, Stein MT. Attention-deficit/hyperactivity disorder evaluation and diagnosis—a practical approach in office practice. Pediatr Clin North Am. 2003;50:1019-48.
21. Sandberg S, Barton J. Historical development. In: Sandberg S (Ed). Hyperactivity Disorders of Childhood. Cambridge: Cambridge University Press; 1996. pp. 1-25.
22. Singhi P, Malhi P. Attention-deficit/hyperactivity disorder in school-age children: approach and principles of management. Indian Pediatr. 1998;35:989-99.

23. Spencer TJ, Biederman J, Harding M, O'Donnell D, Faraone SV, Wilens TE. Growth deficits of ADHD children revisited. J Am Acad Child Adolesc Psychiatry. 1996;5:1460-9.
24. Taylor E, Sandberg S, Thorley G, Giles S. The Epidemiology of Childhood Hyperactivity. London: Institute of Psychiatry; 1989.
25. World Health Organization. International Classification of Diseases, 10th edition. Geneva: WHO Division of Mental Health; 1993.

CHAPTER 9

Disruptive Behavior

Jaydeep Choudhury

■ INTRODUCTION

A child's ability to communicate his or her will and oppose the will of others is crucial to normal development and it is the initiation toward establishing autonomy, creating an identity, and thus setting inner standards and controls. To some extent, defiance and refusal to comply with requests is developmentally normal in children and it marks the normal trend of development. But some children are themselves restricted by the frequency and often the severity of their own defiance and refusal. Disruptive behaviors often first attract notice when they interfere with school performance or family and peer relationships, and frequently intensify over time.

The chapter on disruptive, impulse-control, and conduct disorders is new in the fifth edition of the Diagnostic and Statistical Manual of Mental Disorders (DSM 5), 2013. According to DSM 5, the symptoms go beyond the description of otherwise temperamental children and far beyond common temper tantrums. It is characterized by severe recurrent temper outbursts that are generally out of proportion in intensity or duration to the situation. It occurs on an average three or more times each week for 1 year or more. In between the outbursts, these children display a persistently irritable or angry mood most of the day and nearly every day. This feature is observed by parents, teachers, or peers. According to DSM 5, the diagnosis requires the above symptoms to be present in at least two settings, at home, school, or with peers for 12 or more months. Symptoms must be severe in at least one of these settings. During this period, the child must not have gone through 3 or more consecutive months without symptoms. The onset of symptoms must be before the age of

10 years, and diagnosis should not be made for the first time before the age of 6 years or after 18 years.

Disruptive behavior is categorized into two distinct constellations of symptoms: oppositional defiant disorder and conduct disorder.

▪ OPPOSITIONAL DEFIANT DISORDER

In oppositional defiant disorder, the child's annoying behavior, temper outbursts, and refusal to comply with rules and regulations exceed expectations for these behaviors in children of similar age. The characteristic feature of this disorder is a persisting pattern of negativistic, often hostile, and defiant behavior. But they do not violate the social norms or the rights of others. Normal oppositional behavior peaks between 18 and 24 months. It is considered pathological when the developmental phase persists abnormally or the oppositional behavior recurs considerably more frequently than in most children of similar age. The later normative oppositional stage occurs in adolescence.

Epidemiology

Oppositional defiant, negativistic behavior, in moderation, is developmentally normal in early childhood and adolescence. Oppositional defiant disorder is typically noted between 8 years and adolescent age, but it may begin as early as 3 years. Before puberty, it is more prevalent in boys than girls, but the sex ratio is equal after puberty.

Etiology

Children generally develop a range of strong will, preference, and assertiveness. Parents who adopt an authoritarian type of parenting and resort to extreme ways of expressing and enforcing their will often contribute to the development of chronic struggle with their children, which is then reenacted with other figures of authority. Thus, in these children, what began as a normal effort to establish self-determination may become transformed into a grossly abnormal behavior pattern.

In older children, environmental trauma, illness, or chronic disorders, such as mental retardation, can trigger opposition. This is, in a sense, a defense against helplessness, anxiety, and loss of self-esteem.

Diagnosis
- A definite pattern of angry/irritable mood, argumentative/defiant behavior, or vindictiveness lasting at least 6 months. At least four symptoms from any of the following categories and exhibited during interaction with at least one individual who is not a sibling.

  Angry/irritable mood:
  - Often loses temper
  - Is often touchy or easily annoyed
  - Is often angry and resentful.

  Argumentative/defiant behavior:
  - Often argues with authority figures or for children and adolescents with adults
  - Often actively defies or refuses to comply with requests from authority figures or with rules
  - Often deliberately annoys others
  - Often blames others for his or her mistakes or misbehavior.

  Vindictiveness:
  - Has been spiteful or vindictive.
    Consider a criterion met only if the behavior occurs more frequently than is typically observed in individuals of comparable age and developmental level.
- The disturbance in behavior is associated with disturbance in the individual or others in his or her immediate social context (e.g., family, peer group, work colleagues) or it impacts negativity on social, educational, occupational, or other important areas of functioning.
- The behaviors do not occur exclusively during the course of a psychotic, substance use, depressive, or bipolar disorder. Also, the criteria are not met for depressive mood dysregulation disorder.

Specify Current Severity

Mild: Symptoms are confined to one setting (e.g., home, school, at work, with peer).
Moderate: Some symptoms are present in at least two settings.
Severe: Some symptoms are present in three or more settings.

Clinical Features

The behavior almost invariably starts at home. They may not be present only at school, with other adults or peers. In some children, it may be displayed later outside the home. Typically, the manifestations are most evident in interactions with adults or peers whom the child knows well. Thus, the child may not show any such behavior when examined clinically.

Four refinements have been made to the criteria for oppositional defiant disorder. The symptoms are grouped into three types—angry/irritable mood, argumentative/defiant behavior, and vindictiveness.

Early Warning Signs

- Irritable
- Inattentive
- Impulsive
- Defiance of adults
- Poor social skill
- Lack of school readiness
- Aggression toward peers
- Lack of problem-solving skills.

The manifestations are excessive argumentativeness with adults and loss of temper. They are generally angry, resentful, and get easily annoyed by others. Characteristically, they actively defy an adult's orders or requests and deliberately annoy others. These children do not consider themselves oppositional or defiant; rather they justify their behavior as a result of unreasonable circumstances. They often blame others for their own behavior. The disorder causes more distress to the people around the child than to the child.

In situations when oppositional defiant disorder becomes chronic, it severely interferes with interpersonal relationships and even school performance. Despite adequate intelligence, they perform poorly or fail in school as they do not participate and refuse to take others' help in solving problems. They fail to maintain friendships and perceive human relationships as unsatisfactory.

Secondarily, these children develop low self-esteem, impaired frustration tolerance, depressed mood, and sometimes temper outbursts. Adolescents with oppositional defiant disorder may abuse alcohol and illegal substances. Rarely, oppositional defiant disorder evolves into conduct disorder or mood disorder. Oppositional defiant disorder in which aggression is a prominent feature tends to progress to conduct disorder.

Differential Diagnosis

Oppositional behavior is normal behavior to some extent and also adaptive at specific developmental stages. Thus, these periods of negativism must be distinguished from typical oppositional defiant disorder.

Oppositional defiant behavior occurring temporarily during stress is an adjustment disorder. Oppositional behavior can also be present in conditions such as attention-deficit hyperactivity disorder (ADHD), cognitive disorders, and mental retardation.

Treatment

Family intervention: This is the primary intervention where parents are trained in child management skills.

Behavior therapy: One important component is teaching parents to alter their own behavior to thwart a child's oppositional behavior. In children, behavior therapy focuses on selectively reinforcing and practicing appropriate behavior and at the same time ignoring or not reinforcing undesired behavior.

Psychotherapy: The children should be able to learn strategies to develop mastery in social situations with family and peer. Self-esteem must also be restored.

Elimination of authoritative harsh punitive parenting and augmenting positive parent–child interaction may positively influence the course and outcome of oppositional defiant behavior.

CONDUCT DISORDER

Conduct disorder is characterized by severe repeated acts of aggression that can cause physical harm to themselves and also others and violate the basic rights of others. The enduring set of behavior evolves over time. The following four categories of behavior are demonstrated by children with conduct disorder:
1. Physical aggression or threats of harm to people
2. Destruction of property—self or others
3. Theft or acts of deceit
4. Frequent violation of age-appropriate rules.

Conduct disorder is often associated with other behavioral and psychiatric disorders such as learning disorder, ADHD, and depression.

Epidemiology

Like oppositional defiant disorder, occasional rebellious behavioral outburst and rule-breaking are common in childhood and adolescence. But in conduct disorder, the behaviors that violate the rights of others are repetitive. The disorder is more common in boys. It occurs with greater frequency in children of parents with antisocial behavior and substance and alcohol addiction. It is also affected by socioeconomic factors.

It is worth remembering that oppositional defiant disorder may be a precursor to conduct disorder.

Etiology

Many factors and their interplay contribute toward the development of conduct disorder.

Parental factors: Authoritarian type of parenting with harsh, reprimanding attitude characterized by severe physical and verbal aggression predisposes to children's maladaptive aggressive behavior. Parental negligence, child abuse, parental psychiatric disorders, and alcohol or substance abuse by parents may contribute to the development of conduct disorder in children. Parental divorce may be a risk factor also, but the persistence of hostility and bitterness between divorced parents may be of more importance as an etiologic factor.

Sociocultural factors: Economically, emotionally, and socially deprived children are at a greater risk for the development of conduct disorder. Children born in urban settings, in particular, unemployed parents, and lack of supportive social network may also contribute to the development of maladaptive behavior.

Psychologic factors: Children learn to control their impulse when they are brought up in a favorable environment. When they are in a chaotic, negligent environment, they express poor control of anger, frustration, and sadness.

Neurobiologic factors: There is decreased noradrenergic function as shown by a low plasma level of dopamine β-hydroxylase, an enzyme that converts dopamine to norepinephrine. This is also found in ADHD. Some children may have a high serotonin level also.

Child abuse: Aggressive behavior is often the fallout in children repeatedly exposed to physical or emotional violence or sexual abuse that starts at a young age. Children are also likely to exhibit violence if their caregivers are exposed to violence.

Comorbid factors: ADHD, central nervous system (CNS) dysfunction, and early life extremes of temperament could be the precipitating factors for conduct disorder.

Violence in media and entertainment: Though not a precipitating factor, regular exposure to violence in movies, video games, and other forms of entertainment and relaxation may aggravate violent behavior.

Diagnosis

- A repetitive and persistent pattern of behavior in which the basic rights of others or major age-appropriate societal norms or rules are violated as manifested by the presence of at least three of the following 15 criteria in the past 12 months from any of the categories below, with at least one criterion present in the past 6 months.

Aggression to people and animals:
- Often bullies, threatens, or intimidates others
- Often initiates physical fights
- Has used a weapon that can cause serious physical harm to others (e.g., a bat, brick, broken bottle, knife, gun)
- Has been physically cruel to people
- Has been physically cruel to animals
- Has stolen while confronting a victim (e.g., mugging, purse snatching, extortion, armed robbery)
- Has forced someone into sexual activity.

Destruction of property:
- Has deliberately engaged in fire setting with the intention of causing serious damage
- Has deliberately destroyed others' property (other than by fire setting).

Deceitfulness or theft:
- Has broken into someone else's house, building, or car
- Often lies to obtain goods or favors or to avoid obligations (i.e., "cons" others)
- Has stolen items of nontrivial value without confronting a victim (e.g., shoplifting, but without breaking and entering; forgery).

Serious violations of rules:
- Often stays out at night despite parental prohibitions, beginning before the age of 13 years
- Has run away from home overnight at least twice while living in parental or parental surrogate home (or once without returning for a lengthy period)
- Is often truant from school, beginning before the age of 13 years.

- The disturbance in behavior causes clinically significant impairment in social, academic, or occupational functioning.
- If the individual is of age 18 years or older, criteria are not met for antisocial personality disorder.

Specific types based on age at onset:
Childhood-onset type: Onset of at least one criterion characteristic of conduct disorder prior to age 10 years.

Adolescent-onset type: Absence of any criteria characteristic of conduct disorder prior to age 10 years.

Unspecified onset: Criteria for diagnosis met but not enough information available to determine whether the onset of the first symptom was before or after age 10 years.

Specify severity:
Mild: Few, if any, conduct problems in excess of those required making the diagnosis and conducting problems cause only minor harm to others.

Moderate: Number of conduct problems and effect on others intermediate between "mild" and "severe."

Severe: Many conduct problems in excess of those required to make the diagnosis or conduct problems cause considerable harm to others.

Clinical Features

The symptoms of conduct disorder evolve over time until a consistent pattern develops that violates the rights of others. The usual age of onset of conduct disorder is 10-12 years in boys and 14-16 years in girls.

Aggressive antisocial behavior in children may be manifested by cruel behavior toward peers, bullying, and physical aggression. Toward adults, they may be hostile, defiant, impudent, verbally abusive, and negativistic. Persistent lying, stealing, truancy, physical violence, and vandalism may also be present. Suicidal thoughts and gestures may be present in children and adolescents having conduct disorder who are in conflict and are unable to cope with peers, family members, and law. Sexual behaviors and use of addictive agents such as tobacco, liquor, or other abusive agents begin early.

Children and adolescents with conduct disorder also have poor self-esteem. They usually falsely project an image of toughness. They lack the skill to communicate with others in a socially acceptable manner. They have little regard for feelings for others. They often have impaired social attachment and difficulties in peer relationship. They may befriend much older or younger people or have a very superficial relationship with antisocial people. Though they often feel guilt or remorse for their behavior, they try to put the blame on others. Harsh punishment for unacceptable behavior in children and adolescents with conduct disorder increases their rage and frustration. Juvenile delinquency is often with a fallout of conduct disorder.

Children and adolescents with conduct disorder are most of the time uncooperative and hostile when they are interviewed. Denial and blaming others are common. They become angry if they are questioned repeatedly.

Assessment and evaluation of close family members is an important aspect. Marital disharmony is often present. Children with conduct disorder are more likely to have been unwanted or unplanned babies. Parents of children with conduct disorder, especially the father, may have antisocial personality or various addictions. Close family members of children with conduct disorder may have a similar pattern of impulsive and hostile behavior.

Course of Disease

Conduct disorder is often the progression from oppositional defiant disorder. Progression from conduct disorder to antisocial personality disorder is more likely when symptoms are severe and with childhood onset.

Differential Diagnosis

Isolated acts of antisocial behavior are not conduct disorder. The history of chronology of symptoms must be obtained to determine conduct disorder. Oppositional defiant disorder may be the precursor of conduct disorder.

Mood disorders may manifest with similar features. ADHD and learning disorders are often associated with conduct disorder. About one-third of all children with ADHD have coexisting oppositional defiant disorder, and up to one-quarter have coexisting conduct disorder.

Treatment

Children and adolescents with conduct disorder should be subjected to multimodal treatment. It encompasses behavioral intervention, social skill training, family education and therapy, and pharmacologic intervention. Certain reward systems can be instituted. Nonaggressive behaviors should be properly rewarded.

The family environment should be such that it provides support, but definite rules and expected consequences should be enforced in a gentle way so as not to provoke aggressive behavior. Sometimes, parental psychiatric evaluation may be required to promote parental understanding and prevent psychopathological and environmental stressors.

The school environment is another important domain. Violence and aggression should be reduced in school also. Peer-participant programs, threat assessment, and provision for crisis response initiative should be there in the school.

Behavioral therapy is a key factor as these children have maladaptive response to daily situations. Problem-solving skill should be augmented along with an appropriate reward system. Responsible children and adolescents should be taught self-control and avoidance of the trigger factors of unwanted behavior. The age at which the intervention is started is a determining factor for the outcome; the earlier the treatment is initiated, the better is the outcome.

Pharmacotherapy: Drugs are often needed to treat aggression, and it is an adjunctive treatment for conduct disorder. Pharmacotherapy should be initiated under psychiatric guidance. The choices of drugs are haloperidol, the atypical antipsychotics—risperidone, olanzapine, and the serotonin reuptake inhibitors—fluoxetine, sertraline, and other drugs such as lithium, carbamazepine, or clonidine may be used depending on various manifestations. Pharmacotherapy should be monitored cautiously as all these drugs have various side effects.

INTERMITTENT EXPLOSIVE DISORDER

Intermittent explosive disorder is a condition where the following types of aggression are considered—physical aggression, verbal aggression, and nondestructive/noninjurious physical aggression. The aggressive outbursts are impulsive and/or anger based, and must cause marked distress, cause impairment in occupational or interpersonal functioning, or associated with negative financial or legal consequences. This disorder is often very difficult to diagnose as it is difficult to distinguish this disorder from normal temper tantrums in young children. A minimum age of 6 years or equivalent developmental level is required for diagnosing this disorder.

> **GUIDELINES FOR PARENTS**
> - The target behaviors have to be identified that should be either encouraged or discouraged. These behaviors should be specific, observable, and ideally measurable.
> - Focus on the particular factors that make the behaviors more or less likely to occur. Ways to increase the likelihood of positive behavior and decrease the likelihood of negative behavior should be detected.
> - Adjust the ambient environment. Remove distractions such as television, video screens, and toys and schedule breaks to help him stay alert.
> - Make expectations clear.
> - Give a choice when possible.
> - Give instructions calmly and respectfully. This also helps the child learn to be polite when speaking to others. In turn, they will also learn to listen to calm instructions instead of listening only when you shout instructions several times. Say it once. After you give an instruction, wait a few seconds, rather than repeating what you said.
> - Tell the child what to *do* instead of what *not to do*. If he is jumping on the couch, you want to say, "Please get down from the couch" instead of "Please stop jumping."

BIBLIOGRAPHY

1. Diagnostic and Statistical Manual of Mental Disorders, 4th edition, Text Revision. Washington, DC: American Psychiatric Association; 2000.
2. Diagnostic and Statistical Manual of Mental Disorders, 5th edition. Washington, DC: American Psychiatric Association; 2013.
3. Sadock BJ, Sadock VA. Kaplan and Sadock's Concise Textbook of Child and Adolescent Psychiatry. Philadelphia: Lippincott Williams and Wilkins; 2009.

CHAPTER 10

Feeding and Eating Disorders in Infancy and Childhood

Ketan Bharadva

■ INTRODUCTION

Feeding and eating disorders in young children are a heterogeneous group, usually atypical in presentation, suspected less often, difficult to diagnose firmly, and has less evidence to guide informed treatment decisions. They are long-term disorders, frequently difficult to take care of and requiring prolonged treatment.

A feeding/eating disorder (also called anorexia) of infancy or early childhood is usually primary, but such diagnosis should only be done after ruling out secondary forms, especially in the first few years of life. It is diagnosed when a child appears malnourished, and the problem is not secondarily caused by a medical condition such as cleft palate, cardiac, respiratory, central nervous system or musculoskeletal disorders, airway or head and neck anomalies, and mental retardation. Severe failure to thrive, dysphagia, and signs of aspirations are alerting symptoms indicating a rapid need for diagnostics and evaluation of the safety of oral feeding. It excludes problems of gathering food and getting ready to suck, chew, or swallow it.

As compared to any early childhood disorder, feeding and eating disorders require good skills in both pediatrics and child psychiatry. Being more versed with problems of weight gain/loss, pediatricians are in a better position to evaluate and treat a patient holistically with focus wider than just narrow topic of eating and feeding disorder. It is wise not to underestimate anorexia as in the pediatrician's practice, early detection, initial evaluation, and ongoing management can play a significant role in preventing the illness from progressing to a more severe or chronic state. Increases in the incidence and prevalence of feeding disorders in children have made it increasingly important that pediatricians be familiar with the early detection and appropriate management of eating disorders.

EPIDEMIOLOGY

Anorexia: It is the most frequent reason for taking children to a pediatrician as often it is seen as a "problem" even when it may not be the case. Anorexic eating disorders are on the rise in the last few years, with more cases seen in younger children (up to 0.1–1.4%) than adolescents to experience psychiatric comorbidities, with rarity of bulimia. No sex difference is noted in the prepubertal age. Adolescent girls have a slightly higher prevalence of anorexia nervosa.

A factor that may be contributing to underdiagnosis is that there is also low awareness among the doctors regarding these disorders and lack of consensus regarding the diagnostic criteria and subthreshold disease.

In routine course of development, children self-regulate and may vary their oral intake up to 30% per day with no ill effect on growth. Normal feeding depends on the successful interaction of a child's health, development, temperament, experience, and environment. Altering any of these factors can result in a feeding problem. Up to 10–50% of typically developing young children and up to 80% of those who have developmental disabilities have feeding problems. These may evolve into a feeding disorder, with potential effects on psychomotor and neurological development in 1–5%. They had more psychological problems and somatic complaints and life events in past 1 year. Maternal anxiety disorder increases the risk.

Early age anorexia: It was rarely described in the medical literature. Occasional cases of anorexia at an early age are noted. The number of children with eating disorders has increased steadily from the 1950s onward as well as identification of eating disorders in countries that had not previously been experiencing these problems. Classification of eating disorders in this population also presents unique challenges.

Eating disorders in children are quite common. The classical eating disorders are relatively less common. Nonetheless, cases of prepubertal anorexia nervosa as early as age 7 years have been documented for more than a century. The existence of bulimia nervosa as a manifestation in children is not much documented. On the other hand, overeating/binging episodes have been described, though rarely in male and female children in the course of anorexia nervosa.

Feeding and eating difficulties are documented among the offspring of mothers with eating disorders. Data indicate that mothers with eating disorders express preoccupation with their child's eating, shape, and weight and have many dilemmas about child feeding.

ETIOPATHOGENESIS AND DIAGNOSIS

Anorexia nervosa and bulimia nervosa represent extreme manifestations of weight-control patterns in adolescents. Distinction between organic and nonorganic eating problems is not always clear, especially in infancy. When they occur in preadolescent younger children, they are more often associated with psychiatric or familial dysfunction. But rather than approaching them as psychiatric issues, pediatricians should look at them with developmental perspective in addition to biological, psychological, and social ones. Developmental concerns include family characteristics, parent–child interactions, cognitive development, and oral-motor development.

The most common cause is behavior at mealtimes, such as prolonged stressful mealtimes, food refusal, lack of independent feeding, use of coercion, etc., to increase intake, prolonged breast or bottle feeding, and failure to introduce a variety of tastes/textures/fragrances/colors in the sensitive period before 12 months age. The newest classification also includes the feeding style presented by the caregiver (responsive, controlling, indulgent, or neglectful) and the early in infancy mother–child dyadic pattern classified as a separate cause of feeding disorders. Cesarean delivery, prematurity, neonatal diseases, history of eating disorders in the family, consumption of protein hydrolysates, and treatment with proton-pump inhibitors were highly significant risk factors in children with eating disorders.

The cause of these disorders is often unknown, but they can result from a variety of factors such as:
- Poverty
- Dysfunctional child–caregiver interactions (there is a strong relationship between feeding problems in childhood and eating

disorder in the mother; the mechanisms responsible for this relationship are not understood)
- Parental misinformation about appropriate diet to meet the child's needs
- The psychopathology of the mother, especially of anxiety problems, increases the risk of feeding problems.
- Children with feeding problems have significantly more symptoms of psychological problems, somatic complaints, and experienced more significant life events in the previous 12 months.

Development of feeding is a relational and complex process in a child's environment. The current diagnostic approach, stressing more on an individual child, seems to be fallacious with more concerns in exclusions. But it should be rather inclusive of family and environmental experiences to address the complex process. The general consensus is that these disorders must be considered by taking into account physical, psychological, social, and family factors in origin, assessment, and treatment. There are numerous terminologies for various entities with intersecting attributes. We shall describe them in two ways: Classical DSM 5 (Diagnostic and Statistical Manual of Mental Disorders, fifth edition) categories and nonclassical ones, as below.

CLASSICAL EATING DISORDERS

Anorexia Nervosa

There is increasing literature indicating that anorexia nervosa is common in children with core behavioral, psychological, and physical features similar to those in adults. Children emaciate and suffer starvation quickly. The diagnostic criteria are almost the same as DSM-IV (Diagnostic and Statistical Manual of Mental Disorders, fourth edition), except that the requirement for amenorrhea has been removed.

A. Restriction of energy intake relative to requirements, leading to a significantly low body weight in the context of age, sex, developmental trajectory, and physical health. Significantly low weight is defined as a weight that is less than minimally normal or, for children and adolescents, less than minimally expected.

B. Intense fear of gaining weight or of becoming fat, or persistent behavior that interferes with weight gain, even though at a significantly low weight.
C. Disturbance in the way in which one's body weight or shape is experienced, undue influence of body weight or shape on self-evaluation, or persistent lack of recognition of the seriousness of the current low body weight.

There are two subtypes to be specified:
1. *Binge-eating/purging type:* During the last 3 months, the individual has engaged in recurrent episodes of binge eating or purging behavior (such as self-induced vomiting, misuse of laxatives, diuretics, or enemas).
2. *Restricting type:* During the last 3 months, the individual has not engaged in recurrent episodes of binge eating or purging behavior. Weight loss is accomplished primarily through dieting, fasting, and/or excessive exercise.

Bulimia Nervosa

Childhood cases are uncommon:
A. Recurrent episodes of binge eating. An episode of binge eating is characterized by both:
   1. Eating in a discrete period of time (e.g., within any 2-hour period) an amount of food that is definitely larger than what most individuals would eat in a similar period of time under similar circumstances.
   2. A sense of lack of control over eating during the episodes (e.g., a feeling that one cannot stop eating or control what or how much one is eating).
B. Recurrent inappropriate compensatory behaviors to prevent weight gain, such as self-induced vomiting; misuse of laxatives, diuretics, or other medications; fasting; or excessive exercise.
C. The binge eating and inappropriate compensatory behaviors both occur, on average, at least once a week for 3 months.
D. Self-evaluation is unduly influenced by body shape and weight.
E. The disturbance does not occur exclusively during episodes of anorexia nervosa.

Binge-eating Disorder
A. Recurrent episodes of binge eating.
B. Binge-eating episodes are associated with three or more of the following:
   1. Eating much more rapidly than normal
   2. Eating until feeling uncomfortably full
   3. Eating large amounts of food when not feeling physically hungry
   4. Eating alone because of feeling embarrassed by how much one is eating
   5. Feeling disgusted with oneself, depressed, or very guilty afterward
C. Marked distress regarding binge eating is present.
D. The binge eating occurs, on average, at least once a week for 3 months.
E. The binge eating is not associated with the recurrent use of inappropriate compensatory behavior as in bulimia nervosa and does not occur exclusively during the course of bulimia nervosa or anorexia nervosa.

Rumination Disorder
- Repeated regurgitation of food for a period of at least 1 month following a period of normal eating. Regurgitated food may be rechewed and reswallowed and less often spitted out.
- The disturbance is not due to a gastrointestinal tract (GIT) or other specific medical condition (e.g., esophageal reflux).
- Rumination disorder does not occur specifically during the course of anorexia nervosa, bulimia nervosa, binge-eating disorder, or avoidant/restrictive food disorders. If the symptoms occur exclusively during the course of a different mental disorder, they are sufficiently severe to warrant independent clinical attention.
- In rumination, there is no upset, retching, or disgust and may appear to cause pleasure. The characteristic preparatory movements, often interpreted as voluntary movements, characteristically distinguish this disorder from usual vomiting. It usually starts after 3 months of age and is rare in children and

teenagers. The cause is often unknown. Lack of stimulation of the infant, neglect, and high-stress family situations have been associated with it. It is a potentially fatal syndrome in infants, may narrowly escape surgery when not recognized, and may present as a complicated case from the neonatal intensive care unit (NICU). In some cases, it will disappear on its own. There have been no controlled trials published on any treatment for rumination in eating disorders. Environmental changes and enhanced mothering are described as being critical to correction of problem.

Pica

- Persistent eating of nonnutritive substances for a period of at least 1 month.
- Eating of nonnutritive/nonfood substances, which is inappropriate to the developmental level.
- The eating behavior is not part of a culturally sanctioned practice.
- If the pica occurs exclusively during the course of another mental disorder or medical condition (e.g., mental retardation, pervasive developmental disorder, schizophrenia), it is sufficient to warrant independent attention.

Avoidant/Restrictive Food Intake Disorder

DSM-IV feeding disorder of infancy or early childhood has been renamed avoidant/restrictive food intake disorder (ARFID). ARFID has no such age limitations, and it is distinct from anorexia nervosa and bulimia nervosa in that there is no body image disturbance. The criteria have been significantly expanded as follows:

A. Feeding or eating disturbance (e.g., lack of apparent interest in eating any type of food, avoidance based on the sensory characteristics of food, concern about aversive consequences of eating) which is manifested by sustained failure to meet appropriate nutritional and/or energy requirements associated with one (or more) of the following:
   1. Significant weight loss (or failure to achieve expected weight gain or faltering growth).

2. Significant and multiple nutritional deficiency.
   3. Dependence on enteral feeding or oral nutritional supplements.
   4. Marked interference with normal psychosocial functioning.
B. The disturbance cannot be explained by lack of available food or by an associated culturally sanctioned practice.
C. The eating disturbance does not occur exclusively during the course of anorexia nervosa or bulimia nervosa, and there is no evidence of a disturbance in the way in which one's body weight or body proportions are experienced.
D. The eating disturbance is not attributable to a coexisting medical condition or not better explained by any other mental disorder. When the eating disturbance occurs in the context of another condition or disorder, the severity of the eating disturbance exceeds that routinely associated with the same condition or disorder, and it warrants additional clinical attention.

Elimination Disorders

Elimination disorders exist now as an independent classification in DSM 5 instead of disorders usually first diagnosed in infancy, childhood, or adolescence in DSM-IV.

Other Specified Feeding or Eating Disorders

When the feeding or eating disorders do not meet all the criteria of the diagnostic class described above but cause definite clinical distress or some impairment in social, occupational, or vital areas of functioning. They are mentioned as "other specified feeding or eating disorder" with specific reason such as bulimic tendency or low bulimic frequency.

■ UNCLASSIFIED EATING DISTURBANCES

There is no set system for their definitions or classification, and they may have lot of overlap also. *Others of interest that are not described here are food avoidance emotional disorder, prematurity-related feeding disturbances, feeding problems of children with developmental disabilities, oral-motor sensitivity, etc.*

Food Refusal

Children may refuse food for all kinds of reasons. It seldom lasts long. Infants and children, from a very early age, can control and regulate their own food intake and grow normally, given proper guidance and emotional support from adults. Among young children too, food refusal is now seen as self-restriction secondary to weight concerns and fear of fatness and has led to growth failure. They may not fall under the classical eating disorders. These patients tend to absorb the prevailing cultural values of the society about food and body shape. They noticed first the fattening, then the balanced and healthy characteristics of food, and finally expressed sensory preferences.

Infantile Anorexia

A young child's anorexia may have organic or psychological origin when parent–child relationships are concerned. The most complex and earliest forms often have unspecified etiology. In psychopathological classifications, infantile anorexia is mainly distinguished as follows and there can be early and complex anorexia, mixing an organic vulnerability and a bonding trouble, which can be secondary:

- *Disorders of homeostasis:* These occur during the time period from birth to about 2 months, when basic functional cycles and rhythms of sleep and wakefulness, nursing, and elimination are established. In such cases, a mother's inability or inflexibility to respond to the child's particular needs may disrupt the infant's attempt to establish a regular feeding and, often, sleeping pattern. Temperamental differences, a high level of irritability and oversensitivity to stimulation can give rise to the so-called colicky infant; in others, the integration of the sucking and breathing response may be delayed.
- *Disorders of attachment:* From 2 months onward, it is seen that feeding experience is guided by the infant and mother getting emotionally engaged through body and visual cues. Mothers with depression, character disorders, or deprivation in their own childhood may remain unengaged during feeding due to attachment insecurity. Their children may remain withdrawn,

listless during feedings, or show vomiting, diarrhea, and poor weight gain.
- *Disorders of autonomy and separation:* In the developmental growth, cognitive maturation during 6 months to 3 years is the first separation–individuation disorder phase. When the mother does not respond to the infant's beginning of autonomy, the infant may assert his will and autonomy by refusing to eat in the form of food refusal or rejection. Temperamental children often labeled as those having higher difficulty, irregularity, negativity, dependence, and unstoppable ratings can also present with infantile anorexia.

Feeding Disorder Between Parent and Child

Understanding from the etiopathogenesis and curative point of view are the protracted anorexias here, the relationships in mother-child-surroundings appear disturbed. The degree of mealtime disorganization and the level of maternal strong control and disharmony mediate the association between maternal eating disorder and child feeding disturbance. Generally, the loss or simple reduction of appetite could heal in quick time if the mother would accept willingly the new situation, trusting in a spontaneous resolution. On the contrary, the mother usually forces the infant to take the meal, even if incompletely. On each new attempt, the infant's resistance increases initially passive and then more and more active and effective. Thus, "anorexia for opposition" is established by the conflict between mother and young child that the mother stirs up, to become a loser at the end. In most children, anorexia starts from different causes (illness from minor infections, as a replacement of human milk with the adapted milk, often during weaning) or sometimes without an apparent cause. It progresses after the mother's attempts to force infant to have a meal.

Post-traumatic Eating Disturbances

The children may have food refusal after a traumatic event such as choking or GIT procedures. They may be helped by selective serotonin reuptake inhibitor (SSRI) drugs such as fluoxetine.

Sensitive Periods

There are stages of development when infants are ready to accept advances in taste, texture, and also feeding methods. It may be difficult for feeding development to progress normally if these "sensitive periods" are missed and the corresponding feeding experience is not provided. If children are fed semisolids, which are made pasty by mixers, grinders, and blenders in late infancy, they show transitory delay and difficulty in accepting coarse granular foods later. This issue is more complicated for infants who are fed for prolonged periods of time with nasogastric or gastrostomy feedings. If these children are in transition to oral feedings, it is vitally important that some kind of ongoing oral therapy be maintained. It usually requires a referral to an infant feeding specialist such as an occupational therapist, physical therapist, or speech therapist.

Neophobia

Neophobia is fear of eating new foods. It is a normal attribute of developing children. But if they are given food recurrently in a comfortable, noncoercive, matter-of-fact way, acceptance increases. Exposure to a variety of stimuli through diverse cultures shows a lower incidence of neophobia. Neophobic behaviors are seen at all ages. Not all of them improve with age. New food is introduced often due to social or relational or just for it being new. Restrictive diets with high saturated fats are seen in them with a significantly low overall health eating index score. Neophobics have more of anxiety and maternal neophobia too.

Picky Eating

Pickiness is an unwillingness to eat many familiar foods. There appears to be definite association between a very uninteresting bland diet in the initial few months of life and various food refusals and fussiness about foods later in childhood. Gradual, noncoercive, developmentally appropriate exposure to a wide variety of interesting flavorful foods appears to be proper advice. Parentally reported picky eating is associated with a consistent pattern of inhibited and selective eating beginning in infancy.

Picky eaters eat fewer foods and are more likely to avoid vegetables with poor role model mothers and were breastfed for <6 months. Breastfeeding seems to be protective against picky eating through exposure to a variety of flavors in breastmilk; better mother–child interaction during breastfeeding with balanced control and lesser maternal control on eating.

Picky girls decrease their caloric intake between ages of 3.5 and 5.5 years, whereas all other children increase their caloric intake. Picky children display more parent-reported negative affect than nonpicky children.

Parents should pay less attention to "picky eating" and more to playing as a role model. Positive role modeling in vegetable and fruit eating by mothers reported less pressure on their daughters to eat the same.

Tactile Defensiveness

Tactile defensiveness (TD) children have a fair to poor appetite but choose or have a pronounced aversion toward textures or consistencies, smells, and temperatures of food. They hesitate to eat at off-routine places such as others' houses. They are bad at eating vegetables. They often gag and/or bite their inner lips and cheeks. TD or oral defensiveness can be treated with a team approach.

Night Eating Syndrome

Night eating syndrome is a situation of recurrent episodes of nighttime eating. It may be manifested by eating after awakening from sleep at night or by excessive consumption of food after the evening meal. There is definite awareness of recall of the eating episode. Night eating cannot be explained by various external influences such as changes in the individual's sleep–wake cycle or by existing social norms. It eventually causes significant distress and/or impairment in functioning. The disordered pattern of eating is not like binge-eating disorder and or any other mental disorder, including substance use, and also not attributable to another medical disorder or to an effect of medication.

MANAGEMENT

Each patient with a feeding/eating disorder is unique, so patients with such disorders need a careful evaluation by an experienced multidisciplinary feeding team and recognition and treatment of the leading problem. It needs an interdisciplinary approach with a medical, nutritional, and occupational therapy, social workers, and behavioral evaluation. A diagnosis, including medical, developmental, and behavioral characteristics; the parent; the parent-child relationship; and the social and nutritional context, will help in better treatment planning. The distinguishing features of mild or early stage and established or moderate eating disorders are shown in **Box 1**. A history of rumination should be routinely taken in cases of feeding disorder as it is often attached to shame. Rumination usually lessens by itself; behavior modification, breathing techniques, and gum chewing may help.

A high index of suspicion and aggressive screening will help to prevent delays in diagnosis. Prognosis has been poorly studied, but good outcomes are common with early intervention. Proper therapy of feeding disorders is highly effective, and in cases of children with behavioral feeding difficulties, depending on an underlying cause, the success rate is as high as 60% in complicated preterm infants

BOX 1: Features of mild or early stage and established or moderate eating disorders.

Mild or early stage:
- Mildly distorted body image
- Weight 90% or less of average height
- No symptoms or signs of excessive weight loss
- Use of potentially harmful weight-control methods or exhibit a strong drive to lose weight

Established or moderate eating disorders:
- Definitely distorted body image
- Weight < 85% of average weight for height associated with a refusal to gain weight
- Symptoms or signs of excessive weight loss associated with a denial of the problem
- Use of an unhealthy means to lose weight

to up to 90% in others. The need of tube feeding and swallowing disorders predicts more chances of failure.

The first stage of treatment for mild patients is to establish a weight goal. The criteria for hospitalization are shown in **Box 2**. Ideally, a nutritionist should be involved in the evaluation and treatment of children at this stage. Also, diet journals can be used to evaluate nutrition. Reevaluation by the physician within 1-2 months ensures healthy treatment.

Treatments differ according to the selected etiology. There is no quick cure for the majority.

There is an insufficient quantity of evidence to determine the effects of oral-motor, sensory, and pharmaceutical therapies on functional feeding outcomes in pediatric populations.

Family therapy has emerged with the greatest evidence of efficacy. Besides etiologic therapy, real care to primary anorexia lies in the child's dialogue with parents. Even if the origin is not mainly the relational mother–child dysfunction, parent–child relations require support to avoid aggravation by interactive vicious circles. Maternal characteristics and perceptions of their toddlers' temperament characteristics should be addressed in treatment for infantile anorexia. *Early individualized family-based interventions* for prematurity and other neonatal sickness, during neonatal hospitalization and transition to home, have shown to reduce maternal stress and depression, increase maternal

BOX 2: Criteria for hospitalization.

- Severe malnutrition
- Dehydration
- Electrolyte disturbances
- ECG abnormalities
- Physiological instability
- Arrested growth and development
- Acute food refusal
- Acute medical complications of malnutrition
- Uncontrollable binging/purging
- Acute psychiatric emergencies
- Comorbid diagnosis that interferes with the treatment of the eating disorder

self-esteem, and improve positive early parent–preterm infant interactions.

Behavioral treatments are the pillars of management. They include the Premack principle, time-out plus reinforcement, and negative reinforcement. Behavior modification plans are tailored to reinforce desired behaviors and discourage unwanted behaviors such as gagging and spitting. Apart from enjoying the things eaten during pica, oral stimulation is involved. Hence, alternative ways of developmentally appropriate stimulation (oral and otherwise) that are both positive and reinforcing (e.g., enjoying safe food items and engaging in other highly desirable activities) should help. During systematic desensitization, in a hierarchy of severity starting with the least aversive situation, therapists gradually club an anxiety-provoking food or feeding behavior with a relaxation behavior technique.

Attempts at weight control with higher levels of dietary restraint may promote weight gain in youth at risk for overweight with weight concern and body image dissatisfaction. Rather, there should be positive alternatives such as *encouraging physical activity, promoting acceptance of a variety of low-energy-density foods, and guides to portion sizes.*

Future research should focus on the parent–child interaction process in both mealtime and nonmealtime situations, along with demonstrating parents' and teachers' ability to implement mealtime treatment protocols.

GUIDELINES FOR PARENTS

- Minor eating disorders often can be managed by "responsive feeding." In early infancy, the infants need to be reassured that the discomfort of hunger is overcome by food. They need to be fed directly. On the other hand, parents may need to be trained to recognize and be sensitive to hunger and satiety signals.
- Feed slowly and patiently, and encourage children to eat, but do not force them.
- Minimize distractions during meals.
- Feeding times are periods of learning and love. Talk to children during feeding, with eye-to-eye contact. Parents are taught to recognize their child's hunger and satiety cues and how to create a positive, pleasant feeding environment for their child.

Contd...

Contd...

- New foods should be introduced in a gentle, noncoercive way. Sometimes, food refusal is a common phenomenon. Children sometimes refuse new foods in the first few tries. Spitting out food is often a common behavior, and it should be gently and firmly ignored.
- If children refuse many foods, experiment with different food combinations, tastes, textures, timing of feedings, the position of the person who is feeding, or the type of utensil used to do the feeding and methods of encouragement.
- Daily meals and snacks should be spaced and scheduled at predictable intervals. If the infant firmly protests and chooses not to eat a particular meal, food should not be forced until the next scheduled eating episode. Meals or snacks should be planned at optimum intervals so that the infant does not become overwhelmed with hunger sensation and lose the ability to control his state.
- Sharing and eating with other family members or particularly young children is an effective way to encourage older infants to expand the repertoire of acceptable foods.

BIBLIOGRAPHY

1. Birmingham CL, Firoz T. Rumination in eating disorders: literature review. Eat Weight Disord. 2006;11:e85-9.
2. Berksoy EA, Özyurt G, Anıl M, Üzüm Ö, Appak YC. Can pediatricians recognize eating disorders? A case study of early-onset anorexia nervosa in a male child. Nutr Hosp. 2018;35(2):499-502.
3. Carruth BR, Skinner JD. Revisiting the picky eater phenomenon: neophobic behaviors of young children. J Am Coll Nutr. 2000;19(6):771-80.
4. Celik G, Diler RS, Tahiroglu AY, Avci A. Fluoxetine in posttraumatic eating disorder in 2-year-old twins. J Child Adolesc Psychopharmacol. 2007;17(2):233-6.
5. Chatoor I, Ganiban J, Hirsch R, Borman-Spurrell E, Mrazek DA. Maternal characteristics and toddler temperament in infantile anorexia. J Am Acad Child Adolesc Psychiatry. 2000;39(6):743-51.
6. Chatoor I. Infantile anorexia nervosa: a developmental disorder of separation and individuation. J Am Acad Psychoanal. 1989;17(1):43-64.
7. Chatoor I, Conley C, Dickson L. Food refusal after an incident of choking: a posttraumatic eating disorder. J Am Acad Child Adolesc Psychiatry. 1988;27(1):105-10.
8. Davies WH, Satter E, Berlin KS, Sato AF, Silverman AH, Fischer EA, et al. Reconceptualizing feeding and feeding disorders in

interpersonal context: the case for a relational disorder. J Fam Psychol. 2006;20(3):409-17.
9. Dubedout S, Cascales T, Mas E, Bion A, Vignes M, Raynaud JP, et al. Troubles du comportement alimentaire restrictifs du nourrisson et du jeune enfant: situations à risque et facteurs favorisants. Arch Pediatr. 2016;23(6):570-6.
10. Esparó G, Canals J, Jané C, Ballespí S, Viñas F, Domenèch E. Feeding problems in nursery children: prevalence and psychosocial factors. Acta Paediatr. 2004;93(5):663-8.
11. Falciglia GA, Couch SC, Gribble LS, Pabst SM, Frank R. Food neophobia in childhood affects dietary variety. J Am Diet Assoc. 2000;100(12):1474-81.
12. Flight I, Leppard P, Cox DN. Food neophobia and associations with cultural diversity and socio-economic status amongst rural and urban Australian adolescents. Appetite. 2003;41(1):51-9.
13. Forcada-Guex M, Pierrehumbert B, Borghini A, Moessinger A, Muller-Nix C. Early dyadic patterns of mother-infant interactions and outcomes of prematurity at 18 months. Pediatrics. 2006;118(1): e107-14.
14. Galloway AT, Fiorito L, Lee Y, Birch LL. Parental pressure, dietary patterns, and weight status among girls who are "picky eaters". J Am Diet Assoc. 2005;105(4):541-8.
15. Galloway AT, Lee Y, Birch LL. Predictors and consequences of food neophobia and pickiness in young girls. J Am Diet Assoc. 2003;103(6):692-8.
16. Gosa MM, Carden HT, Jacks CC, Threadgill AY, Sidlovsky TC. Evidence to support treatment options for children with swallowing and feeding disorders: a systematic review. J Pediatr Rehabil Med. 2017;10: 107-36.
17. Kerzner B, Milano K, MacLean Jr WC, Berall G, Stuart S, Chatoor I. A practical approach to classifying and managing feeding difficulties. Pediatrics. 2015;135(2):344-53.
18. Kreipe RE. Eating disorders among children and adolescents. Pediatr Rev. 1995;16(10):370-9.
19. Marranzini M, Paesetto AG. Anorexic and pseudoanorexic child. Pediatr Med Chir. 1995;17(6):545-58.
20. O'Brien S, Repp AC, Williams GE, Christophersen ER. Pediatric feeding disorders. Behav Modif. 1991;15(3):394-418.
21. Phalen JA. Managing feeding problems and feeding disorders. Pediatr Rev. 2013;34(12):549-57.
22. Poinso F, Viellard M, Dafonseca D, Sarles J. Infantile anorexia: from birth to childhood. 2006;13(5):464-72.

23. Rosen DS. Eating disorders in children and young adolescents: etiology, classification, clinical features, and treatment. Adolesc Med. 2003;14(1):49-59.
24. Rozzell K, Moon DY, Klimek P, Brown T, Blashill AJ. Prevalence of eating disorders among US children aged 9 to 10 years: data from the Adolescent Brain Cognitive Development (ABCD) study. JAMA Pediatr. 2019;173:100-1.
25. Rybak A. Organic and nonorganic feeding disorders. Ann Nutr Metab. 2015;66(5):16-22.
26. Sadeh-Sharvit S, Levy-Shiff R, Feldman T, Ram A, Gur E, Zubery E, et al. Child feeding perceptions among mothers with eating disorders. Appetite. 2015;95:67-73.
27. Shunk JA, Birch LL. Girls at risk for overweight at age 5 are at risk for dietary restraint, disinhibited overeating, weight concerns, and greater weight gain from 5 to 9 years. J Am Diet Assoc. 2004;104(7):1120-6.
28. Smith AM, Roux S, Naidoo NT, Venter DJL. Food choices of tactile defensive children. Nutrition. 2005;21(1):14-9.
29. Watkins B, Lask B. Eating disorders in school-aged children. Child Adolesc Psychiatr Clin N Am. 2002;11:185-99.

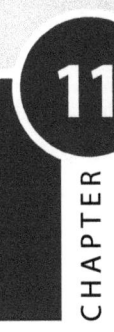

Elimination Disorders (Urinary Incontinence and Encopresis)

Nandita Chatterjee

URINARY INCONTINENCE

INTRODUCTION

In the fetus, voiding occurs by reflex bladder contraction and an infant has coordinated, reflex voiding 15-20 times a day. As the child grows up it is natural for him to gain control over bladder evacuation, during day and night, through several steps, which include the following:
- Awareness of bladder filling
- Cortical inhibition of reflex bladder contractions
- Ability to consciously tighten the external sphincter to prevent incontinence
- Normal bladder growth
- Motivation by the child to stay dry.

Toilet training begins at 2-4 years and by 5 years of age 90-95% are nearly completely continent during the day and 80-85% are continent at night. Girls typically acquire bladder control before boys, and bowel control is typically achieved before urinary control.

A delay in attaining bladder control by day results in daytime incontinence, and inadequate control at night leads to enuresis. Both, though common entities, are not socially well acceptable, thus causing much distress and agony to the child and parents.

DAYTIME INCONTINENCE

Daytime incontinence is a common occurrence in children. About 92% of children are dry by day at age 5 years and 96% are dry by

7 years, although 15% have significant urgency at times. At 12 years, 99% are dry during the day.

Etiology

Daytime urine incontinence can reflect several pathological processes disrupting the systems involved in continence. The causes include the following:
- *Neurological lesions:* Cortical, spinal, or peripheral nerves
- Anatomical anomalies of ureter, urinary bladder, urethra, and labia
- Excessive urine production with diabetes mellitus, diabetes insipidus, and sickle cell disease with reduced urine concentration
- Bladder wall irritability due to infection, calcuria, or constipation
- Emotional stress
- Functional voiding disorders.

The most common cause of daytime incontinence is a pediatric unstable bladder, also termed uninhibited or overactive bladder, bladder spasms.

Pathophysiology

According to the etiology, the pathophysiology also varies greatly as per the various groups.

Neurological Condition

- Loss of cortical control due to brain lesions and intermittent alteration of consciousness, as in epilepsy. It interrupts the cortical regulation of continence.
- Spinal cord lesions, such as tethered cord or other dysraphism can interfere with bladder control.
- Pudendal nerve injury or peripheral neuropathies, as in long-standing diabetes mellitus can impair involuntary sphincter contraction necessary for urine holding.

Anatomical Abnormalities

- Labial adhesions can limit urination due to small opening, with urine accumulation into the pocket behind the fused labia which

slowly leak out after voiding. Stagnant urine predisposes children to urinary tract infections (UTIs). Topical estrogen creams lyse the adhesions.
- Vaginal reflux occurs commonly in obese or younger girls who fail to fully spread the labia while voiding. Urine refluxes from redundant folds into the vagina and later leaks. Children should spread the labia widely while urinating (by dropping the underwear to the ankles or sitting backward on the toilet).
- Ectopic ureters inserted just distal to the external urethral sphincter can lead to continuous dribbling of urine. It is more common in girls than in boys.
- Posterior urethral valves can present with continuous dribbling due to bladder outlet obstruction.
- Stress incontinence results from insufficiency of the intrinsic urinary sphincter in girls and presents as leakage of urine during Valsalva maneuvers.

Excessive urine production: Seen with diabetes mellitus, diabetes insipidus, sickle cell disease with reduced urine concentration, volume overload, and diuretic agents often leads to dribbling. Excessive urine production can overwhelm an otherwise functional lower urinary tract.

Bladder wall irritability: It may lead to incontinence. UTI and calcuria may thus produce incontinence. Constipation commonly causes incontinence, apparently because the stool mass irritates the bladder and decreases its storage volume.

Emotional stress: Post-traumatic stress disorder, sexual abuse, or other major life changes, can lead to regressive behaviors such as incontinence.

Functional voiding disorders: These are a heterogeneous group of disorders that account for daytime incontinence in otherwise healthy children. Typically, the findings on physical and neurological examinations are normal. The independent preschooler is more interested in his or her environment, often ignoring the body's signal to void. Children with attention deficit hyperactivity disorder (ADHD) may have a higher incidence of dysfunctional voiding symptoms, perhaps related to inattention to body signals.

Functional voiding disorders can be categorized as follows:
- *Pediatric unstable (overactive) bladder:* It reflects excessive bladder irritability. A pediatric unstable bladder is smaller than normal and exhibits strong uninhibited contractions. These children typically exhibit urinary frequency, urgency, and urge incontinence. To suppress the urge to urinate, children hold the perineum, cross their legs, or squat on their heels (Vincent curtsy). If the child is picked up while squatting, an immediate accident ensues. Many children indicate that they do not feel the need to urinate, even just before they are incontinent. In girls, voiding cystourethrography (VCUG) often shows a dilated urethra, "spinning top deformity", and narrowed bladder neck with bladder wall hypertrophy. The urethral finding results from inadequate relaxation of the external urinary sphincter. In addition, constipation is common.
- *Giggle incontinence:* Giggle incontinence is a condition typically affecting girls between 7 and 15 years of age and is characterized by complete emptying of the bladder while laughing and usually comes with other daytime symptoms (urgency, hesitancy, and urge incontinence). The pathogenesis is thought to be sudden relaxation of the urinary sphincter. Anticholinergic medication and timed voiding rarely are effective. The most effective treatment is methylphenidate administration.
- *Underactive bladder:* This is characterized by infrequent voiding and the need to increase intra-abdominal pressure to urinate; urodynamic studies typically show detrusor underactivity. Affected patients are typically girls whose incontinence is triggered by physical activity. Children may delay the first morning void and avoid using the school toilet. Urine infections, constipation, and encopresis are commonly associated.
- *Hinman syndrome (detrusor sphincter dyssynergia):* This is a rare but serious disorder, characterized by infrequent urination, urge incontinence, recurrent UTIs, constipation, and encopresis. It involves failure of the external sphincter to relax during voiding in children without neurologic abnormalities. Children with this syndrome, typically exhibit a staccato stream. Evaluation often reveals vesicoureteral reflux, a trabeculated bladder, and a decreased urinary flow rate with an intermittent pattern.

Bladder imaging shows a thickened bladder wall with reflux and hydronephrosis. Urodynamic studies confirm incoordination between the bladder and the external urinary sphincter, resulting in detrusor contraction in the face of a narrowed sphincter. In severe cases, hydronephrosis, renal insufficiency, and even end-stage renal disease can occur. The pathogenesis of this syndrome is thought to involve learning abnormal voiding habits during toilet training. The treatment may include anticholinergic and α-blocker therapy, timed voiding, treatment of constipation, behavioral modification, and encouragement of relaxation during voiding. In some cases, botulinum toxin injection into the external sphincter can provide temporary relief.

- *Voiding postponement:* It is a behavioral problem, similar to functional voiding disorders. Affected children are often preschoolers who delay urination and assume holding postures until "the last minute." They may restrict fluid to avoid urinating. Underactive bladder is characterized by infrequent voiding and the need to increase intra-abdominal pressure to urinate; urodynamic studies typically show detrusor underactivity. Affected patients are typically girls whose incontinence is triggered by physical activity. Children may delay the first morning void and avoid using the school toilet. Urine infections, constipation, and encopresis are commonly associated.
- *Daytime frequency syndrome of childhood:* Some children, aged 4–6 years, after becoming toilet trained, have an abrupt onset of severe urinary frequency, voiding as often as every 10–15 minutes during the day, without dysuria, UTI, daytime incontinence, or nocturia. This is seen commonly in boys. This condition is termed "pollakiuria". It is functional problem, with no anatomical defect. Symptoms often occur just before a child starts kindergarten or if there are stress-related problems in the family. Occasionally, pinworms can cause these symptoms. The condition is self-limited, and symptoms generally resolve within 2–3 months.

Clinical Features

Important points in the history include the pattern of incontinence, including the frequency, the volume of urine lost during incontinent episodes, whether the incontinence is associated with urgency or giggling, whether it occurs after voiding, and whether the incontinence is continuous. In addition, the frequency of voiding and whether there is nocturnal enuresis (NE), a strong, continuous urinary stream, or sensation of incomplete bladder emptying should be assessed. A voiding diary with timing, presence of urgency, hesitancy, dysuria, quality of stream, hematuria, straining, and squatting may suggest etiology. Other urologic problems, such as UTIs, reflux, neurologic disorders, or a family history of duplication anomalies should be assessed. Bowel habits also should be evaluated, because incontinence is common in children with constipation or encopresis, or both. Back pain and gait abnormalities with incontinence suggest spinal cord disease.

Triggering psychological events, family response to a child's incontinence and the emotional impact of incontinence on the child must be assessed. Ask both the caregiver and the child about sexual or physical abuse.

A detailed physical examination is essential. Elevated blood pressure might reflect renal dysfunction; fluid overload may indicate renal failure or congestive heart failure. Palpation of the abdomen allows identification of constipated stool masses, and bladder percussion may find distention from outlet obstruction or neurogenic disease. Examination of the back can detect vertebral anomalies or cutaneous markers of spinal dysraphisms, such as hemangiomas or hair tufts. Neurologic examination of the perineum involves assessment of the sacral reflexes including anal and cremasteric reflexes in boys. Rectal examination may be performed in the cooperative child to confirm sphincter tone and the extent of constipation. Neurologic examination of the lower extremities can detect abnormalities related to spinal cord disease (altered strength or gait, diminished muscle stretch reflexes, and upgoing toes).

Investigations

A urinalysis and culture should be performed to check for infection. A random specific gravity of <1.002 (or <1.025 after 12 hours of fluid restriction) suggests inability to concentrate urine and is confirmed with serum electrolyte determinations and osmolality. Glucosuria likely indicates diabetes mellitus; nitrites, or white blood cells suggest a UTI. In some children, assessing the postvoid residual urine volume or urinary flow rate is appropriate. Imaging is reserved for children who have significant physical findings, a family history of urinary tract anomalies, UTIs, or those who do not respond to therapy appropriately.

A renal ultrasonogram with or without a voiding cystourethrogram is indicated. Urodynamics may be helpful if there is evidence of neurologic disease or if empirical therapy is ineffective.

Management

In most cases, history, unremarkable physical examination, and normal urinalysis suggest that the voiding disorder is functional or behavioral. Treatment of constipation often resolves urinary symptoms. For children with concomitant daytime and nighttime symptoms, address daytime symptoms first, and then the night symptoms, which may remit after daytime symptoms are treated.

Behavioral Approaches

All behavioral approaches require active participation of the child. The child is expected to attempt to void at regularly scheduled times every 2-3 hours, regardless of the sensation of the need to go. Positive reinforcement encourages motivation. A wrist alarm watch that sounds at set intervals minimizes child-parent conflict, optimizes a child's sense of achievement, and may serve as an additional reward for compliance with the plan. In school, the assistance of the teacher to encourage the child to go to the washroom at routine intervals is essential. Regular voids can be scheduled around natural breaks in the day, such as meals, recess, and snack. Arranging to use a private (nurse's or staff) washroom can improve program adherence.

Stressful family dynamics must be addressed; resolution may take weeks to months. Parents may be frustrated with the child's incontinence, and their negative affect may become an obstacle that prevents the child from overcoming this problem. Instruct families not to punish the child; the disorder is neither the fault of the child nor under his or her voluntary control. Eliminate arguing and disparaging remarks when the child has an accident. Accidents should be handled in a matter-of-fact manner, with the child taking responsibility to change his or her clothes after wetting. Motivating strategies, such as a sticker chart for bathroom visits, can help motivate and empower the reluctant child. With significant family stress, a period of days to weeks of "cooling off" is recommended before interventions begin, when no discussion of accidents is allowed. Referral to family therapy is indicated at times.

Children with functional incontinence may benefit from urge containment exercises to increase the functional capacity of the bladder and to avoid detrusor contractions at low urine volume. During urination, the child stops and starts the urinary stream by contracting the muscles of the pelvic floor. Measurement of the volume of urine voided at the beginning of therapy and at intervals of the treatment course may document improvement.

Medication

Oxybutynin is an antispasmodic, anticholinergic medication approved by the Food and Drug Administration (FDA) for treatment of overactive bladder. The short-acting preparation is approved for children older than 5 years; initial dosing is 2.5 mg twice daily, which can be titrated to 5 mg three times a day. The long-acting preparation is dosed at 5 mg once a day, titrated to 20 mg once a day. Tolterodine is not FDA approved for children but is often used in children intolerant to oxybutynin.

Anticholinergic agents can be used at the beginning of therapy with behavioral approaches in children whose symptoms are severe or socially debilitating and can be added in those with urge symptoms failing to respond to several weeks of behavioral interventions. The effect of medication should be evident within a few days, and dosage can be titrated while observing closely for anticholinergic side effects.

Anticholinergic medications and behavioral therapy may be tried for 6 months and then medication is slowly tapered during a few weeks while maintaining behavioral interventions. If symptoms recur, a course of therapy is repeated, after which the persistently symptomatic children need to be referred for a urologic evaluation.

Intensive Evaluation and Treatment

Children with neurologic signs suggesting spinal cord abnormalities should be evaluated with magnetic resonance imaging of the lumbosacral spine to assess for tethering or other abnormalities. Lack of improvement after a few months of behavioral or medical therapy should prompt further investigation of underlying emotional needs and difficulties with compliance. These children should be referred to a pediatric urologist for investigation of unrecognized organic disease.

The initial therapy of acquired or congenital anatomic abnormalities of the lower urinary tract is timed voiding every 1.5-2 hours and anticholinergic therapy with oxybutynin chloride, hyoscyamine, or tolterodine. Constipation and UTIs also must be addressed. This treatment program is usually prolonged and should be interrupted periodically to determine its continued need. An alternative to pharmacologic therapy is biofeedback, in which children are taught pelvic floor exercises, because there is evidence that daily performance of these exercises may reduce or eliminate unstable bladder contractions. In some children, treatment with an α-blocker such as terazosin or doxazosin may aid in timed voiding. Children not responding to therapy should be evaluated endoscopically and urodynamically to rule out other possible forms of bladder or sphincter dysfunction.

ENURESIS (NOCTURNAL INCONTINENCE)

Enuresis is defined as urinary incontinence during sleep in children older than 5 years of chronological or mental age. According to the International Children's Continence Society (ICCS), NE is an intermittent loss of urine during sleep characterized as a symptom and a condition. The diagnosis of enuresis is made when urine is voided twice a week for at least 3 consecutive months or the bed-wetting causes significant distress to the child.

Classification

Children with enuresis, without any definite medical or psychological causes, can be grouped into two categories with distinct clinical features and etiological factors. Monosymptomatic enuresis (MSE) where night wetting occurs without other urinary tract symptoms and nonmonosymptomatic enuresis where urinary tract symptoms, such as urgency, hesitancy, frequency, or daytime incontinence coexist with the night wetting.

Enuresis may also be classified as primary, where the child has never been dry at night and secondary, where children present with symptoms after a period of at least 6 months of dry nights. The former is more common while the latter is seen in 20-30% cases.

Incidence

Incidence of enuresis and parental concern, thereof, are similar across the globe. It occurs in about 15-20% of 5 years old with a 15% annual spontaneous remission rate. About 0.5-3% remains enuretic as adolescents and adults. Boys are more commonly affected (60%) than are girls.

Genetics

Enuresis is a heritable disorder, usually autosomal dominant. Four chromosomes have been linked to the trait, in particular, chromosomes 12 and 13, but no specific genes have been identified yet. Family history is positive in 50% of cases. If one parent is affected, the risk that a child is affected approximates 44%; if both parents are affected, that risk nears 77%. Approximately, 30% of cases are sporadic.

Physiology of Nocturnal Continence

Nocturnal continence is a result of maturation of multiple systems in the body. The simultaneous changes include the following:
- Diminution of urine production during sleep mediated by antidiuretic hormone
- Increased bladder capacity
- Neurologic development leading to increased functional bladder capacity. Normally, these changes are complete by 5 years of age.

Pathophysiology and Pathogenesis

Absence of the above adaptations and maturations in a child leads to NE.

Monosymptomatic enuresis results from the complex interaction of three physiological processes, nocturia (excessive night-time urine production); reduced nocturnal functional bladder capacity, provoking detrusor contraction at lower than expected volumes and difficulties with arousal, preventing the child from appropriately responding to the stimulus to urinate. Nocturnal calciuria is also being considered as a contributing factor for enuresis, and thus it is a potential target for therapy.

The pathogenesis of primary NE is multifactorial and includes the following:
- Delayed maturation of the cortical mechanisms that allow voluntary control of the micturition reflex.
- Reduced antidiuretic hormone production at night, resulting in an increased urine output.
- Enuretic children are more difficult to arouse than those with normal bladder control.
- Medical disorders, such as nocturnal epilepsy and obstructive sleep apnea, can also present with bed-wetting.
- Constipation can cause bed-wetting because of decreased bladder capacity and increased irritability.
- Secondary enuresis may be associated with pinworm infestation.
- Association with use of psychoactive medications, such as selective serotonin reuptake inhibitors, valproate, and risperidone has also been reported.
- Organic factors, such as UTI or obstructive uropathy, are uncommon causes of enuresis.
- Enuresis can be due to psychological trauma, such as child abuse, witness to violence, or other extraordinary stress.
- In the majority of affected children, enuresis resolves with age, suggesting developmental and maturational factors in its pathogenesis.

There is increasing evidence on the association of monosymptomatic nocturnal enuresis (MNE) with sleep disorders and obstructive sleep apnea. Although there is insufficient data to conclude that sleep disorders are not the cause of NE and they may be comorbidities.

Clinical Features

A detailed history and physical examination is of paramount help. A detailed history should be obtained, especially with respect to fluid intake at night, compensatory polydipsia (found in diabetes insipidus, diabetes mellitus, and chronic renal disease), pattern of NE, and passage of worms. History of snoring, abnormal breathing patterns while asleep, and abnormal night-time events (seizures or parasomnias) suggest definite diagnoses. Psychological triggers should be asked for.

A complete physical examination should include palpation of the abdomen and rectal examination after voiding to assess the possibility of a chronically distended bladder. The child with NE should be examined carefully for neurologic and spinal abnormalities.

Investigations

A urinalysis is essential, particularly to assess for concentrating defects (specific gravity and osmolality), infections (pyuria and bacteriuria), and glucosuria. If there are no daytime symptoms and if the physical examination and urinalysis are normal and culture is negative, further evaluation for urinary tract pathology generally is not warranted. A renal ultrasonogram is reasonable in an older child with enuresis or in children who do not respond appropriately to therapy.

Management

The basic three elements of the therapeutic process include: First stage—assessment of the way in which a child urinates; Second stage—treatment of bladder dysfunctions; Third stage—learning to wake up in order to urinate.

Monosymptomatic Nocturnal Enuresis

Active treatment should be avoided in children younger than age of 6 years. Children who are developmentally 7 years old and interested in ending bed-wetting are candidates for intervention.

Initial treatment involves demystification, particularly for young children with MSE. Parents should be counseled about the self-limiting nature of the problem and its excellent prognosis. Clarify that enuresis is not volitional, the child does not have full control over the symptoms, punishment, or reprimands have no role in the management of the disorder.

Simple behavioral strategies are safe and effective in some children with enuresis. Visual imagery at bedtime, to picture a full bladder and how they will wake up and go to the bathroom in response, has been found to be useful. They imagine waking up to a dry bed.

Some common initial interventions include limiting excessive fluids (particularly those with caffeine, calcium, and sodium) in the evening hours and waking the child to urinate as the parents go to bed.

The child should be responsible for helping with wet linens as a way to be "in charge of himself", rather than as punishment. Sticker charts can be motivating; the child is offered a sticker or a star for a dry night or for helping with wet linens. Helping the child and family manage the incontinence so that the child's self-worth and family relationships are maintained is vital. Emphasis is on success and competence.

For older children or those whose symptoms cause family or social distress, further therapy is indicated. If the child snores and the adenoids are enlarged, referral to an otolaryngologist should be considered. Medical disorders such as sleep apnea and epilepsy require appropriate referral. Constipation management often ameliorates symptoms. Children with a history of trauma should be referred for mental health evaluation and treatment.

If there is no decrease in wet nights following a few weeks of simple strategies, consider additional interventions that promote arousal in the setting of a full bladder, increased functional bladder capacity, or reduced volume of urine produced at night.

Alarm Therapy

Numerous studies, including randomized controlled trials, support the use of alarm therapy in NE and indicate overall efficacy approximating 68%. A typical alarm has a moisture sensor (activated when it is exposed to a small amount of urine) attached to the child's underwear. As the child urinates during sleep, the alarm sounds or vibrates. Many children initially sleep through the alarm, requiring parents to wake the child and walk the child to the bathroom to complete voiding, then during the following weeks, the child begins to wake at the sound of the alarm. Within a few months of consistent alarm use, the child begins waking spontaneously to urinate when the bladder is full or may sleep through the night without urinating. A sticker reward initially is helpful. The alarm should be used until the child completes one full month of uninterrupted dryness. Treatment with alarm therapy is more effective in children with monosymptomatic than with polysymptomatic NE. Alarm therapy is generally required to continue for 3-6 months. If no improvement occurs within 2 months, pharmacotherapy or combination therapy should be considered. Relapse occurs in about 50% of children when alarms are stopped but often responds to a repeated treatment course.

Pharmacotherapy

- *Desmopressin:* It is an analog of antidiuretic hormone is approved for use in children over 6 years of age with NE. Administration of desmopressin before bedtime reduces urine production at night, counteracting the nocturia. Desmopressin oral tablet formulation can be used daily with a dosage of 0.2-0.6 mg at bedtime, or on an as needed basis for camp or sleepovers. The use of desmopressin intranasal preparation is no longer recommended due to the high risk of hyponatremic seizures. Use of desmopressin tablets should be interrupted during acute illnesses that may lead to fluid and/or electrolyte imbalance.

    Lack of response after 2-3 months of desmopressin calls for reevaluation, particularly for symptoms of constipation, mechanical dysfunction, or daytime voiding dysfunction. Combination therapy, with use of both an alarm and desmopressin simultaneously for up to 3 months, is often considered after failure of monotherapy, but supporting evidence for this practice is limited.

- *Anticholinergics:* Anticholinergics such as oxybutynin chloride has been used in some children with primary NE, but the response rate is low. It can be helpful in cases of reduced functional bladder capacity at night or for a child with comorbid daytime voiding symptoms (i.e., urgency). A night-time dose of the short-acting preparation may be given with the option of changing to the long-acting preparation if enuresis occurs later in the night. Long-term administration is relatively safe, but monitoring for postvoid urine residuals should be considered. Furthermore, constipation induced by anticholinergic agents can worsen enuresis.

- *Imipramine:* It has been used sparingly in conjunction with desmopressin in recalcitrant cases, at a lower dose of 10–25 mg at bedtime for children older than 6 years, increased by 25 mg/day, after 1 week, to a final dose that should not exceed 2.5 mg/kg/day or 50 mg at bedtime for 6–12 years old, 75 mg for children older than 12 years. The mechanism of action appears related to anticholinergic and central nervous system effects. Given the potential for cardiac toxicity, screening, and follow-up electrocardiography and plasma drug level determinations are recommended.

Alternative and Complementary Therapy

Trials on electrotherapy have been conducted as an alternative method to treat patients with overactive bladder, using ambulatory transcutaneous parasacral electrical stimulation (TCPSE). Studies have shown that 63% of the patients symptomatically resolved completely and 20% improved significantly. There are weak evidences in support of the use of hypnosis, psychotherapy, acupuncture, and chiropractors. Trials were characterized by small size and weak methodology.

Approach to Nonresponders

Children who do not respond to enuresis therapies may benefit from taking a treatment break for a few months. There is a chance of 15% yearly rate of spontaneous resolution. If difficulties persist, urologic referral is indicated to assess the anatomy and function of the lower urinary tract. In general, daytime bladder symptoms should be treated before addressing night-time symptoms.

ENCOPRESIS

■ INTRODUCTION

Encopresis and toileting failure are common problems in children. The Diagnostic and Statistical Manual of Mental Disorders-5 (DSM 5) defines encopresis as "repeated passage of feces into inappropriate places (e.g., clothing or floor). Most often this is involuntary but occasionally may be intentional. The event must occur at least once a month for at least 3 months, and the chronological age of the child must be at least 4 years (or for children with developmental delays, a mental age of at least 4 years). The fecal incontinence must not be due exclusively to the direct physiological effects of a substance (e.g., laxatives) or a general medical condition except through a mechanism involving constipation."

■ INCIDENCE

The incidence varies with age, affecting approximately 2.8% of 4 years old, 1.5% of 7–8 years old, and 1.6% of 10–11 years old. Constipation and toileting refusal, with encopresis is common in preschool children. Although these problems often cause a great deal of stress to children and families, most cases are not the result of an organic illness and are curable with appropriate and diligent treatment. However, many children with encopresis are also vulnerable to developmental, behavioral, and emotional problems.

■ CLASSIFICATION

The subtypes include encopresis with constipation and overflow incontinence (retentive encopresis) and encopresis without constipation and overflow incontinence (nonretentive encopresis). About two-thirds of encopresis cases are of the retentive type and associated with chronic constipation. Primary encopresis persists from infancy onward, whereas, secondary encopresis appears after successful toilet training. In children younger than 4 years of age, the male to female ratio for chronic constipation is 1:1, whereas, in the school-aged child, encopresis is more common in males.

ETIOLOGY

Encopresis is a complex disorder with multiple etiological factors which may be physical, environmental and behavioral. The primary cause is a physical predisposition to constipation, reduced bowel regularity and ineffective evacuation. In some cases, there may be a history of painful bowel movement with subsequent withholding. Children with attention deficit disorder, obsessions and compulsions, and oppositional behavior are more prone to encopresis. Children with attention deficit disorder may be less attuned to body signals around toileting and may have trouble establishing a regular toilet routine. Environmental factors such as lack of access to the toilet, disorganized home setting, and exposure to trauma or violence can contribute to the development of encopresis. However, a majority of children with encopresis do not have a history of emotional disturbance.

PATHOPHYSIOLOGY

A child who is toilet trained or in the process of toilet training has the ability to keep the external anal sphincter closed until he or she has the opportunity to release. However, if a child develops constipation because of either diet changes or stool withholding, stool remains in the rectum. As a result, more water is absorbed; it becomes harder and subsequently more difficult to pass. This results in pain with defecation, and more withholding ensues. The rectum dilates as more stool collects and the muscles and nerve fibers stretch and do not function appropriately leading to poor control of the external anal sphincter and inability to sense the urge to defecate as the reflex arc becomes less sensitive. When the child squeezes the external anal sphincter to retain stool, some stool may be ejected into the underwear, resulting in staining. Children may also have leakage of wet stool that makes its way past the harder bolus of stool, or they may have complete stool accidents resulting from inability to appropriately control defecation.

Eventually, watery content from the proximal colon may percolate around hard retained stool and pass per rectum unperceived by the child. This involuntary encopresis may be mistaken for diarrhea.

TOILET TRAINING

Toilet training typically occurs from 2.5–3 years of age. Children typically reach the developmental milestones needed for toilet training between 18 and 30 months of age. The development of night-time bowel continence is usually followed by daytime bowel continence, then daytime urine continence, and last, night-time urine continence.

The current model of toilet training, endorsed by the American Academy of Pediatrics, is a child-centered process emphasizing developmental readiness as a precursor to toilet training. As part of this approach, three factors must be in place. The developmental and physiological skills (motor, language, and social skills) needed for toileting, the ability to understand instruction and the motivation to perform the task. A child must have the motor skills needed for ambulating, sitting, and assisting with removal of clothing, which are usually attained by the age of 18 months. To maintain continence, a child must have voluntary control of the bowels and bladder (usually emerging at 9 months) and then be aware when he or she needs to defecate (usually attained at 18 months). The child must have a way of indicating to caregivers that she or he needs to use the toilet. Cognitively, the child must understand that certain things go in certain places. Socially, the child needs to recognize the behavior of others and possess the motivation to attain continence.

A step-by-step approach is used to introduce model and facilitate appropriate toileting behavior. Use of a comfortable potty seat, regular sitting habits on the seat, preferably 20–30 minutes after meals (gastrocolic reflex increases the urge to defecate) and a reward on successful defecation is often effective. Children learn how to toilet train at different rates. Research shows that constipation and difficult temperament traits are associated with challenges in toilet training.

TOILET REFUSAL

Toileting refusal is a unique form of encopresis and it presents its own challenges to treatment. These children are averse to toileting and tend to hold back defecation. In young children who are resistant to toileting, toilet training should be discontinued for a period of few months and the child returned to diapers. The child should be assessed for constipation and treated appropriately before continuing with training. Medical evaluation for any contributing organic causes is suggested.

Management involves a behaviorally based program to desensitize a child's toileting aversion by decreasing anxiety around toileting. Start with whatever portion of toileting a child is willing to perform, set simple goals and reward the child on attaining the goal, before setting the next goal, till toilet training is achieved.

TOILET TRAINING IN SPECIAL SITUATION

Some children have developmental conditions that make toilet training more challenging. For example, children with chronic illness, children in daycare, children with developmental disabilities, and those with neurologic impairment may take longer or need special guidance to master toileting. A child with developmental delay may have difficulty making the connection between the urge to defecate and the social need to hold. Some children may have difficulty understanding the concepts of being wet and dry.

Toilet training can be particularly challenging in children with autism spectrum disorders because of decreased social and communication skills as well as behavioral rigidity. Children with autism spectrum disorders may be overly sensitive to the sensation of defecating, and they may not know to communicate the urge to void. They are also more prone to anxiety around toileting. If the child uses a picture exchange communication system or other communication system, this should be appropriately incorporated into training. This might include the development of a story or picture sequence that demonstrates toileting instruction. If the child suffers from firm stools that might increase resistance to defecation, medications can be used for softening the stools.

In children who have a physical disability, such as a spina bifida or cerebral palsy, neurologic factors may make it more difficult or impossible for a child to maintain continence. Stool softening agents should be used when needed. Timed sittings can help to keep a child dry in-between sittings and possibly allow the child to wear underwear, which may be important socially for the child.

Catheterization may also be an appropriate option and, in some cases, medically necessary. There are also other medical therapies that may be helpful, such as medications to reduce bladder spasms or to induce longer periods of dryness and surgeries to allow independence with toileting.

CLINICAL FEATURES
History

Some patients do not present with encopresis until school age, but many have had a history of stool withholding or initial toileting refusal. Some children may have had a history of mild soiling such as smearing and are not identified as having encopresis until the condition progresses to more frequent or larger accidents or their soiling affects their functioning with peers or in other settings.

In some children, parents can target a specific illness or other situation that may have immediately preceded withholding behavior. Ask about frequency of symptoms, whether there are entire bowel movement accidents or just staining, consistency and size of stool, and ease of passage. Ask about the frequency of stool accidents. Most children soil between 3 and 7 PM or specifically after or on the way home from school. Soiling at school is usually a marker of a more severe problem. Very rarely do children soil during sleep. Children with significant withholding may soil just as they fall asleep when they finally relax. However, nocturnal soiling can also be a sign of seizures.

Questions about urine accidents are also important. Children with constipation may have urine accidents caused by bladder spasms resulting from pressure to the bladder. Girls with encopresis are also at risk for UTIs from contamination or poor hygiene. Diet history should include intolerances or allergies to any foods. Past medical history should review any concerns about growth; short stature may be a clue to thyroid disease as a cause of constipation. A history of weight loss soon after introduction of solids may be a clue for celiac disease. The neurologic history should include questions about clumsiness or newly acquired lower extremity problems, which might be present in the case of a tethered cord. History of explosive stools after retention or thin-caliber stools may indicate

Hirschsprung disease. The family history should include questions about constipation, encopresis, colitis, irritable bowel syndrome, thyroid disease, or similar concerns. Social history should include screening for history of trauma or ongoing trauma. History of sexual or physical abuse is also important.

Physical Examination

General physical examination should include a look at the overall appearance, including physical habitus and growth parameters, possible dysmorphism, and behavioral and social interaction. Systemic examination needs focus on assessment of the abdomen, genitourinary, and neurologic systems. Abdominal examination may reveal fullness, distention or a nontender sausage-shaped mass in the lower left quadrant. The absence of this finding does not rule out constipation and may be difficult to appreciate in a child who is overweight or cannot tolerate an abdominal examination. The neurologic examination needs to be thorough including assessment of gait as well as lower extremity reflexes and strength. Increased reflexes or decreased tone could signal a spinal cord abnormality.

Examination of the perianal region should include position of the anus, evidence of soiling, signs of trauma, such as scarring, tears, or reduced rectal tone. In girls, the distance between the posterior fourchette and the anus should be at least one-third the distance between the posterior fourchette and coccyx. In boys, the distance between the scrotum and anus should be half the sacrococcygeal distance. A rectal examination should be performed. Increased rectal tone with a history of small-caliber stools and delayed passage of meconium may be a sign of Hirschsprung disease. Decreased rectal tone might be a sign of neurologic concern, such as spinal cord tethering or anomaly, although decreased tone can also be seen with prolonged constipation. Digital rectal examination should also include assessment of the rectal content. A large amount of stool in the rectum has a high positive predictive value for the presence of fecal retention, although absence of stool in the rectum does not rule out fecal retention. Intact neurologic sensation of the anus can be tested by eliciting the anal wink reflex, which involves lightly touching the anus with a cotton swab; this should result in closing of the sphincter. A cremasteric reflex in boys is another way to test lower sacral function. The causes of fecal incontinence are given in **Table 1**.

TABLE 1: Causes of fecal incontinence.

Disorder		History/Physical finding
Malformations	• Anal stenosis	• Abnormality on inspection and examination of the anus
	• Partial imperforate anus	
	• Neurogenic	
	• Occult spinal dysraphism	• Increased lower extremity tone
	• Tethered cord	
Neoplasia	Tumor	Neurologic signs, back pain, difficulty walking up stairs and incontinence of recent onset
Endocrine-metabolic	• Multiple endocrine neoplasia III	• Variable presentation
	• Thyroid disorder	• Constipation, weight gain, lack of energy, cold intolerance
	• Electrolyte imbalance	• Variable presentation, depending on electrolyte affected
Neuromuscular	• Muscular dystrophy	• Presents in boys aged 3–5 years; lower extremity proximal muscle weakness
	• Hirschsprung disease	• Constipation from birth followed by explosive stools; delayed passage of meconium, thin-caliber stools
Medications		Variable presentation
Sexual abuse		Physical signs of trauma or history of abuse
Diarrheal disease	Celiac disease	Constipation or diarrhea with growth concerns

INVESTIGATION

In most cases, children presenting with constipation and encopresis do not require routine laboratory evaluation or imaging. However, if there is clinical suspicion of an organic cause, further investigation is warranted. Laboratory testing might include thyroid function studies and determination of calcium, magnesium, and electrolyte values depending on history and examination findings. If the history is unclear and physical examination does not confirm constipation, abdominal X-ray may be helpful to determine the amount of retained stool. A baseline X-ray can also be useful to have as a reference after a clean out is performed. For children who present with urinary incontinence as well as constipation, urinalysis, and urine culture may be useful. Constipation can result in pressure on the bladder and may also lead to UTI. If a child has any lower extremity symptoms, lumbosacral spinal films and lumbosacral magnetic resonance imaging may be useful to rule out a tethered cord or spinal dysraphism. If there is increased rectal tone and a history of inconsistent explosive stools, anal manometry may be useful to rule out Hirschsprung disease.

TREATMENT

Once the diagnosis of encopresis is confirmed by thorough history and physical examination, a multimodal treatment program ensues. This requires both medical management of the underlying constipation, if present and behavioral intervention to encourage the child to use the toilet regularly. In fact, resolution of encopresis is most dependent on diligent adherence to a regular sitting regimen. Treatment plan for patient with encopresis is shown in **Figure 1**.

Education

Encopresis can be emotionally overwhelming for a child and family. The child is often punished or continually reprimanded for the accidents before medical advice is sought. The first step in treatment is parental education to explain the cause and process of encopresis, emphasizing on physical factors, predisposition to constipation, and emotional or temperamental traits in some cases. Emphasize to the

Family education
Clean out with
• Day 1: Bisacodyl tablet
• Day 2: Bisacodyl suppository
• Day 3: Enema
Repeat the cycle 4 times (total 12 days)
OR
Osmotic laxative with stimulant
Maintenance
Osmotic laxative, titrated dose for soft stool

Fig. 1: Treatment plan for patient with encopresis.

family that this is not the child's fault and explain the relapsing and remitting course of this disorder both before and after treatment.

Clean Out

In children with constipation, intervention includes the clean out of retained stool and a regimen to maintain regular passage of stool so as not to exacerbate the underlying problem. In most cases, this clean out can be performed at home. For less severe constipation, a child may benefit from a daily medication to soften the stool, such as an osmotic laxative or lubricant in conjunction with a mild-to-moderate bowel stimulant to encourage stool passage until there is clean out. This less intensive approach is milder and will take longer than the aggressive clean out. For severe constipation enemas alone or in conjunction with oral cathartics may be useful. Enemas are not recommended in children younger than 5 years or in children with a history of abuse or trauma. For severe constipation, a child may require reexamination or repeated abdominal radiography to confirm the clearance of stool.

Initially, accidents may appear to increase with the introduction of a clean out regimen. For children who attend school, one option is to use an agent to soften the stool during the week and add a stimulant on the weekends in hopes of decreasing the likelihood of an accident during the school day.

In a majority of cases, hospitalization or inpatient treatment is never necessary. Aggressive outpatient treatment with a clear treatment plan is typically appropriate. Hospitalization itself can be traumatic and further add to the problem and therefore should be avoided if at all possible. Only severe cases, such as extreme abdominal distress, risk of obstruction, vomiting of feculent material, or extreme parental noncompliance, necessitate hospitalization.

Maintenance

Once clean out is achieved or if a child does not require a full clean out, the next step is maintenance therapy with mineral oil or polyethylene glycol without electrolytes or osmotic laxatives, such as lactulose or stimulants such as senna-based products, at a lower dose than for clean outs. The goal of maintenance therapy is to encourage regular evacuation of soft bowel movements and to prevent recurrence of constipation. Often, medications need to be titrated to effect. The dose may change over time and with a change in diet. Polyethylene glycol without electrolytes can also be safely used up to 12 months. As the constipation resolves, children can be slowly weaned off of medications as tolerated. The length of use depends on need as well as on the safety of the medication used. The prolonged use of stimulants and enemas should be avoided because of the side effects and potential for dependence.

Diet

Parents should encourage high-fiber foods including fruits, vegetables, and whole grains as well as fluids. For very mild cases of constipation, diet changes or a fiber supplement alone may be all that is required.

Behavioral Plan

The behavior component of treatment is very essential. A child requires a regimen of regular sitting on the toilet for two reasons. First, to encourage the evacuation of stool and second, to help the child become comfortable with using the toilet. Initially, a child may be resistant to sitting on the toilet due to a fear or aversion to use of the toilet and the painful act of defecation.

The behavior plan includes motivating and rewarding a child for sitting on the toilet. The best time to sit is 20–30 minutes after meals as the gastrocolic reflex encourages defecation. It may also be practiced in the morning or directly after school. Depending on the age of the child, she or he should be encouraged to sit on the toilet one to three times a day for 5-10 minutes at a time. The child may have a specific toy, book, or desired object during that time. Reward is very useful in implanting the task. If the child does not perform the task, she or he should not be punished or reprimanded. The child should be gently reminded that if she or he does not complete the task, she or he will not receive the reward.

Regular scheduled visits with a provider are key to maintain motivation, to clarify the plan, and to provide encouragement. Often, it is easier for a child to perform the task for the provider rather than for a parent. If there is a great deal of conflict or resistance, consider eliciting the aid of a psychologist or behavioral specialist.

Other Therapies

Parents often seek complementary and alternative therapies for their children, but the literature is not extensive in regard to complementary and alternative treatment of encopresis. Use of prokinetics or acupuncture is also of no proven value. Some reports suggest improvement in some children on tricyclic antidepressants, though there is not enough data to warrant regular use of these drugs.

■ OUTCOME

Encopresis tends to be a relapsing and remitting disorder. Increased soiling and accidents are common during times of stress, for example. Most children will improve and many will have resolution of symptoms with treatment. The cure rate is variable but has been reported as 30-50% by 1 year and 48-75% by 5 years. Outcomes vary, depending on the medical complexity of the case as well as other emotional and psychosocial factors involved. The longer condition is present, the greater impact on child and family functioning and overall treatment. It is important, therefore, to recognize and to treat this disorder as soon as possible. This also includes helping parents anticipate challenges to toilet training.

The principles for successful toilet training include recognition of readiness skills and following a stepwise process that recognizes individual developmental, behavioral, and temperamental variation. Management of toilet refusal includes ensuring soft stools and using a stepwise approach with positive behavioral strategies. Encopresis is common in the pediatric population and may or may not be associated with constipation, withholding, or toilet refusal. Encopresis is rarely caused by organic illness, and careful history and physical examination are usually sufficient to rule out organic disease. Management of encopresis includes treatment and alleviation of constipation and the use of a structured sitting program with positive behavioral strategies.

GUIDELINES FOR PARENTS

- Medication for maintenance therapy titrated to maintain soft daily stool with minimum leak.
- Behavioral plan including daily sitting with developmentally appropriate reward.
- Discussion of diet changes including increasing fiber and water content
- Encourage increasing activity.
- Regular visits with provider to reinforce the plan and continually educate the family.

BIBLIOGRAPHY

1. Aceto G, Penza R, Coccioli MS, Palumbo F, Cresta L, Cimador M, et al. Enuresis subtypes based on nocturnal hypercalciuria: A multicenter study. J Urol. 2003;170:1670-3.
2. Baker SS, Liptak GS, Colletti RB, Croffie JM, Di Lorenzo C, Ector W, et al. A medical position statement of the North American Society for Pediatric Gastroenterology and Nutrition. Constipation in infants and children: Evaluation and treatment. J Pediatr Gastroenterol Nutr. 1999;29:612-26.
3. Barroso Jr U, Lordêlo P, Lopes AA, Andrade J, Macedo Jr A, Ortiz V. Nonpharmacological treatment of lower urinary tract dysfunction using biofeedback and transcutaneous electrical stimulation: a pilot study. BJU Int. 2006;98:166-71.
4. Blum NJ, Taubman B, Nemeth N. During toilet training, constipation occurs before stool toileting refusal. Pediatr. 2004;113:e520-2.
5. Boris NW, Dalton R. Enuresis. In: Kliegman RM, Stanton BF, Geme III JW, Schor NF, Behrman RE, (Eds). Nelson Textbook of Pediatrics, 19th edition. Philadelphia: Elsevier Saunders; 2011. p. 75.
6. Boris NW, Dalton R. Enuresis. In: Kliegmen RM, Stanton BF, St. Geme JW, Schor NF, Behrman RE, (Eds). Nelson Textbook of Pediatrics, 19th edition. Philadelphia: Elsevier Elsevier Saunders; 2011. pp 74-5.

7. Brazelton TB, Christophersen ER, Frauman AC, Gorski PA, Poole JM, Stadtler AC, et al. Instruction, timeliness and medical influences affecting toilet training. Pediatr. 1999;103:1353-8.
8. Brazelton TB. A child-oriented approach to toilet training. Pediatrics. 1962; 29:121-8.
9. Brooks RC, Copen RM, Cox DJ, Morris J, Borowitz S, Sutphen J. Review of the treatment literature for encopresis, functional constipation, and stool-toileting refusal. Ann Behav Med. 2000;22:260-7.
10. Casale A. Daytime wetting: Getting to the bottom of the issue. Contemp Pediatr. 2000;17:107.
11. Fritz G, Rockney R, Bernet W, Arnold V, Beitchman J, Benson RS, et al. Practice parameter for the assessment and treatment of children and adolescents with enuresis. J Am Acad Child Adolesc Psychiatry. 2004;43:1540-50.
12. Glazener CM, Evans JH, Cheuk DK. Complementary and miscellaneous interventions for nocturnal enuresis in children. Cochrane Database Syst Rev. 2005;(2):CD005230.
13. Glazener CM, Evans JH, Peto RE. Alarm interventions for nocturnal enuresis in children. Cochrane Database Syst Rev. 2005;(2):CD002911.
14. Glazener CM, Evans JH. Simple behavioural and physical interventions for nocturnal enuresis in children. Cochrane Database Syst Rev. 2004;2:CD003637.
15. Hjalmas K, Arnold T, Bower W, Caione P, Chiozza LM, von Gontard A, et al. Nocturnal enuresis: An international evidence based management strategy. J Urol. 2004;171:2545-61.
16. Jain S, Bhatt GC, Goya A, Gupta V, Dhingra B. Obstructive Sleep Apnea in Children with Nocturnal Enuresis. Indian Pediatr. 2018;55(5):433-4.
17. Joinson C, Heron J, Butler U, von Gontard A; Avon Longitudinal Study of Parents and Children Study Team. Psychological differences between children with and without soiling problems. Pediatr. 2006;117:1575-84.
18. Kroll P, Zachwieja J. A system for the treatment of nocturnal enuresis in children. Minerva Urol Nefrol. 2017;69(3):293-99.
19. Loening baucke V. Constipation and encopresis. In: Lifschitz CH (Ed). Pediatric Gastroenterology and Nutrition in Clinical Practice. New York: Marcel Dekker; 2001. pp. 551.
20. Loening-Baucke V. Encopresis. Curr Opin Pediatr. 2002;14:570-5.
21. Loening-Baucke V. Polyethylene glycol without electrolytes for children with constipation and encopresis. J Pediatr Gastroenterol Nutr. 2002;34:372-3.
22. Nazir R, Schonwald A. Urinary Function and Enuresis. In: Carey WB, Crocker AC, Coleman WL, Elias ER, Feldman HM (Eds). Developmental-Behavioural Pediatrics, 4th edition. Philadelphia: Elsevier; 2009. pp. 610-8.

23. Nazir R, Schonwald A. Urinary Function and Enuresis. In: Carey WB, Crocker AC, Coleman WL, Elias ER, Feldman HM (Eds). Developmental-Behavioural Pediatrics, 4th edition. Philadelphia: Elsevier; 2009. pp. 602-9.
24. Neveus T, von Gontard A, Hoebe P, Hjalmas K, Bauer S, Bower W, et al. The standardization of terminology of lower urinary tract function in children and adolescents: report from the Standardization Committee of the International Children's Continence Society. J Urol. 2006;176:314-24.
25. Reisner SH, Sivan Y, Nitzan M, Merlob P. Determination of anterior displacement of the anus in newborn infants and children. Pediatr. 1984;73:216.
26. Robson WL. Diurnal enuresis. Pediatr Rev. 1997;18:407-12.
27. Rockney RM, McQuade WH, Days AL. The plain abdominal radiograph in the management of encopresis. Arch Pediatr Adolesc Med. 1995;149:623.
28. Schonwald A, Rappaport L. Consultation with the specialist. Encopresis: Assessment and management. Pediatr Rev. 2004;25:278-82.
29. Schonwald A, Sherritt L, Stadtler A, Bridgemohan C. Factors associated with difficult toilet training. Pediatr. 2004;113:1753-7.
30. Tsuji S, Takewa R, Ohnuma C, Kimata T, Yamanouchi S, Kaneko K. Nocturnal enuresis and poor sleep quality. Pediatr Int. 2018;60(11):1020-3.
31. von Gontard A, Schaumburg H, Hollmann E, Eiberg H, Rittig S. The genetics of enuresis: A review. J Urol. 2001;166:2438-43.

CHAPTER 12

Tic Disorders

Jaydeb Ray, Jaydeep Choudhury

■ INTRODUCTION

Tics are abnormal movements or vocalizations that most commonly affect the muscles of the face and neck. They may also present as eye blinking, head jerking, grimacing, lip smacking, and tongue thrusting. Motor tic is a typical condition in which a part of the body moves repeatedly, quickly, suddenly, and uncontrollably. Typical vocal tics include throat clearing, snorting, grunting, and coughing. Tics can occur in any body part, such as face, neck, shoulders, trunk, hands, or legs. Children and adolescents manifest tic disorders that usually occur after a stimulus or in response to an uncontrollable internal urge. Tics are essentially a tension-relieving habit disorder. Generally, tics begin in early childhood or sometimes in adolescence with a stable or fluctuating course during childhood that generally wanes in adolescence.

A unique aspect of tics, relative to other movement disorders, is that they are suppressible by the child for short periods if made conscious or reprimanded. It can be controlled voluntarily, yet it is irresistible. Tics are never associated with transient inability to interact, unlike petit mal epilepsy. Tics disappear when the child is asleep, unlike dystonias and dyskinetic movements. Rarely, tics are precipitated in a child on stimulant medication like methylphenidate for attention-deficit hyperactivity disorder (ADHD).

■ EPIDEMIOLOGY

Up to 20–25% of children may be diagnosed with a tic disorder and it is most often in the school-age period. Tourette's disorder is less common but may affect up to 4% of school-age children. Males are more often affected than females. All races and ethnic groups are affected. Tic disorders, however, are known to run in families.

ETIOLOGY

Neuroanatomic Factors
Though no definite causes of tics have yet been established, considerable evidence points to disinhibition of several pathways in the brain connecting muscular movement, vocalization, and cognitive and emotional functions. There is indirect evidence of dopamine system involvement also.

Genetic Factors
Genetic studies indicate that tic disorder is often inherited, although the exact gene or genes are not yet determined. Family members with a child with tic disorder may be affected by obsessive-compulsive disorder (OCD). Chronic motor tics and Tourette's syndrome are probably different manifestations of an autosomal dominant gene with high penetrance.

Immunologic Factors
Pediatric autoimmune neuropsychiatric disorders associated with streptococcal infection (PANDAS) is a group of disorders recently recognized as a clinical entity which remitted after 1 month of treatment. Recent group A beta-hemolytic *Streptococcus* infection should be considered in a child who presents with a sudden explosive onset of tics or obsessive-compulsive symptoms.

CLINICAL FEATURES
Most tics are essentially mild and hardly noticeable. However, in some cases, tics are frequent and often severe and can affect many aspects of a child's life.

Tic disorders are classified as follows:
- *Transient:* Lasting >4 weeks but less than a year
- *Chronic:* Lasting >1 year
- *Tourette's disorder:* This is the most unusual tic in children.

The disorders are distinguished from one another based on three criteria—the child's age at onset, the duration of the disorder, and the number and variety of tics.

Transient Tic Disorder

Transient tic disorder is the most common tic disorder. It may affect up to 10% of children during the early school years. The diagnostic criteria for transient tic disorder as per the Diagnostic and Statistical Manual of Mental Disorders, Fifth Edition (DSM 5) are as follows:

- Single or multiple motor and/or vocal tics (i.e., sudden rapid, recurrent, nonrhythmic, stereotyped motor movements or vocalizations)
- The tics occur many times a day, nearly every day for at least 4 weeks, but for no longer than 12 consecutive months.
- The onset is below the age of 18 years.
- The disturbance is not due to the direct physiologic effects of a substance (e.g., stimulants) or a general medical condition (e.g., Huntington's disease or postviral encephalitis).
- Criteria have never been met for Tourette's disorder or chronic motor or vocal tic disorder.

The onset is generally between 6 and 10 years of age. It usually begins before the age of 12 years. Transient tic disorder can be distinguished from chronic tic disorder and Tourette's disorder only by observing symptom progression over time. It is impossible to predict at the outset whether the tics will disappear spontaneously, progress, or eventually become chronic. Probably the best approach for transient tics initially is to ignore them as much as possible. In the majority of situations, they disappear on their own. Giving much attention to mild or infrequent tics may also cause undue stress to the child. But if the tics are severe enough to cause impairment in the child's social, academic, or emotional function, then appropriate neurologic and psychiatric evaluation and management is recommended.

Chronic Motor or Vocal Tic Disorder

Rarely some tics do not go away. Tics which last 1 year or more are called chronic tics. Chronic tics are usually single or multiple motor or vocal tics but not both and generally involve one or two muscle groups. They affect <1% of children with tics. The diagnostic criteria for chronic motor or vocal tic disorder as per DSM 5 are as follows:

- Single or multiple motor and/or vocal tics (i.e., sudden rapid, recurrent, nonrhythmic, stereotyped motor movements or vocalizations), but not both, have been present at some time during the illness.
- The tics occur many times a day, nearly every day, or intermittently throughout a period of >1 year and during this period there was never a tic-free period of more than 3 consecutive months.
- The onset is below the age of 18 years.
- The disturbance is not due to the direct physiologic effects of a substance (e.g., stimulants) or a general medical condition (e.g., Huntington's disease or postviral encephalitis).
- Criteria have never been met for Tourette's disorder.

Chronic tic disorder is a complex condition. It is characterized by multiple motor and sometimes vocal tics. Simple tics are focal movements involving one particular group of muscles; complex tics are sequential patterns of movement that involve more than one muscle group or sometimes resemble purposeful movements. Characteristics of simple and complex motor and vocal tics are shown in **Table 1**.

Tourette's Disorder

Tourette's disorder is an unusual verity and most severe form of tic disorder, also known as Gilles de la Tourette's syndrome. More children exhibit this disorder than adults. It occurs three times more often in boys. The onset of the motor component of Tourette's disorder generally occurs by the age of 7 years, and vocal tics emerge later by about 11 years of age.

Prodromal behavioral symptoms such as irritability, attention difficulties, and poor frustration tolerance are usually evident before or coincide with the onset of tics. The first symptom of Tourette's disorder usually is involuntary movements (tics) of the face, arms, limbs, or trunk. These tics are often frequent, repetitive, and rapid. The most common first symptom is a facial tic (eye blink, nose twitch,

TABLE 1: Characteristics of simple and complex motor and vocal tics.

Simple tics	Complex tics
Eye blinking or eye rolling	Jumping excessively
Grimaces: Nose, mouth, tongue, or facial (nose twitch, nasal flaring, chewing lip, teeth grinding, sticking out tongue, mouth stretching, lip licking)	Spinning
Head jerks or movements (neck stretching, touching chin to shoulder)	Touching objects or people
Shoulder jerks/movements (shoulder shrugging, jerking a shoulder)	Throwing objects
Arm or hand movements (flexing or extending arms or fingers)	Repeating others' action (echopraxia)
Coughing repeatedly without any physical cause	Obscene gestures (copropraxia)
Throat clearing, grunting	Repeating one's own words (palilalia)
Sniffing, snorting, shouting	Repeating what someone else said (echolalia)
Humming	Obscene, inappropriate words (coprolalia)

or grimace). It is then replaced or added to by other tics of the neck, trunk, and limbs. These tics may also be complicated, involving the entire body, such as kicking and stamping. Other symptoms such as touching, repetitive thoughts and movements, and compulsions can occur sometimes.

All patients with Tourette's disorder have involuntary movements, and some have verbal tics also. These verbal tics usually occur with the movements. Later, they may replace one or more motor tics. The vocalizations include grunting, throat clearing, shouting, and barking. Echo phenomena are also reported, although less frequently. These include repeating words or phrases of others (echolalia), repeating one's own words, and repeating movements of others. The verbal tics may also be expressed as coprolalia which is the involuntary and repetitive use of obscene language. But neither echolalia nor coprolalia is necessary for the diagnosis of Tourette's disorder. Coprolalia usually begins in early adolescence and occurs in about one-third of patients. Mental coprolalia, in which a person thinks of a sudden socially unacceptable thought or obscene word, can also occur. In some cases, physical injuries have resulted from severe tics.

Obsessions, compulsions, attention difficulties, impulsivity, and personality problems have also been associated. While attention difficulties usually precede the onset of tics, obsessive-compulsion symptoms often occur after their onset. Many tics have an aggressive and often sexual component that may result in serious consequences for the patient. Tics actually resemble a failure of involuntary censorship, both conscious and unconscious, with increased impulsivity and inability to inhibit a thought from being put into action.

The diagnostic criteria for Tourette's disorder as per DSM 5 are as follows:
- Both multiple motor and one or more vocal tics have been present at some time during the illness, although not necessarily concurrently. (A tic is a sudden, rapid, recurrent, nonrhythmic, stereotyped motor movements or vocalizations.)
- The tics occur many times a day (usually in bouts), nearly every day or intermittently throughout a period of >1 year and during this period there was never a tic-free period of more than 3 consecutive months.
- The onset is below the age of 18 years.
- The disturbance is not due to the direct physiologic effects of a substance (e.g., stimulants) or a general medical condition (e.g., Huntington's disease or postviral encephalitis).

The following are confirmatory but are not essential for the diagnosis of Tourette's disorder:
- Coprolalia (involuntary use of obscene words)
- Copropraxia (involuntary obscene gesturing)
- Echolalia (involuntary repetition of sounds from self or others)
- Echopraxia (involuntary imitation of the movements of others)

Punishment or scolding by parents or teachers and teasing by the peer group will not help the child to control the tics. Actually, it will hurt the child's self-esteem and increase their distress. Parents can help these children to become more relaxed by making sure that they are not overscheduled and by not being overly critical.

Some tics disappear by early adulthood and some may continue. Children with Tourette's disorder may also have problems with attention and learning disabilities.

DIAGNOSIS

Diagnosis is made by evaluation of the history of onset and evolution of symptoms and by observation of clinical features. Blood test may be needed to rule out Wilson's disease or other metabolic disorders. Throat swab culture may be done if streptococcal throat infection is suspected. Antibodies against group A streptococci may be measured if PANDAS is the suspected diagnosis.

DIFFERENTIAL DIAGNOSIS

Tics may resemble other movement disorders, including stereotype disorders, dystonia, chorea, ballism, and myoclonus. Differential diagnosis of tics is given in **Table 2**.

TREATMENT

Most cases of mild tics do not require medical treatment and disappear on their own over time. It is recommended that family members should try to ignore simple tics, since teasing or other unwanted attention may make the tics worse. The first step in determining the most appropriate treatment for tic disorder is consideration of the child's or adolescent's overall functioning. A visit to a specialist doctor is recommended under the following circumstances:

- If the tics appear to persist for beyond 1 year.
- The child is falling behind in school because of the tics.
- The child's relationships with peers and adults outside the family are affected by the tics.
- The child cannot carry out activities of daily living (self-feeding, bathing, getting dressed, etc.).
- The child has fallen, injured himself, or developed other physical problems because of the tics.

TABLE 2: Features of the movement disorders that may resemble tics.

Tics	Stereotype disorders	Dystonia	Chorea	Ballism	Myoclonus
Sudden, repetitive, stereotyped, nonrhythmic movements or vocalizations	Patterned, nonpurposeful movement	Co-contraction of agonist and antagonist muscles, causing an abnormal twisting posture	Continuous, flowing, nonrhythmic, nonpurposeful movement	Forceful, flinging, large amplitude choreic movement	Sudden, quick, shock-like movement
Usually start after 3 years of age	Usually start before 3 years and resolve by adolescence	More common in adults	–	–	–
Decrease when focused. Increase when stressed, anxious, fatigued, or bored	Occur when the child is excited	Worsens during motor tasks	Worsens during motor tasks	Worsens during motor tasks	–
Comorbid conditions include obsessive-compulsive disorder and attention-deficit hyperactivity disorder (ADHD)	Common in children with mental retardation or autism	–	Can occur after streptococcal infection	Can occur after streptococcal infection	–
Preceded by a premonitory urge or sensation	Possibly preceded by an urge	Not preceded by an urge	Not preceded by an urge	Not preceded by an urge	Not preceded by an urge
Temporarily suppressible	Suppressible	Not suppressible	Partially suppressible; can incorporate into semi-purposeful movements	Partially suppressible	Not suppressible

- Other family members have or have had tic disorders.
- The child has recently had an episode of streptococcal throat infection or other streptococcal infections.
- The child has been diagnosed with OCD, ADHD, or depression.
- The tics have started suddenly.

The management plan of tics should be determined after discussing with the family members about their feelings about therapy and medications and considering the severity of the condition. Family education is the mainstay of appropriate treatment. Children should not be unwittingly punished for their tics. Before initiating therapy, a neurologist's consultation may be sought to rule out any neurological condition and a psychiatrist's consultation may be taken to rule out Tourette's disorder. The management strategies are behavior therapy and medication.

The approaches to tic treatment are:
- Provide the child and mainly the family with basic guidelines for managing tics.
- Help alleviate environmental stress and other potential triggers of tics.

The recommended treatment for mild-to-moderate symptom is comprehensive behavioral intervention for tics (CBIT). The primary component of CBIT is habit reversal training (HRT). HRT consists of tic awareness and competing response training. Awareness training and competing response training are practiced in treatment sessions of one tic at a time. Usually, treatment can be completed in approximately 8–12 sessions.

Medication is the treatment of choice for the management of more severe symptoms. Many medications are available. No particular medication can completely eliminate tics and many have substantial side effects. Before initiating medical treatment, one must consider the following:
- Whether moderate or severe symptom is present.
- Whether there is significant functional interference.
- Whether there are significant social disruption despite efforts to optimize the social environment for the child?

Individuals respond differently to the various types of medications and frequently it takes some time until the optimal

TABLE 3: Medicines with tic-suppressing effects.

Medication	Starting dose	Target dose
Haloperidol	0.25–0.5 mg/d	1–4 mg/d
Pimozide	0.5–1 mg/d	2–8 mg/d
Risperidone	0.25–0.5 mg/d	1–3 mg/d
Fluphenazine	0.5–1 mg/d	1.5–10 mg/d
Ziprasidone	5–10 mg/d	10–80 mg/d
Clonidine	0.025–0.05 mg/d	0.1–0.3 mg/d
Guanfacine	0.5–1 mg/d	1–3 mg/d
Botulinum toxin	1–20 units/kg	30–300 units

treatment for each individual is achieved. Medicines should be used under the supervision of a pediatric psychiatrist. The first-line pharmacologic agent for tic suppression generally is an alpha-adrenergic medication, unless the tics are severe. A trial of alpha-adrenergic medication (clonidine or guanfacine) for at least 2–3 months is to be given. Second-line agents include typical and atypical antipsychotics. Haloperidol and pimozide have shown efficacy in reducing tics in some patients as have risperidone and ziprasidone. The emergence of serious side effects is a risk for both typical and atypical antipsychotics. Botulinum toxin injection has been found to be effective for motor and vocal tics. Botulinum toxin and implantation of deep brain stimulators are invasive options and generally are reserved for severe, treatment-resistant tics. The medication is started at a low dose and must be slowly increased until the tics are reduced or until side effects are encountered. The usual side effects are reversible. Various medicines with tic-suppressing effects are listed in **Table 3**.

▪ PROGNOSIS

The prognosis for most tics and tic disorders is good. In the majority of cases, the tics diminish in severity and eventually disappear as the child grows. Even in Tourette's syndrome, about 85% of children find that their tics diminish or go away entirely during or after adolescence. Tics that persist beyond the teenage years, however,

usually become permanent. Factors associated with a poorer prognosis for all tic disorders include the following:
- History of complications during the child's birth
- Chronic physical illness in childhood
- Physical or emotional abuse in the family or a history of family instability
- Exposure to anabolic steroids or cocaine
- Comorbid psychiatric or developmental disorders

> **GUIDELINES FOR PARENTS**
> - If the child does not seem to be aware of the tics but they are apparent to others, it may be helpful to initiate a supportive discussion about the tics to raise the child's awareness.
> - If the child is aware of the tics, it can be helpful to inquire directly if the tics are causing any concerns, for example, head or neck aches, other bodily symptoms, or any worries or embarrassment about them.
> - Even if the tics are not causing the child any distress or impairment in functioning, it can be reassuring to him or her to know of your awareness and interest in how he or she is experiencing the symptoms.
> - Most tics do not interfere with activities of daily living and are less problematic during focused, pleasurable activities.
> - Since anxiety and stressful or new situations can temporarily increase tics, it is helpful to encourage relaxation and fun. Usually, quiet places and reduction in stimulation, excitement, or anxiety will facilitate reduction of the symptoms. Allowing the child to exit the classroom for brief periods can be helpful in reducing tics.
> - Development of simple relaxation techniques, such as breathing exercises, can be helpful.

BIBLIOGRAPHY

1. Beers MH, Berkow R. The Merck Manual of Diagnosis and Therapy. Whitehouse Station, NJ: Merck Research Laboratories; 2002.
2. Bernard BA, Stebbins GT, Siegel S, Schultz TM, Hays C, Morrissey MJ, et al. Determinants of quality of life in children with Gilles de la Tourette syndrome. Mov Disord. 2009;24(7):1070-3.
3. Deckersbach T, Rauch S, Buhlmann U, Wilhelm S. Habit reversal versus supportive psychotherapy in Tourette's disorder: a randomized controlled trial and predictors of treatment response. Behav Res Ther. 2006;44:1079-90.
4. Diagnostic and Statistic Manual of Mental Disorders, 5th edition. Washington DC: American Psychiatric Association; 2013.

5. DSM-IV. Diagnostic and Statistical Manual of Mental Disorders, 4th edition. Text Revision. Washington, DC: American Psychiatric Association; 2000.
6. Dure LS, DeWolfe J. Treatment of tics. Adv Neurol. 2006;99:191-6.
7. Freeman R. Tic disorders and ADHD: answers from a world-wide clinical dataset on Tourette syndrome. Eur Child Adolesc Psychiatry. 2007;16(Suppl. 1):15-23.
8. Harris E, Wu SW. Children with tic disorders: how to match treatment with symptoms. Curr Psychiatr. 2010;9(3):29-34.
9. Maini B, Bathla M, Dhanjal GS, Sharma PD. Pediatric autoimmune neuropsychiatric disorders after *Streptococcus* infection. Indian J Psychiatry. 2012;54:375-7.
10. Marras C, Andrews D, Sime E, Lang AE. Botulinum toxin for simple motor tics: a randomized, double-blind, controlled clinical trial. Neurology. 2001;56(5):605-10.
11. Porta M, Maggioni G, Ottaviani F, Schindler A. Treatment of phonic tics in patients with Tourette's syndrome using botulinum toxin type A. Neurol Sci. 2004;24(6):420-3.
12. Porta M, Sevello D, Sassi M, Brambilla A, Defendi S, Priori A, et al. Issues related to deep brain stimulation for treatment-refractory Tourette's syndrome. Eur Neurol. 2009;62(5):264-73.
13. Robertson MM. Tourette syndrome, associated conditions and the complexities of treatment. Brain. 2000;123(3):425-62.
14. Sallee F, Kurlan R, Goetz C, Singer H, Scahill L, Law G, et al. Ziprasidone treatment of children and adolescents with Tourette's syndrome: a pilot study. J Am Acad Child Adolesc Psychiatry. 2000;39(3):292-9.
15. Sallee F, Nesbitt L, Jackson C, Sine L, Sethuraman G. Relative efficacy of haloperidol and pimozide in children and adolescents with Tourette's disorder. Am J Psychiatr. 1997;154:1057-62.
16. Scahill L, Erenberg G, Berlin C, Budman C, Coffey BJ, Jankovic J, et al. Contemporary assessment and pharmacotherapy of Tourette syndrome. NeuroRx. 2006;3(2):192-206.
17. Scahill L, Leckman J, Schultz R, Katsovich L, Peterson BS. A placebo-controlled trial of risperidone in Tourette syndrome. Neurology. 2003;60:1130-5.
18. Shapiro E, Shapiro A, Fulop G, Hubbard M, Mandeli J, Nordlie J, et al. Controlled study of haloperidol, pimozide and placebo for the treatment of Gilles de la Tourette's syndrome. 1989;46:722-30.
19. Stefl M. Mental health needs associated with Tourette syndrome. Am J Public Health. 1984;74:1310-3.
20. Woods DW, Miltenberger RG. Habit reversal: a review of applications and variations. J Behav Ther Exp Psychiatry. 1995;26:123-31.

CHAPTER 13

Sleep Problem

Jaydeep Choudhury

■ INTRODUCTION

Good sleep is essential for physical and psychological well-being. A proper sleep pattern makes the mind alert, which is critical for good academic performance and learning skills. Children's sleep is affected by the age of the child, day of the week (depends on school day or weekend), and the place where the child lives. In western countries, children are mainly solitary sleepers; they sleep alone in their own designated bed. In India and many South East Asian countries, co-sleeping with parents in a common bed is common. Ideally, a child should sleep in a cool, quiet, comfortable, well-ventilated room with minimal light. Television should not be kept in the bedroom and children must not watch television or any other light-emitting screens before going to bed. Small children should be put to sleep by lullaby or bedtime stories.

Sleep problem is actually a sleep pattern that is unsatisfactory or a cause of concern to the parent, child, or physician. As families vary in their sleeping habits and have varied conception of children's sleeping habits, the interpretation of proper sleep also varies. A pattern which is of great concern to a family may be inconsequential or trivial to another. Most of the sleep-related problems are temporary and self-limited. Professional help is generally sought when the child's sleep problem causes parental sleeplessness.

Children with neurodevelopmental and behavioral disorders are at an increased risk of sleep problems. They may experience exacerbation of emotional and cognitive disturbances. It has been observed that children with autism have shorter total sleep time with decrease in rapid eye movement (REM) sleep. Differences in sleep architecture are seen in children with attention-deficit hyperactivity disorder (ADHD).

PATTERNS OF NORMAL SLEEP

Childhood years are characterized by changes in initiation, timing, organization, and structure of sleep. Neonates sleep most of the day except when they are hungry. The 24-hour rhythm is usually established between the ages of 3 and 6 months. Normally, the total sleep duration decreases from an average of 14 hours per day at 6 months of age to an average of 8 hours at 16 years of age. A gradual increase in the duration of nighttime sleep occurs during the first 1 year after birth with a decreasing trend of daytime sleep. Sleep duration declines about 10 minutes per year from 9 until 18 years of age. Children generally sleep less on school days than on weekends and vacations. Girls sleep a little more than boys. Children from wealthy households sleep a little longer. Obese children usually sleep less. Children like adults sleep more in winter than in summer.

There is no fixed duration that one should sleep. Sleep requirement varies according to sleep practices and environmental demands and are probably regulated by genes. Short sleepers spend 4–5 hours per day in sleep and still feel fresh and energetic. Long sleepers sleep for 10–12 hours a day.

CONSEQUENCES OF POOR SLEEP

Regular poor quality and short duration sleep is associated with a range of psychosocial and physical disturbances in children. Other than daytime sleepiness, these children may suffer from impaired attention, memory consolidation, creativity, learning and academic performance, increased impulsivity, aggression, and hyperactivity. So, a sleep-deprived child may have poor school performance. It has been observed that persistent short sleep duration is also associated with an increased risk of overweight and obesity in children.

TYPES OF SLEEP PROBLEMS

The following are the types of sleep-related problems:
- *Dyssomnias:* Disorders of initiating and maintaining sleep
- *Hypersomnias:* Excessive sleepiness
- *Parasomnias:* Abnormal activity or behavior during sleep.

EVALUATION

A complete sleep history is the main guiding factor. A comprehensive sleep diary for 2 weeks helps in the analysis of the child's sleep problem. Detailed medical, developmental, and behavioral history should also be taken. Physical examination should include assessment for tonsil or adenoid enlargement, sinusitis with postnasal drip, bronchial asthma, gastrocolic reflux, abdominal colic, and examination of the central nervous system (CNS).

COMMON SLEEP PROBLEMS
Sleep Terror

Sleep terror is generally seen in children between 4 and 12 years of age, and it is episodic in nature. There may be a history of sleep terrors in the family also. It is characterized by a state of confusion and partial arousal usually during the first third of night sleep time, in the transition from nonrapid eye movement (NREM) stage 3 or 4 to light sleep. It usually lasts for a few minutes, occasionally for about 30 minutes. Sleep terrors are associated with autonomic activities such as tachypnea, tachycardia, sweating, mydriasis, confusion, tremulousness, and vocalization. A state of terror or intense fear is reflected in facial expression. Uncontrollable moaning, shouting, screaming, and agitation may accompany. Sleep terrors rarely occur in isolation. Some children may start walking or running during an episode. There may be associated somniloquy, night awakenings, and separation anxiety. Any attempt to wake up the child during such episode may exacerbate the child's sleep disturbance. The episodes generally end abruptly and the child rapidly returns to normal deep sleep. Children with sleep terror have poor recall of their dream content and are often difficult to arouse.

Sleep terrors are a reflection of CNS immaturity. Most children outgrow sleep terrors. Precipitating factors are fever, sleep deprivation, and some drugs such as antihistaminics, bronchodilators, and antireflux medication.

Management

Sleep terror is usually a self-limiting disease. Parental reassurance and proper guidance are essential. Proper sleep hygiene should be followed. Children should have proper sleep as sleep deprivation is a usual precipitating factor. Children should go early to bed. Stress, if any, should be relieved. Short-acting benzodiazepines such as clobazam or lorazepam may be given for 3–6 months if there is a danger of self-harm. Long-term use may induce tolerance.

Nightmares

Contrary to sleep terror, nightmares occur in the last phase of REM sleep. These are usually seen in 6- to 10-year-old children and are precipitated by a previous traumatic or stressful event. Nightmares are characterized by disturbing dreams followed by postevent anxiety and refusal to go to sleep. Contrary to sleep terrors, here, the child remembers the dreams and is consolable. Proper sleep hygiene is the mainstay of treatment. Violent and frightening television programs just before bedtime should be avoided.

Night Time Fears

Childhood fears to some specific objects such as ghosts, storms, darkness, cockroaches, flying insects, and lizards are normal. These fears may manifest in various ways, like resistance in going to sleep and even as frightening dreams. Fear of darkness may be alleviated by low night light. Other fears may be countered by parental support and good bedtime stories.

Somnambulism

Somnambulism or sleepwalking is generally seen in the age group of 4–8 years. Sometimes, a child walks in sleep in a dazed confused state with eyes open and reacts to external stimuli. It is an altered state of consciousness or impaired judgment. The child does not appear to recognize the surrounding person. Though the child makes simple or complex acts during the episode, he does not recall them. Sleep deprivation or febrile illness may be the precipitating factors. Somnambulism is associated with the risk of safety concern for the child. The condition can be managed by avoidance of sleeplessness, anticipatory arousal, and benzodiazepines or tricyclic antidepressants.

Somniloquy

Somniloquy or talking during sleep is a common feature in the general population, seen in children as well as in adults. It is seen in both NREM and REM sleep. It is a benign condition and often features legible sentences with meaning and good recall. It can coexist with other parasomnias such as somnambulism and night terrors.

Confusional Arousals

Confusional arousals are common in children. The child suddenly wakes up, utters a few words or cries inconsolably. It appears as if the child is not able to recognize people around and again falls asleep. The episodes build slowly and last longer, even 30 minutes. This is generally seen in the transition from one stage to another stage of sleep.

Bruxism

Bruxism is the forceful grinding or rhythmic clenching of teeth including rhythmic movements of the mandible during sleep. It is seen in >50% of children and also in the adult population. The onset may be in adolescence, also when there is a sleep timing problem and delayed sleep phase disorder. There is no confirmatory evidence of the belief of bruxism as the manifestation of worm infestation. Emotional or psychological factors may contribute to bruxism. Severe bruxism may precipitate temporomandibular disorders and it may require orthodontic treatment.

Delayed Sleep Phase Disorder

Delayed sleep phase disorder is a type of dyssomnia where there is a delay in initiation of sleep beyond socially acceptable or desired bedtime, which leads to difficulty in and delayed waking up. It is commonly seen in the adolescent years. It is usually associated with daytime sleepiness. In this situation, the sleep–wake schedule is progressively delayed by 2 or more hours beyond the scheduled bedtime and it leads to difficulty in daily activities.

The treatment plan should be to gradually shift the bedtime by 15 minutes. Melatonin, 1 mg and gradually increased up to 3 mg, when given 1 hour before the desired time of onset of sleep is effective in altering the sleep phase. But a proper sleep environment should also be maintained.

Behavioral Insomnia of Childhood

The causes of insomnia in children are numerous. There are two types of behavioral insomnia of childhood (BIC): One is sleep onset association type and the other is limit setting type. BIC is more common in the preschool and older age group. It occurs in 10–30% of the childhood population.

Insomnia by definition is difficulty in initiation or maintenance of sleep causing impairment in functioning areas occurring at least 3 nights a week for >3 months despite adequate opportunity to sleep. The usual causes and approach are as below.

Poor sleep hygiene: It is believed to play a vital role in many insomnia problems. Sleep hygiene is a constellation of sleep-related behaviors that promote appropriately timed and effective sleep. This includes sleeping in an environment which is comfortable and conducive to sleep, regular, and appropriate scheduling of daily and sleep-related activities, calming atmosphere and appropriate practices in the presleep period, and particularly avoiding things which are physiologically arousing and stimulating (late daytime napping, stimulants such as caffeine, and activities such as excessive and inappropriately timed use of electronic media).

Psychophysiological insomnia: It is characterized by heightened arousal, both cognitive and somatic, around the sleep onset phase which is generally associated with sleep-incompatible associations, which can prevent the onset of sleep. Here, the habit of lying awake in bed for extended periods has become a learned behavior and it will persist beyond the presence of the root cause, for example, even after the source of stress or trauma has passed.

Idiopathic insomnia: It is a lifetime pattern of sleep difficulties. It is considered to arise as a result of genetically determined or certain congenital abnormalities, which cause atypical functioning of the brain-based sleep and/or arousal systems.

Paradoxical insomnia: It is a state of severe sleep disturbance which is not corroborated by objective evaluation of sleep.

Insomnia due to another mental disorder: Various coexisting psychiatric conditions can be associated with insomnia.

Insomnia due to a medical condition: Several medical conditions are associated with insomnia such as epilepsy, persistent cough, and any painful physical conditions affecting breathing or mobility.

Insomnia due to a drug or substance: Many drugs, substances, or their withdrawal can be associated with insomnia in a variety of ways.

Neurobehavioral and Neurocognitive Effects

Insufficient and poor-quality sleep results in the following:
- Behavioral manifestations of sleepiness in children are varied. These range from those that are classically "dozing" or "sleepy," such as yawning, rubbing eyes, and/or resting the head on a desk, to various externalizing behaviors, such as increased impulsivity, hyperactivity, and aggressiveness, to mood lability and inattentiveness.
- Daytime sleepiness and behavioral dysregulation can affect neurocognitive functions in children, especially the functions involving learning and memory consolidation and also those associated with the prefrontal cortex (e.g., attention, working memory, and other executive functions).
- Affect mood (irritability, decreased positive mood, poor affect modulation).
- Obstructive sleep apnea syndrome (OSAS), sleep-disordered breathing (SDB) (i.e., OSAS and snoring).
- Restless legs syndrome (RLS) and periodic limb movement disorder (PLMD).
- Other postulated health outcomes include potential deleterious effects on the cardiovascular, immune, and various metabolic systems, including glucose metabolism and endocrine function. There is also an increase in accidental injuries. There may be secondary effects on parents (e.g., maternal depression).

GENERAL MANAGEMENT

Sleep problem is often not a disease, and many healthy children may also suffer from sleep-related disorders. Sleep hygiene is the most important aspect of the management of sleep problems. Though sleep habits are relative and vary in different families to a great extent, proper sleep habits should be inculcated in all children from an early age. The main components of sleep hygiene are as follows:

- Proper and consistent time to go to sleep and wake up
- Proper environment—comfortable bed, dark quiet room
- Electronic gadgets such as television, computer, tabs, gaming systems, and smartphones should be restricted
- Avoidance of caffeine-rich food and beverages in the evening and night
- Avoidance of play and exercise before bedtime
- Positive reinforcement—various age-appropriate strategies may be beneficial.

Other nonpharmacological therapies are extinction and graduated extinction, fading, scheduled waking, sleep restriction, and light therapy. Parents can play a vital role in the management of sleep problems in children. Sharing bed with small children or bedtime stories may solve many sleep-related problems.

Referral to a sleep medicine behavioral specialist or pediatric sleep clinic may be required under the following circumstances:

- Unsatisfactory response in the child
- Failure of adherence by caregivers to the behavioral interventions
- Insomnia in patients with medical, psychiatric, or neuro-developmental comorbidities
- Insomnia accompanied by significant daytime sleepiness
- Pharmacotherapy being considered
- Suspected additional sleep diagnoses, such as sleep-related breathing disorders, RLS, or circadian-based disorders.

Pharmacological therapies should be reserved as the last resort. But drugs should only be an adjunct to behavioral therapy. Melatonin as a drug is the synthetic form of the hormone produced by the pineal gland and is a commonly used pharmacologic treatment for insomnia in children. It is particularly appropriate for children with sleep disturbance due to circadian phase delay.

It is efficacious and generally very well tolerated both in special pediatric populations, such as children with ADHD or autism, and in typically developing children. No significant long-term adverse effects have been identified with melatonin use. Antihistamines such as diphenhydramine are sometimes used as sedatives in pediatric practice. They may be useful in acute situations such as sleeplessness related to travel or illness. But they are rarely appropriate for managing a chronic sleep problem because tolerance tends to develop.

> **GUIDELINES FOR PARENTS**
> - Proper sleep hygiene should be inculcated in all children from a *very early age*.
> - Appropriate environment and consistent bedtime are crucial for proper sleep.
> - Screen time should be restricted before bedtime.
> - Parental support can cure many sleep problems.
> - Drugs are rarely required.

BIBLIOGRAPHY

1. American Academy of Sleep Medicine. International Classification of Sleep Disorders, 3rd edition. Darien, IL: American Academy of Sleep Medicine; 2014.
2. Bharti B, Mehta A, Malhi P. Sleep problems in children: a guide for primary care physicians. Indian J Pediatr. 2013;80:492-8.
3. Bhatia MS, Gupta R. Common sleep disorders. In: Gupte S (Ed). Recent Advances in Pediatrics–19, Hot Topics. New Delhi: Jaypee Brothers Medical Publishers; 2010.
4. Chhangani B, Greydanus DE, Patel DR, Feucht C. Pharmacology of sleep disorders in children and adolescents. Pediatr Clin North Am. 2011;58:273-91.
5. Owens JA, Moturi S. Pharmacologic treatment of pediatric insomnia. Child Adolesc Psychiatr Clin N Am. 2009;18:1001-16.

CHAPTER 14

Mood Disorder

Saheli Misra

■ INTRODUCTION

Behavioral problems have increased in the society with the increase of small family structures, where individual children are getting more attention. Hence, their problems are addressed better. The behavioral problems in children will differ from adults in the following aspects:
- The child is in the process of development; hence, it is important to determine whether the problems arising are deviations from normal development. For example, temper tantrums are normal in children up to 5 years of age.
- The ongoing process of change during adolescence and the play of hormones may predispose the youth to behave differently, hindering proper assessment of the adolescent.
- Inability of a child to tell the examiner their problems as they are often limited in their ability to verbalize.

Mood disorders such as depression occur in children of all ages but are more common with increasing age. Though the normal developmental process influences the features of depressive disorder, the core features are similar in children, adolescents, and adults. Children and adolescents with depressive disorders usually are irritable and withdrawn from family and peers with academic deterioration. It often leads to social isolation.

■ EPIDEMIOLOGY

Mood disorder among preschool children is rare. The prevalence rate of major depression was reported as 1.4% using Diagnostic and Statistical Manual of Mental Disorders, fourth edition (DSM-IV) based diagnosis from parental responses in preschool children.

About 3.5% of children and teenagers between the ages of 5 and 17 years suffer from depression, and the rate increases with age. Depressive disorders are as high as 18.2% for girls and 7.7% for boys by the age of 17 years, causing morbidity and even mortality. The prevalence of early onset bipolar disorder is rare and reported to be 1% in older adolescents. The gender difference, though not present in childhood, is present in teens among girls. The prevalence of bipolar disorder and disruptive mood regulation disorder is estimated at 0.8–4.3% in children.

Indian studies are few, and they report a prevalence of depression in 0.1% children in the 4–16-year age-group in a Bengaluru-based community sample. A clinic-based study in Chandigarh and Delhi reports 1.2% and 3–6%, respectively, in 2–12-year age-group.

ETIOLOGY

Genetic

Two genes have been identified as incurring vulnerability for depressive disorder. The *MAOA* gene is responsible for functioning of the monoamine oxidase enzyme. The second is the serotonin transporter gene (*5-HTT*).

Familial

Mood disorders in children tend to cluster in the same families. A mother with depression is a strong predictor for a child developing a mood disorder. If both the parents suffer from depression, the chance of the child suffering from depression is four times. A strong family history of attention-deficit hyperactivity disorder (ADHD) exists in bipolar disorder.

Biological

There are biological abnormalities in prepubertal children with depression. There is alteration in neurotransmitters and hormones, but the exact role is yet to be established.

Neuroimaging

Magnetic resonance imaging (MRI) of more than 100 children with mood disturbances reports low frontal lobe volumes and a high ventricular volume. Since the frontal lobe has multiple connections with limbic system and basal ganglia, it is involved in the neuropathology of mood disorders. In bipolar disorder, there is a dysfunction in neural circuit in the amygdale, striatal, thalamic, and prefrontal structures of the brain.

Endocrine
Thyroid function studies have found low free thyroxine levels in depressed adolescents though the thyroid-stimulating hormone levels are normal.

Social
The social causes include parental neglect, parental disharmony, or any sad event such as the death of a near and dear one.

Psychological/Cognitive
The thought process of a child is maladjusted such that the child has automatic negative thoughts (*Teacher is mad because I did something wrong*) along with self-critical and highly negative views of oneself (*I have no friends because I'm bad in studies*).

Behavioral
Lack of social skill causes negative feedback with negative perception. They constantly seek reassurance from others.

CLINICAL FEATURES
- Irritable, oppositional, and negative; refusing to do work in school; and have severe emotional outburst at home and school
- Children with unexplained physical complaint, headache, or stomachache, where a medical cause cannot explain the disability
- Hyperactive, impulsive, motor-driven children who tear up the world around them

The first two depict depression, while the third describes bipolar disorder.

Disruptive Mood Dysregulation Disorder

This disorder may be identified in individuals who have persistent irritability or anger and recurrent episodes (on average three times per week) of developmentally inappropriate verbal or behavioral dyscontrol. The symptoms start before the age of 10 years, the diagnosis is made between the ages of 6 and 18 years, and the disorder causes significant impairment.

Persistent Depressive Disorder

Under Diagnostic and Statistical Manual of Mental Disorders, fifth edition (DSM 5), persistent depressive disorder requires a duration of 1 year in children and only two (or more) depressive symptoms.

Premenstrual Dysphoric Disorder

Specific symptoms are seen in teens in the week before menstruation, which subside with the onset of menstruation. The main symptoms include mood swing, irritability, anxiety or tension as well as additional symptoms mounting to at least five symptoms.

Bipolar Disorder

Depression and mania may not alternate in children. The manic phase may not appear until years later. This disorder is found to be more common in adolescence and youth, where the primary symptoms are irritability and grandiosity.

DIAGNOSIS

Evaluating a child or an adolescent for depression can be time consuming. Hence, various screening methods are used. These include psychosocial evaluation, questionnaires, and structured interviews.

The DSM 5 criteria are used to classify mood disorder as shown in **Flowchart 1**. The types of depressive and bipolar mood disorders are shown in **Flowchart 2**.

The following are the diagnostic criteria as per DSM 5:
- A prominent and persistent period of depressed mood or markedly diminished interest or pleasure in all, or almost all, activities that predominates in clinical practice

Mood Disorder

Flowchart 1: Classification of mood disorder.

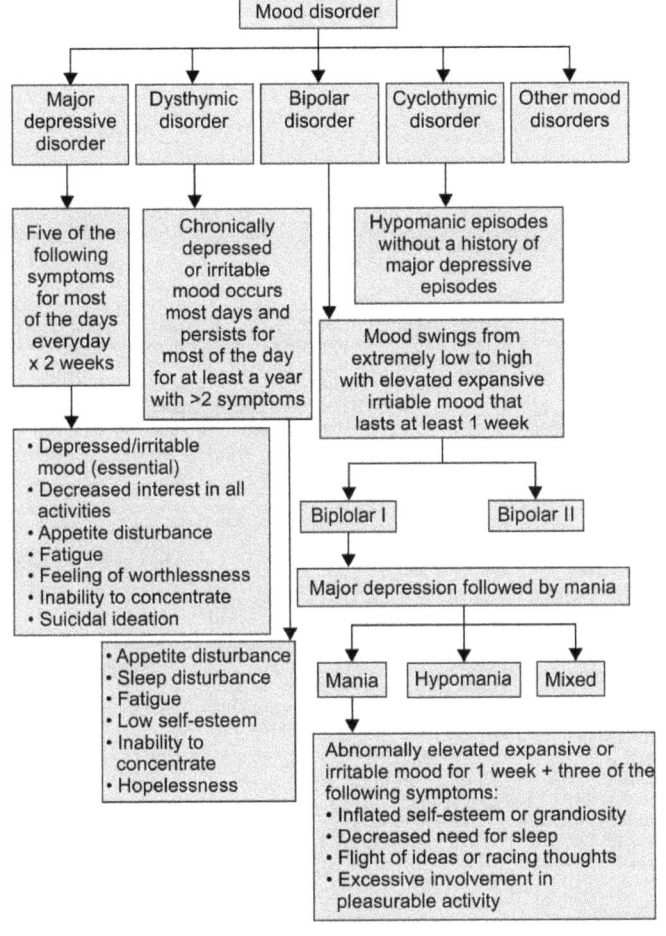

- There is evidence from the history, physical examination, or laboratory findings that the disturbance is the direct pathophysiological consequence of another medical condition.
- The disturbance is not better explained by another mental disorder (e.g., adjustment disorder, with depressed mood, in which the stressor is a serious medical condition).
- The disturbance does not occur exclusively during the course of a delirium.

Mood Disorder

Flowchart 2: Types of depressive and bipolar mood disorders.

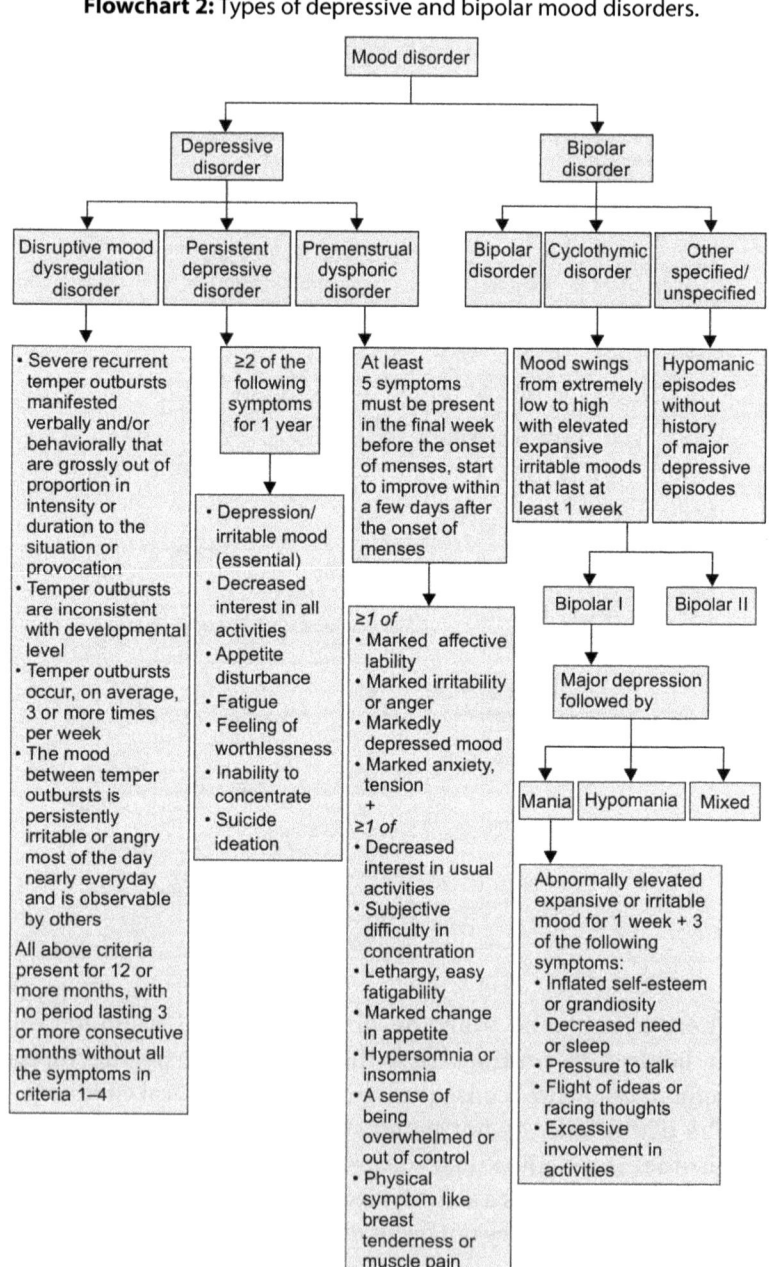

TABLE 1: Diagnostic tests.

Physiologic	Neurophysiologic
• Complete blood count • Serum electrolyte • Liver function • BUN • Lead level • Iron studies • Thyroid function • Toxicology screen for lead and mercury • Genetic testing	• Electroencephalogram • Neuroimaging MRI

(BUN: blood urea nitrogen; MRI: magnetic resonance imaging)

TABLE 2: Differential diagnosis.

Psychiatric disorder	Medical disorder	Depression secondary to medication
Anxiety	Hypothyroidism/hyperthyroidism	Beta blocker
ADHD	Anemia	Corticosteroid
SLD	Inflammatory bowel disorder	Neuroleptics
Substance abuse	Lupus/collagen disorder	
Eating disorder	Stroke/tumor/CNS disorder	
	HIV/hepatitis	
	Premenstrual dysphoria	

(ADHD: attention-deficit hyperactivity disorder; CNS: central nervous system; HIV: human immunodeficiency virus; SLD: specific learning disorder)

- The disturbance causes clinically significant distress or impairment in social, occupational, or other important areas of functioning.

In addition, physiologic tests and neuropsychologic tests **(Table 1)** are also required. When required, a projective personality test is done.

DIFFERENTIAL DIAGNOSIS

Psychiatric and medical conditions mimic depressive disorder in children and adolescents **(Table 2)**. Often, most of these disorders present as comorbid conditions with depression. ADHD, conduct disorder, and anxiety disorder coexist with bipolar disorder in children.

■ TREATMENT

Depression

Cognitive behavioral therapy (CBT), interpersonal psychotherapy (IPT), supportive interventions, and behavioral family interventions help to reduce mood problems in children.

Cognitive Behavioral Therapy

This therapy helps children to develop coping strategy but the effect is not long lasting.

Interpersonal Psychotherapy

This therapy helps to identify interpersonal conflicts that are causing distress and provides support strategies to address these conflicts. It is effective with depressed adolescents.

Supportive Intervention

The child or adolescent is encouraged to expose themselves to a situation in order to understand the factor causing the stress. The intervention is dependent on the success of the therapist to engage the child.

Behavioral Family Interventions

This involves the parents and assists them to address the child's problem. The parent–child relationship needs to be addressed when the root of the cause lies in the family.

Pharmacotherapeutic Agents

Selective serotonin reuptake inhibitors (SSRIs) are widely accepted as first-line intervention for depression. The usual rule is to start at a low dose, such as 5–10 mg of fluoxetine or its equivalent, and to increase the dosage gradually over 4–6 weeks to 20 mg before effectiveness can be appreciated. The drug dosages are shown in

TABLE 3: Drug dosage.

Name	Strength	Starting dose	Target dose	Side effects
Fluoxetine	20 mg/5 mL, 10, 20	2.5–10	20–60	GI symptoms, restlessness
Sertraline	25, 50, 100	12.5–25	50–100	GI symptoms, restlessness
Citalopram	10, 20, 40	2.5–10	20–40	GI symptoms, restlessness
Valproate	100, 200, 100 mg/5 mL	20 mg	Serum level	Liver dysfunction, alopecia, pancreatitis
Lamotrigine	25, 50, 100	25	200	Rash
Risperidone	0.25, 0.5, 1, 2, 3, 4	0.25 bd	1–2	Weight gain, EPS, galactorrhea
Olanzapine	2.5, 5, 10, 15, 20	2.5 bd	10–20	Weight gain

(EPS: extrapyramidal symptoms; GI: gastrointestinal)

Table 3. The American Academy of Child and Adolescent Psychiatry allows progression from one SSRI to another, if the first agent is ineffective. Sertraline and citalopram have been effectively tried in children.

Clearly, for the treatment of resistant depression, consultation with a child psychiatrist who is an expert in mood disorders is necessary. Medications are used after psychotherapy has been availed and failed to show optimal result. Occasionally, they may be used hand in hand.

Bipolar Disorder

Trials have shown valproate to be effective in the treatment of mania in childhood. A trial of lamotrigine in the treatment of bipolar depression in youth provides support for its use in children and adolescents. Risperidone may be effective in controlling mania in children. Olanzapine is another drug that has undergone trial for the treatment of both mania and depression in bipolar disorder in children.

Family focused psychoeducational treatment with mood stabilizers have shown improvement over a year.

PROGNOSIS AND OUTCOME

About 90% of major depression remits in 1.5-2 years after onset, with 6-10% persisting beyond. Relapse occurs 6 months to 1 year after withdrawal of treatment at a rate of 34-50%. Recurrence has been reported in studies of children and adolescents followed for 3-8 years at 54-72%. The predictors for relapse and recurrence are younger age at onset, increased severity of index episode, increased stressors, poor compliance, female, strong family history, and conflict with parents. Dysthymia lasts from 3 to 4 years. It may progress to depression within 2-3 years. Bipolar depression is estimated to occur in 20-40% children and adolescents within 5 years of diagnosis of major depression. 70% of bipolar disorder recovers from their index episode within 2 years.

> **GUIDELINES FOR PARENTS**
> It is important to get help for children and teens when they:
> - Are persistently unhappy
> - Are irritable without provocation
> - Lose interest in their favorite activities

BIBLIOGRAPHY

1. Diagnostic and Statistical Manual of Mental Disorders, 5th edition. Washington DC: American Psychiatric Association; 2013.
2. Emslie GJ, Mayes T, Kennard BD, Hughes JL. Pediatric mood disorders. In: Stein DJ, Kupfer DJ, Schatzber AF (Eds). Textbook of Mood Disorders. Washington, DC: The American Psychiatric Publishing Inc.; 2006. pp. 573-602.
3. Kowatch RA, Emslie GJ, Wilkaitis J, Dingle AD. Mood disorders. In: Sexson SB (Ed). Child and Adolescent Psychiatry, 2nd edition. Massachusetts: Blackwell Publishing Ltd; 2005. pp. 132-53.
4. Lack CW, Green AL. Mood disorders in children and adolescents. J Pediatr Nurs. 2009;24:13-25.
5. Mullen S. Major depressive disorder in children and adolescents. Ment Health Clin. 2018;8(6):275-83.
6. Sadock BJ, Sadock VA. Mood disorders and suicide. Kaplan and Sadock's Concise Textbook of Child and Adolescent Psychiatry. Philadelphia: Lippincott Williams and Wilkins; 2009.
7. Tang MH, Pinsky EG. Mood and affect disorders. Pediatr Rev. 2015;36(2):52-61.

CHAPTER 15

Anxiety Disorder

Ranjana Chatterjee, Mandira Roy

■ INTRODUCTION

Anxiety has been described as a dysphoric, aversive feeling. It is made up of the following:
- *Physiological symptoms*: Sweaty palms, "butterflies" in the stomach
- *Behavioral signs*: Such as avoidance
- *Cognitive components*: Like "I am going to fail and everyone will laugh at me."

Fear and anxiety are a common part of the human condition. Though these two terms are used interchangeably, they are essentially different. *Fear* is defined as an emotional response to a real or perceived imminent threat. *Anxiety* is the anticipation of a future threat. They are age-typical transitory states in a developing child, and in many situations, they are adaptive and protective in that they signal danger and prepare the child to face the challenging situation.

In general, children become anxious or fearful at some time in their lives, typically during childhood transitions, such as shifting to another neighborhood, starting a new school, attending camps, taking tests, or participating in different social activities. The majority of youth move out of such anxious episodes without any disruption to their lives, but around 10–20% of them experience moderate-to-severe anxiety symptoms that affect their academic, social, and emotional development. The degree of distress, impairment of functioning, and/or interference with daily life activities decide what is "normal" adaptive response or it needs intervention. But the exact landmark where normal anxiety ends, and clinical anxiety begins remains obscure.

EPIDEMIOLOGY

As a group, anxiety disorders are the most common psychiatric disorders of childhood. Epidemiologic data suggest that they occur in 10–30% of all children and adolescents approximately, though the incidence varies with different types of anxiety disorder. It is one of those mental health issues that may present earliest, even in infancy. Anxiety disorder can be missed in young children due to its nonspecific variable presentations. Various researches suggest that children with anxiety disorder can have an increased likelihood of other psychiatric comorbidities such as hyperactivity disorder, oppositional defiant disorder, language disorder, and depressive disorder. Interestingly, different types of anxiety can also coexist.

Data from a cohort of behaviorally inhibited infants followed longitudinally revealed that both a family history of anxiety disorders and maternal overinvolvement predicted later clinically significant anxiety problems.

ETIOPATHOGENESIS

Anxiety disorder evolves with multifactorial causation. Genetics, epigenetics, biochemistry, and environment all contribute to the development of anxiety disorders. Most adolescents and adults seem to have a biological vulnerability to stress, making them more susceptible to environmental stimuli than the rest of the population.

Origin of Anxiety

To understand the mechanism of the origin of anxiety, we need to know the different types of stressors. Though the word "stress" has negative connotations, according to various psychological forums, we need a certain amount of stress to function, especially when we are learning new things, appearing for some competitive sports, writing time-bound exams, or giving a stage performance. This healthy or positive level of stress is called *eustress*. This acts as a protective and adaptive response to the challenges we are facing in our daily life. For the developing child, various age-typical fears such as social anxiety and fear of darkness are good examples of eustress. Now, when the stress-coping mechanism does not function well, it leads to *distress*, which is negative stress. This is where the anticipatory preoccupation with an imaginary threat begins to evolve and manifests as anxiety disorder.

The rate of functional development is greater during childhood and adolescence than at other times of life. Knowledge concerning "normal" fears and anxieties at each developmental stage is vital when attempting to ascertain whether or not a child suffers from an anxiety disorder. Anxiety that is typical for a preschooler may be atypical if experienced by an adolescent. As a consequence of developmental experiences of children along with their increasing cognitive abilities, the content of their fears and anxieties changes over time. The focus generally shifts from concrete, external fear to internalized abstract anxieties. Thus, an infant generally gets afraid of strangers, loud noises, and unexpected environmental stimuli, while children fear separation from their parents, insects, and darkness. Between the ages of 4 and 6 years, predominant fears include clowns, kidnappers, ghosts, and monsters. Around the age of 6 years, fears of bodily injury, shame, failure, and death develop. These may continue into early adolescence. At 10 or 11 years of age, fears regarding social comparison, physical appearance, personal conduct, and school examinations may predominate.

Developmental Factors

Progression of anxiety can be seen throughout developmental ages over the lifespan. Age-appropriate transitory anxieties can be perfectly normal for a certain age, but their persistence beyond a certain age can be a manifestation of a disorder. Infants who are excessively apprehensive and hesitant to novel stimuli grow as behaviorally inhibited toddlers who lack the excitement of exploring a new surrounding and are at a greater risk of developing anxiety symptoms. These children can also continue to be anxious as adults.

Anxious cognitive pattern in childhood can lead to cognitive distortion as adolescents and adults. There can be hypervigilance for essentially neutral stimuli, overinterpretation of potential threats from neutral stimuli, lack of ability to ignore a threat when harm is not expected, and faulty termination of mental preparedness for an anticipatory threat when required.

Neurobiological Factors

An important pathway in the development of fear and anxiety is the cortico-amygdala circuit. Amygdala plays an important role in pairing an unconditioned stimulus with a conditioned stimulus. The hippocampus and prefrontal cortex (PFC) are implicated in learning. An imbalance in the amygdale-PFC network, specifically elevated amygdala activity, and decreased PFC are regarded as hallmark of anxiety disorder. This imbalance is maximum in the developmental stage of adolescence, which may explain the emergence of anxiety disorders in the pubertal age group.

Multiple studies explored and suggested that imbalance of neurotransmitters may contribute to anxiety disorders. The neurotransmitters that are associated with anxiety disorders are gamma-aminobutyric acid (GABA), serotonin, dopamine, and epinephrine. Serotonin is considered to be specifically important in feelings of well-being, and deficiencies are highly related to anxiety and depression. Stress hormones such as cortisol also play a significant role. Genetic analysis studies have linked different variants of the serotonin transporter (*5-HTT*) gene to have an effect on the brain's response to anxiety-producing stimuli.

Genetic Factors

Up to 50% of children with panic disorder and 40% of patients with generalized anxiety disorder (GAD) have close relatives with the disorder.

Obsessive-compulsive disorder (OCD) is strongly related to a family history of a similar problem. Close relatives of people with OCD are around nine times more likely to develop OCD. Ongoing researches are trying to identify specific genetic factors that might particularly contribute to an inherited risk. Of specific interest are genes that regulate specific neurotransmitters, including serotonin and glutamate. Recent research has suggested that the *SLC1A1* gene, which is associated with glutamate regulation, may play an important role in early onset OCD in boys. Research is also beginning to pinpoint regions on specific chromosomes (1, 3, 7, 6, 9, and 15) that may contain genes linked to OCD.

Although family genetic studies have shown that there may be some genetic vulnerability to stressors and developing anxiety disorders, there is no single genetic test that can identify patients at risk of anxiety disorders. Children develop a particular anxiety disorder at specific developmental stages. For example, separation anxiety disorder (SAD) and specific phobias are generally seen in children under the age of 9 years, whereas GAD, social anxiety, OCD, and panic disorders often appear in mid-childhood through adolescence. Acute stress disorder and post-traumatic stress disorder can occur at any age.

Environmental Factors

Environmental and social factors play an important role in the development of anxiety disorder. Various twin studies show a significant direct environmental transmission of anxiety from parents. Parenting style is found to be a critical component of environmental factor. Anxious, overprotective, and overly critical authoritarian parenting can suppress the spontaneous expression of fear and anxiety in children. Overprotective parenting that focuses strictly on avoiding dangers for the children may itself instill fear and attenuate child's brave and exploratory behaviors. Child abuse by parents and other relatives, and frequent punishments in school can also be very important reasons for anxiety disorder.

Clinical Manifestation

Children may exhibit symptoms of anxiety quite differently than adults. The presence of symptoms of anxiety or stress does not always decipher that the child has an anxiety disorder.

Children and adolescents can present with a variety of clinical symptoms, e.g., avoidance of certain activities such as school, camps, homework, and parties; some somatic issues such as headache or abdominal pain, sleep problems, bad dreams, poor scholastic performances, anger issues, or oppositional behaviors; eating disorders; and depressive symptoms. Certain phobias may even lead to self-injurious or suicidal behaviors, especially in adolescent.

■ TYPES OF ANXIETY DISORDERS

The main categories of anxiety disorder are described here. The Diagnostic and Statistical Manual of Mental Disorders, 5th edition (DSM 5), 2013 chapter on anxiety disorder no longer includes OCD, post-traumatic stress disorder, or acute stress disorder, which was there previously in DSM-IV, 1994.

Separation Anxiety Disorder

Children aged 18 months to 5 years generally get anxious with the thought of being detached from their parents. They cry, get nervous, and often throw tantrums when separated from their caregivers. Separation anxiety is a protective, natural, developmental phase that typically persists till the preschool years. However, for a very small percentage of children, separation remains a terrifying experience even when they are older. When separated from their parents or family members they are most attached to, these children fear that they themselves or a parent will be harmed or that they will be abandoned or kidnapped. The anxiety may be severe enough to cause school refusal. They may avoid playing outside, going to parties, or participating in other developmentally appropriate activities. Though SAD is most common in children between the ages of 7 and 9 years, according to DSM 5, it can be diagnosed at any age, even after 18 years. The typical signs of SAD include the following:

- Episodes of nagging cry, clinging, or tantrums while separating from a parent/caregiver
- Refusal to attend school or sports activities without the parent
- Complaints of somatic symptoms such as abdominal pain or nonspecific pains before school or outing
- Demands that a parent be present until the child falls asleep

Generalized Anxiety Disorder

All children experience anxiety from time to time, but some children experience constant and unrelenting worry, and in that case, a diagnosis of GAD should be considered. Adolescents with GAD seem to worry about everything related to family members, school grades, performance in sports and other activities, relationships, health, and society at large. They are often found to be perfectionists who spend countless hours and energy on school projects, considering minute details, with the fear of making a mistake, performing poorly, or failing in test. They are so preoccupied with their racing thoughts that they actually become clumsy and make silly mistakes. The typical signs of GAD include the following:

- Overthinking and worrying about a range of day-to-day activities or issues
- Extreme reactiveness to minor setbacks. For example, they get very anxious before any kind of performance, and if some unpredictable delay or obstacle happens, it makes them overwhelmed.
- Physiological signs of anxiety, such as trouble relaxing, being easily fatigued, difficulty falling or staying asleep, irritability, and movements of legs, hands, eyelids, and lips.

Social Anxiety Disorder

Humans are social beings. Social understanding starts developing as early as 6 months in infants, and then real social exposure happens at play school, park, and family functions. Children are expected to interact with friends and adults and develop adaptive, essential social skills and cultural values.

Generally, children or adolescents enjoy social interaction if it appeals to their interest and they fit in well. It helps them to learn some soft skills to navigate this world confidently. However, a small percentage of them develop social anxiety disorder, which is characterized by an intense fear of negative judgment by others that results in anxiety in social situations. This type of anxiety leads to withdrawal from social interactive situations and avoidant behavior. The duration of the condition should be persisting for 6 months or more. Children with social anxiety disorder are interested in developing social relationships, but their intense anxiety prevents them from doing so, resulting in self-isolation. The typical signs of social anxiety disorder include the following:

- Intense fear of doing something embarrassing, saying the wrong thing or being judged by others
- Avoidance behavior, including not making or sustaining eye contact, answering in brief sentences, or fumbling

- Limited participation in school activities, such as refusing to answer questions or read aloud in class, skipping lunch with friends, and avoiding performance situations and group interactions
- Limited participation in any kind of enjoyable social activity, such as finding excuses not to attend sleepovers, parties, and camps, and refusing to make phone calls or initiate social contact with others
- Fear of interacting with strangers manifesting as an inability to order in a restaurant, approach a teacher, or ask an adult for assistance

Specific Phobia

Fears of cockroaches in the storeroom or monsters under the bed are a natural part of a child's development, as are fears of strangers, heights, darkness, and loud noises. Such fears are considered protective and adaptive; children typically outgrow them over the course of time, and normally it does interfere with their daily life. However, some children experience persistent and intense fears; they may cry, freeze, or cling when they are in a threatening situation or near the feared object. The most commonly seen phobias include fear of animals, insects, reptiles, and birds; some environmental conditions include fear of heights, closed spaces, thunderstorms, deep water and darkness, blood and injections, doctors and other healthcare staff, and hospitals.

Children with phobias are often preoccupied with fear, and it may significantly hamper their quality of life. For example, if a child has phobia of darkness, he may keep lights on always, seek presence of some adults, and cling to them; it may hamper his sleep.

The typical signs of a specific phobia include the following:

- The child may have had a prior upsetting exposure to the feared object or conditions.
- Individuals in the child's immediate surroundings, such as parents or other close family members, have similar fears (e.g., mother is afraid of spiders).
- When the child gets exposed to or anticipates exposure to the phobic situation, it becomes extremely distressing for him.

He gets angry, cries, gets freeze reaction, clings to an adult, and refuses to approach the situation.
- The child's fear persists in spite of support and encouragement from others and does not diminish in intensity.

Panic Disorder with or without Agoraphobia

Panic disorder and agoraphobia are unlinked in DSM 5 as a substantial number of individuals with agoraphobia do not experience panic symptoms.

Panic attacks are characterized by an intense and sudden onset of fear followed by a range of physiological and cognitive symptoms such as palpitation, breathlessness, and the belief that one is dying.

Agoraphobia is the anticipatory anxiety about being in a particular situation where the youth might have a panic attack and may not be able to easily escape, escape without embarrassment, or in which he/she may feel helpless. Panic attacks and agoraphobia are not very common in childhood but can emerge in adolescence and are similar to panic disorder with or without agoraphobia in adults. Panic attacks and agoraphobia can be commonly seen in an adolescent with neurodevelopmental disorders such as autism spectrum disorder.

Post-traumatic Stress Disorder

Children or adolescents may experience traumatic events at any point of time. This includes experiences such as witnessing the death of a parent, grandparents, or family member; experiencing a natural disaster; or being physically or sexually abused. Although most children are resilient and recover from such trauma within a few weeks to months, some of them experience a range of psychological, behavioral, and cognitive symptoms that persist over an extended period of time. This indicates the presence of acute stress disorder or post-traumatic stress disorder.

Obsessive–Compulsive Disorder

As per DSM 5, 2013, anxiety disorder no longer includes OCD. It has been included in trauma and stressor-related disorders. But OCD is discussed here due to a close relationship among them.

In day-to-day life, some children require a bit more structure and routine than other children. They are more comfortable when they have a specific set of routines or when their belongings are placed as per their choice. However, during late childhood and early adolescence, 0.5–1% of youth exhibit these and similar behaviors to an extreme degree and may develop OCD.

Obsessive–compulsive disorder is characterized by persistent thoughts or urges that compel the child to take some repetitive actions, which in turn causes distress and exhaustion to the child (obsessions), followed by some rituals intended to get relief from this distress (compulsions). OCD can produce significant interference in the youth's daily life activities, such as in school, family chores, and social activities. The typical signs of OCD include the following:

- Persistent and intrusive thoughts or impulses for certain situations
- Repetitive behaviors or mental rituals to soothe the discomfort or anxiety experienced by the thoughts, images, or impulses
- The child or adolescent may have awareness that these obsessions and compulsions are senseless or "silly"; even then, he or she feels compelled to engage in the rituals. It means that they most often have insight about their own compulsions, and their awareness is preserved.

▪ MANAGEMENT

Cognitive-behavioral Therapy for Anxiety Disorders

Cognitive-behavioral therapy (CBT) is an evidence-based treatment approach that combines skill development with generating alternate perspectives. It includes a variety of methods designed to teach the child or adolescent to cope with anxiety. CBT uses concrete skills that allow the child to approach and remain in situations that previously induced anxiety. The main components of CBT for children with anxiety disorders include the following:

- *Psychoeducation:* Educating the child and family about the nature of anxiety and what factors can trigger and maintain anxiety.
- *Monitoring:* Increasing awareness of anxiety and recognition of early warning signs so that anxiety can be predicted and prevented at the earliest.

- *Relaxation training:* Teaching the child a range of coping skills to increase the child's control over unexpected arousal and to break the connection between arousal and anxiety.
- *Cognitive retraining:* Teaching the children alternative and adaptive ways of thinking to increase control and decrease arousal and anxiety.
- *Problem solving:* Providing a concrete approach to solving everyday problems so that they can become skilled at managing unexpected events and thus decrease arousal and anxiety.
- *Assertiveness training:* Training them verbal and nonverbal skills designed to express themselves in adaptive ways, including skills for handling teasing or bullying.
- *Exposure and response prevention:* Increasing the child's ability to approach feared objects or situations without using rituals to cope.
- *Relapse prevention:* Teaching them skills so that they can maintain gains after treatment has ended.

Treatment methods are selected based on the child's symptoms and problems and are delivered in sequence, with a new component presented when previous skills have been mastered. Careful consideration of the child's developmental age ensures that the child can effectively learn and apply a variety of skills. Parents are an integral part of treatment, and they are also taught many of the same skills that the child learns so they can help the child learn to manage his or her anxiety.

Screening for parental depression or anxiety is to be done. Individual or group CBT is of benefit. Parents should be counseled and told to remain calm in the face of child's anxiety. Systematic desensitization is a form of behavior therapy that exposes the child to the fear-inducing situation or object while a simultaneously relaxation technique for anxiety management is to be taught.

Pharmacotherapy has a definite role in the problem of anxiety disorders. But controlled trials suggest that CBT may lead to somewhat higher response rates, greater symptom reduction levels, and more durable treatment gains than medication alone.

Anxiety is a common experience for the children; most often, professional intervention is not required. If anxiety is so severe that your child cannot do expected tasks, however, then intervention may be indicated. Untreated anxiety can lead to depressive disorder and other psychological problems that can persist even into adulthood. However, anxiety problems can be treated effectively, especially if detected early. Even with all interventions, some degree of anxiety may persist but without disturbing the daily life activities.

GUIDELINES FOR PARENTS

Although professional intervention may be necessary, the following list may be helpful to parents in working with the child at home:
- It is to be remembered that anxiety is not willful misbehavior but reflects an inability to control it. Therefore, be patient and be prepared to listen. Being overly critical, impatient, or cynical will only make the problem worse.
- To maintain realistic, attainable goals and expectations for the child. Often, anxious children try to please adults and will try to be perfect if they believe it is expected of them.
- To maintain a consistent, but flexible, routine for homework, chores, and activities.
- To accept mistakes as a normal part of growing up, and that no one is expected to do everything equally well. Every effort is to be praised and reinforced, even if success is less than expected.
- If the child is worried about an upcoming event, such as giving a speech in class, practice it often so that confidence increases, discomfort decreases, and the anxiety reaches a level that is manageable.
- Parents are advised to listen to and talk with the child on a regular basis and to avoid being critical. Being critical may increase pressure to be perfect, which may be contributing to the problem in the first place.
- All discussions are to be taken seriously. Avoid giving too much advice. Instead, be there to help and offer assistance as requested.
- Parents should not assume that the child is being difficult or that the problem will go away. They have to seek help if the problem persists and continues to interfere with daily activities.

BIBLIOGRAPHY

1. Abellarte MJ, Ginsburg GS, Walkup JT, Riddle MA. The treatment of anxiety disorders in children and adolescents. Boil Psychiatry. 1999;46:1567-78.
2. Anxiety disorders: causes. [online] Available from https://www.nimh.nih.gov/health/topics/anxiety-disorders.
3. Chansky T. Freeing Your Child from Obsessive-Compulsive Disorder: A Powerful, Practical Program for Children and Adolescents. New York: Three Rivers Press; 2000.

4. Dacey JS, Fiore B. Your Anxious Child: How Parents and Teachers Can Relieve Anxiety in Children? San Francisco: Jossey-Bass; 2000.
5. Helping Children at Home and School II: Handouts for Families and Educators. [online] Available from http://www.nmha.org. [Accessed August, 2013].
6. King NJ, Bernstein GA. School refusal in children and adolescents: a review of the past 10 years. J Am Acad Child Adolesc Psychiatry. 2001;40:787-94.
7. Manassis K. Keys to Parenting Your Anxious Child. New York: Barrons; 1996.
8. McClure-Tone EB, Pine DS. Clinical features of anxiety disorders. In: Sadock BJ, Sadock VA, Ruiz P (Eds). Kaplan and Sadock's Comprehensive Textbook of Psychiatry, volume I, 9th edition. Philadelphia, PA: Lippincott Williams and Wilkins; 2009. pp. 1844-55.
9. Stafford B, Boris NW, Dalton R. Anxiety disorders. In: Behrman RE, Kilegman RM, Jenson HB (Eds). Nelson Textbook of Pediatrics, 19th edition. Philadelphia: Saunders; 2011. pp. 81-4.

16 Somatic Symptoms and Related Disorders

Mandira Roy

■ INTRODUCTION

Children are by nature socially underdeveloped in terms of their ability to communicate, especially when it comes to expressing emotions and feelings. Psychosomatic conditions affecting them are those that present often very real symptoms but usually have a limited physiological basis.

■ WHAT IS SOMATIC SYMPTOM DISORDER?

Somatic symptom disorder is characterized by one or more physical symptoms that are accompanied by excessive thoughts, feelings, and/or behaviors related to the somatic symptoms, which may or may not be explained by any recognized general medical illness. These symptoms cause significant discomfort or distress to the child and caregivers.

"Somatoform disorders" were first described formally in the Diagnostic and Statistical Manual of Mental Disorders, 3rd edition (DSM 3) in the year 1980. As the term "somatoform" was a neologism, it was difficult to understand. Another relatively easier term that was being used during that time was "medically unexplained symptoms" (MUS), but this term also generated conflicts among clinicians. These issues were addressed in DSM-IV-TR (published in the year 2000) where psychosomatic disorders were classified in multiple groups such as somatization disorder, undifferentiated somatoform disorder, hypochondriasis disorder, and pain disorders. All these groups had significant overlapping features and lacked clarity. Terms such as "somatoform" and "somatization" created much confusion. The criteria mentioned in DSM-IV-TR lacked sensitivity in the pediatric population.

In 2013, DSM 5 was released with much anticipated revision on psychosomatic disorders. DSM 5 reconceptualized these disorders and classified them into simpler discrete entities where functional impairments are also considered. DSM 5 classified the illnesses that were previously called "somatoform disorders" as *somatic symptom and related disorders (SSRDs)*. SSRDs that are mostly encountered in children and adolescents include *somatic symptom disorder, conversion disorder, factitious disorder, illness anxiety disorder,* other *specified or unspecified somatic symptom disorders*, etc. It removed all other existing nomenclatures such as functional disorder and psychosomatic disorder which were being used interchangeably among clinicians.

Dilemma of Diagnosing Somatic Symptom and Related Disorders

- SSRDs most of the time present to primary care physicians or pediatricians or to some subspecialists and rarely to psychiatrists. This leads to specialty-oriented diagnosis.
- Diagnosing SSRDs in children and adolescents is one of the most difficult challenges faced by a pediatrician. These disorders in children not only are a burden to themselves and their parents but also frustrate the pediatrician investigating such cases with a battery of tests which invariably yield inconclusive results. Parents are unhappy when all the investigations are unable to pinpoint the cause and often doubt the competency of the physician managing such a child, and this often results in "doctor shopping" in search for an answer to the bodily symptoms of their children. This adds a lot of burden to the health care system in terms of not only money but also man-hours. Refusing to acknowledge the emotional link to such disorders often impairs acceptance of appropriate management. This "brick wall of resistance" of parents for acceptance of the nature of these illnesses is a difficult hurdle to cross.
- Pediatricians on the other hand should not be overzealous in diagnosing SSRDs, ignoring ruling out organic causes, particularly in younger children < 5 years of age.
- According to DSM 5, somatic symptoms do not exclude the presence of a general medical illness. Both may coexist, leading to diagnostic confusions.

EPIDEMIOLOGY

Almost all the available evidences suggest a sharp progressive rise in mental health issues among children and adolescents. According to a cross-cultural study by the World Health Organization (WHO), nearly 20% of primary care patients are affected by multiple somatoform symptoms. Many of the symptoms are transient, but a sizeable minority becomes persistent. In fact, social, emotional, or behavioral problems can constitute up to 25% of visits in a pediatric practice, and it has been estimated that as many as 68% of children who present for medical treatment have psychological factors associated with somatic complaints. Prevalence of SSRDs varies greatly due to heterogeneity of symptoms, multiple criteria of classification, and study methodology.

Although SSRDs are common in children and adolescents, they are rare in children <5 years of age. The symptoms peak during the age of 7 years for boys and at ages of 6 and 16 years for girls. In children, the most common symptoms are pain in the abdomen and headache that frequently meet the criteria for SSRDs.

ETIOLOGY

The etiology of SSRDs is still not fully understood, but evidence supports an interaction of physiological, psychological, and interpersonal factors. Although the lack of organic pathology is the central feature of SSRDs, there is some evidence of autonomic and neuromuscular dysregulation in patients with somatic symptoms, such as heart rate reactivity, respiratory dysregulation, and smooth muscle contractions. It seems probable that some of these physiological processes contribute to the complaints. However, evidence is still inconclusive, and even less is known about the specificity of physiological processes in somatoform symptoms.

Biobehavioral Continuum of Diseases

This is a biopsychosocial model of diseases that was put forth by Wood BL, et al. (2000) conceptualizes that all diseases have biological and psychosocial influences that vary across a spectrum. For example, on somatic extreme, it contains functional abdominal pain and on biologic end, it contains congenital heart disease. This concept challenges the traditional medical model which considers biological and somatic disorders as completely separate entities. This model prevents the mind-body dichotomy in clinicians and helps to understand somatic symptoms in a comprehensive manner.

Psychosocial Factors

Several psychosocial factors may lead to somatic symptoms in children and adolescents.

- *Developmental factors*: Children and adolescents can have poor awareness of their own emotions, and managing difficult emotions can be challenging for them without proper tender guidance from adults, especially parents and relatives.
  Children develop somatic symptoms as a *coping mechanism*, a kind of valve used to manipulate their immediate surroundings so that they become most comfortable and anxiety free for them. This process is known as "primary gain." If this behavior is allowed and accepted by parents leading to complete avoidance of the uncomfortable stressor, it can lead to "secondary gain." Children with anxiety and uncomfortable emotions may assume that physical symptoms are given more serious attention and that extra attention tends to reinforce their symptoms.
- *Cognitive and perceptual distortions:* Somatic symptoms may arise from unrealistic obsession toward maintaining health, especially in patients with illness anxiety disorder. Perception of bodily sensations can be distorted that causes catastrophic interpretation influenced by vague cultural beliefs and psychological distress. Benign physiological sensations can be amplified due to lower pain threshold.
- *Difficulties with self-expression:* Some children and adolescents can have difficulties to express emotional distress in words (alexithymia) and may resort to express them through physical symptoms.
- *Psychiatric comorbidity:* There is an association between somatic symptoms and preexisting psychiatric illnesses such as depressive and anxiety disorders. These problems can be familial also.

- *Trauma:* Physical, emotional, or sexual abuse can cause somatic symptoms.
- *Family environment:* Potential stressors within the family can be an important and commonly encountered etiology. These are transitions within the family systems, death of a close member, divorce of parents, domestic violence, birth of a sibling, punishments by parents, gender bias, and physical or mental abuse.
  - *Financial:* Hardship affecting families has been empirically related to the children's hardship, on accounts of material and economic resources. It has also been related to nonmaterial circumstances such as their social relations with parents and peers. Furthermore, it has been shown that young people tend to worry about economic problems in the family. In this way, financial problems can work as a stressor in children's lives, while they are simultaneously afforded fewer coping resources to deal with the resulting stress.
  - *Adult guidance:*
    - *Lack of adult contact and guidance:* Work and stress limit the amount of "quality time" spent together within the family. Structure and guidance are security for children. Therefore, any situation where there is a breakdown of this structure, there is considerable stress on the child.
    - *Excessive use of gadgets:* Children are curious by nature and want information from adults, to know what is expected of them. Many children have a tough time at home after school. Parents work, are absent, and a feeling of guilt makes it hard for parents to place "normal" demands on their children. Children no longer need to take part in household work ending up sequestering themselves in front of the computer, TV, or games console. Excessive use of social media can lead to immense peer pressure and stress in adolescents.
  - *Parental response:* In some families, physical symptoms are given more attention than any mental stress. For example, pain in the abdomen or headache is given serious attention than fear and panic. So, children can obtain sympathy

for somatic symptoms. Interestingly, excessive parental protective response can also cause somatic symptoms.
- *School environment:* There is a close association between stressors in school environment, psychosomatic symptoms, and psychological complaint in school-going children. Therefore, the changes in the school environment over time may be important in understanding why increasing numbers of school children report these symptoms. Psychosocial aspects of the working environment have been linked to many aspects of health in adults, including pains of various kinds. The school environment is in many ways equivalent to the working environment for children of school age but has been much less extensively investigated in relation to health outcomes. Multiple factors in the school or work environment are potential stressors. They are as follows:
  - Harassment and fear of academic failure have been identified as major stressors in the school environment with the closest association with recurrent nonspecific pain.
  - Bullying can cause significant damage to self-esteem and confidence. Troubled relationship with peers and teachers and the demands of school work have been identified as important facets in this respect. This can lead to school avoidance.
  - Aspects of the physical work environment such as peace and quiet, and the quality of maintenance of facilities, have been found to be stress factors in studies of adults' health, but have not been often studied as school stressors, though these factors are likely to be influential in the mental health of a child, e.g., some children may not like to use toilets in school and can present with urinary symptoms or pain symptoms.

Genetic Factors

There are some schools of thoughts which believe that psychosomatic conditions are genetically linked. High anxiety seems to be passed on behaviorally in families and though there is little evidence to suggest that anxiety is passed on through genetic instinct, it cannot entirely be ruled out. Studies suggested that

TABLE 1: Factors that influence childhood vulnerability to psychosomatic illnesses.

Psychological	• Hypersensitivity to bodily sensations • General tendencies toward worry and anxiety
Biological	• Genetic pain traits • Physiological reactivity • Illness or injury • Female sex
Social environment	• Socioeconomic status • Media • School environment
Family	• Parent psychopathology • Social learning • General functioning
Developmental	• Fund of illness knowledge • Physiological and cognitive development

some aberrant neural pathway within the autonomic nervous system and hypothalamic–pituitary axis can cause increased pain sensitivity. Migraine or tension-type headache or chronic pain may be associated with progressive loss of gray matter densities in structures registering pain sensations such as anterior cingulated cortex and somatosensory cortex.

Studies on monozygotic and dizygotic twins confirm genetic contribution to somatic symptoms and depressive and anxiety disorders.

Table 1 shows the various factors that influence childhood vulnerability to psychosomatic illnesses.

■ CLINICAL FEATURES

Psychogenic symptoms are common among children and adolescents, and every pediatric subspecialty has its share of symptoms that can be labeled as "functional."

Gastrointestinal (GI) system: It is the most commonly involved system. Symptoms include vomiting, dysphagia, bloating, abdominal pain, and diarrhea.

Cardiorespiratory system: Noncardiac chest pain is traditionally referred to as "musculoskeletal" chest pain but is probably psychogenic. Other symptoms include shortness of breath and cough.

Nervous system and pain disorder: Pain syndromes for which a psychogenic component is likely to occur include tension headaches, abdominal pain, chronic back pain, limb pain, and rectal pain. Although the perception of pain is by definition entirely subjective, it is extremely difficult and perhaps impossible to designate any particular pain as "psychogenic." It could even be argued that all pain is psychogenic, and thus psychogenic pain is one of the most "uncomfortable" diagnoses to make. In addition to isolated symptoms, some syndromes are considered to be at least partially psychogenic by some and possibly entirely psychogenic (i.e., without any organic basis) by others. These controversial yet sophisticated diagnoses include fibromyalgia, fibrositis, myofascial pain, chronic fatigue, and irritable bowel syndrome. Psychogenic symptoms are relatively also common in neurology.

Functional neurological symptom disorder presents with symptoms such as paralysis, mutism, visual symptoms, sensory symptoms, movement disorders, gait or balance problems, and pain.

Psychogenic nonepileptic seizure (PNES) is an important and commonly encountered somatic symptom which has been studied widely and misdiagnosed often.

Ear, nose, and throat (ENT): Psychogenic globus and dysphonia can be presenting symptoms in adolescents.

Ophthalmology: It can present as ptosis or blindness.

Other than these system-wise involvements, SSRDs can present as a combination of various symptoms along with excessive anxiety regarding recovery and establishing health. These symptoms can follow some prototypes in children and adolescents. These are described in DSM 5 and have individual criteria for diagnosis. Few common SSRDs in pediatric patients from DSM 5 are shown in **Box 1**. DSM 5 criteria for diagnosing somatic symptom disorder are shown in **Box 2**.

BOX 1: Few common somatic symptom and related disorders (SSRDs) in pediatric patients from the Diagnostic and Statistical Manual of Mental Disorders, 5th edition (DSM 5).

> *Somatic symptom disorder:* This involves a person having a significant focus on physical symptoms, such as pain, weakness, or shortness of breath that results in major distress and/or problems functioning
>
> *Illness anxiety disorder:* This is a persistent fear of having a grave medical illness. A person with this disorder pays excessive attention to health. He or she can become easily alarmed by anything that might be interpreted as a sign of illness, including normal sensations, bodily functions, and mild symptoms. Previously, it was called hypochondriasis but the term is obsolete now. For example, normal peristaltic gut can seem as a severe life-threatening problem
>
> *Functional neurologic disorder or conversion disorder:* In this variety, the patient complains of neurological symptoms that cannot be explained by a neurological disease or other medical conditions. However, the symptoms are real and cause significant distress. As for example, paralysis of limbs, swallowing difficulties, astasia abasia, or other gait problems
>
> *Factitious disorders or by proxy:* In this disorder, the patient falsely identifies himself or herself as sick by inducing some injury or disease associated with identified deception. This behavior cannot be explained by any other mental condition. For example, producing menstrual blood as hematemesis
> In a relatively rare situation, a person (adult caregiver) can bring a child (victim) inducing some injury or illness for medical attention. Here, the adult needs treatment
>
> *Psychological factors affecting other medical conditions:* This condition is associated with a medical condition, especially severe illness or chronic illness

■ DIAGNOSIS

Establishing diagnosis of somatic symptoms in children is challenging. The chances of misdiagnosis in these cases are very high. The average delay in the diagnosis of PNES usually remains long. Studies have reported that around 80% of PNES patients receive antiepileptic drugs unnecessarily before the proper diagnosis, indicating that the index of suspicion for psychogenic symptoms may not be high enough. Though this fact is true

BOX 2: The Diagnostic and Statistical Manual of Mental Disorders, 5th edition (DSM 5) criteria for diagnosing somatic symptom disorder.

- One or more somatic symptoms that are distressing or result in significant disruption of daily life
- Excessive thought, feelings, or behaviors related to the somatic symptoms or associated health concerns as manifested by at least one of the following:
  - Disproportionate and persistent thoughts about the seriousness of one's symptoms
  - Persistent high level of anxiety about health symptoms
  - Excessive time and energy devoted to these symptoms or health concerns
- Although any one somatic symptom may not be continuously present, the state of being symptomatic is persistent (typically >6 months)

Specify if:
With predominant pain (previously known as pain disorder in DSM-IV-TR): For individuals whose somatic symptoms involve pain predominantly

Persistent: A persistent course is characterized by severe symptoms, marked impairment, and long duration (>6 months)

for PNES, it is applicable to other psychosomatic symptoms as well. SSRDs are, in general, diagnosed by exclusion. Therefore, psychogenic symptoms are most certainly underdiagnosed.

When to Suspect an SSRD?

A number of "red flags" are useful in raising the suspicion that "seizures" may be psychogenic rather than epileptic. The helpful historical features are as follows:

Resistance to antiepileptic drugs: This is usually the reason for referral to the epilepsy center, and most patients with psychogenic nonepileptic events have received them for some time before the correct diagnosis is made.

Frequency: They usually have a very high frequency of seizures (multiple daily episodes) that are completely unaffected by antiepileptics.

Triggers: These cases have specific triggers that are unusual for epilepsy (e.g., stress, getting upset, pain, certain movements, sounds), especially if they are alleged to consistently trigger a seizure.

Circumstances: The attacks may occur under various circumstances. Psychogenic events tend to occur in the presence of an audience, and occurrence in the physician's office or waiting room is particularly suggestive of psychogenic events. Similarly, psychogenic events tend not to occur in sleep, although they may seem to be reported as doing so. The presence of fashionable diagnoses, such as fibromyalgia and chronic pain, could also be a suggestive clue. Similarly, a florid review of systems, especially written lengthy lists of symptoms or diagnoses, should raise the suspicion.

The basic principles of diagnosing SSRDs are as follows:
- To investigate thoroughly not to miss any major organic pathology
- To establish a psychological causation of the somatic symptoms
- General medical illness and SSRDs are not mutually exclusive and may coexist.

ASSESSMENT

Patients suffering from somatic symptom disorders most frequently come to a pediatrician than a psychiatrist. So, it is important for the pediatricians to take a thorough history and do a detailed physical examination and judicious workup rather than stamping a diagnosis of psychogenic origin. It may cause unnecessary stigmatization and avoidance of seeking consultation by the family. Serious attention should be given to both medical and psychosocial aspects by the practitioner and the family.

Medical history: It should be elicited to identify a coexisting medical or psychological illness. History of sleep is very important. Most of the time, somatic symptoms are absent during sleep. Children and adolescents with chronic medical illnesses can present with somatic symptoms and excessive reaction to those symptoms or behavioral issues. There can be family history of chronic medical or psychological illness such as anxiety or depression. History of multiple consultation and workup regarding the same set of complaints (doctor shopping) and not getting any relief can suggest the possibility of SSRDs.

Somatic Symptoms and Related Disorders | 237

Psychosocial evaluation: SSRDs require psychiatric consultation at the earliest. The psychosocial aspect of the disease needs careful attention by the physician. Assessing the risk factors or stressors within the family or in the school environment must get identified as soon as possible. Especially in a case of child abuse, it is very important to protect the child from its immediate environment. Many times, the child or adolescent may not open up in the presence of their family; in that case, a psychologist can be of great help in bringing out the stressors or risk factors by talking to them separately. Diagnosis is based on particular DSM 5 criteria for individual illnesses as shown in **Box 2**.

Detailed systemic physical examination: It is important to find out any associated organic illness. Somatic symptoms without any positive physical signs are highly suggestive of the psychogenic origin. Certain points in neurological examination can give a clue to psychosomatic disorders manifesting with neurological abnormalities. For several, neurological symptoms, signs, or maneuvers have been described to help differentiate organic from nonorganic symptoms; for example, limb weakness is often evaluated by Hoover's test. Other examples include looking for "give way" weakness and alleged blindness with preserved optokinetic nystagmus. More generally, the neurologic examination often tries to elicit symptoms or signs that do not make neuroanatomical sense, e.g., facial numbness affecting the angle of jaw, gait with astasia-abasia, or tight roping. While evaluating events which closely mimic seizures, these can be initially suspected in the clinic on the basis of history and examination.

Judicious workup: Diagnosis of psychogenic symptoms requires an extensive and costly diagnostic workup to exclude even the most unlikely etiology. This results in a large number of tests, procedures, and treatments, increasing costs, and risk of complications. Even when a psychogenic etiology is suspected early on, good medical practice mandates exclusion of possible organic causes. When all evaluations are unrevealing and if the psychological profile fits, then a psychogenic etiology is entertained. The main problem is that when all tests are negative and the diagnosis of a psychogenic origin is only one of elimination, the level of certainty is relatively low; that is, the doubt of missing an organic pathology always remains. In this situation, it is beneficial to counsel family and maintain proper communication in each and every step. Cost of diagnosis and benefit from the diagnosis must be kept in mind for establishing the balance.

Suggestibility: It is a useful diagnostic technique which can be used to diagnose these conditions. This is the essential principle behind provocative techniques. When symptoms are caused by unconscious psychological causes, suggesting a change in symptoms may induce that change. Suggestibility is a feature of SSRDs. As for example, in psychogenic movement disorders where diagnosis rests solely on phenomenology, response to placebo or suggestion is considered a diagnostic criterion for definite psychogenic mechanism. Likewise, in most specialties, response to placebo is the only method that may allow a positive diagnosis of psychogenic symptoms as opposed to just diagnosis of exclusion, although this technique is a topic of much ethical debate.

TREATMENT

The way to handling this situation might be by opting for the biopsychosocial model (biobehavioral continuum) to explain such illnesses right from the onset when the doctor is suspicious of this cause. It is best to explain to the parents at the outset that both organic and psychological causes are being considered during diagnosis, and they can be invited to actively participate in the pursuit to find the underlying etiology.

Principles of Treatment
- Explain to patients that the symptoms are perceptible and familiar to the doctor.
- Provide a positive explanation, including how behavioral, psychological, and emotional factors may exacerbate physiologically-based somatic symptoms.
- Offer opportunity for the discussion of patient's and family's worries.

- Give practical advice on coping with symptoms and encourage return to normal activity and work.
- Identify and treat comorbid conditions such as depressive and anxiety disorders.
- Discuss and agree on a treatment plan.
- Follow-up and review.

Multidisciplinary Approach

Once the diagnosis is confirmed, a multidisciplinary rehabilitative approach ought to be the treatment of choice for children exhibiting chronic physical problems. Well-organized treatment plans, positive family/team alliance, and good aftercare are the most robust facilitators of improvement. Characteristics of treatments reported to have good outcome rates include close liaison between mental health and pediatric professionals, an attitude of belief in the child from staff, and moving the family toward a psychological understanding at their own pace. Multidisciplinary rehabilitation approaches also explicitly acknowledge the veracity of the symptoms, emphasizing the necessary involvement of both mind and body in the recovery process, while also allowing young people to "save face" through prompting physical recovery as the primary goal; graded physical exercise, along with participation in sports and extracurricular activities, should be suggested. Medical home model is one such model for multidisciplinary rehabilitation.

Family-focused Cognitive-behavioral Therapy

Family-focused cognitive-behavioral therapy links thoughts, feelings, and behaviors, which includes activity scheduling, pacing, establishment of a sleep routine, modification of negative and unhelpful thinking, and relapse prevention, and has also been incorporated into rehabilitation approaches. Therefore, once the diagnosis of a psychosomatic disorder is made, a child should be referred to appropriate mental health services so that cognitive behavioral therapy can be instituted. *Biofeedback* therapy has often also been found to be helpful in managing these children, but support from family members and friends is crucial for managing a child with psychosomatic problems.

Comorbid Conditions

In psychosomatic conditions where depression is found as a comorbid condition, this needs to be screened for and treated for a good outcome by mental health professionals. Pharmacotherapy is to be considered for treating depression and anxiety disorders or any other psychiatric comorbid conditions.

Pediatricians play a pivotal role in ensuring the appropriate care of children with SSRDs, by not only identifying these children but also actively managing them along with mental health professionals for both treatment and long-term follow-up. The understanding of the interplay between biological, psychological, interpersonal, and medical factors in the predisposition, precipitation, and perpetuation of functional somatic symptoms allows convincing explanations to be provided to ailing children, adolescents, and their families, as well as facilitating the planning of effective treatment to diminish the detrimental effects of such disorders on young people's lives.

> **GUIDELINES FOR PARENTS**
> - Acknowledge that the child's pain is real. Do not attempt to challenge the reality of the symptoms.
> - There is a possibility of undiagnosed organic disease.
> - Identify social or interpersonal reinforcement factors for the symptoms.
> - Minimize the reinforcement of sick role.
> - The daily activities such as school attendance should be continued.
> - A rehabilitative approach should be started and continued.
> - Encourage cognitive skill, self-monitoring, and relaxation training.

■ BIBLIOGRAPHY

1. Bensing JM, Verhaak PFM. Somatisation: a joint responsibility of doctor and patient. 2006;367:452-4.
2. Bould H, Collin SM, Lewis G, Rimes K, Crawley E. Depression in pediatric chronic fatigue syndrome. Arch Dis Child. 2013;98:425-8.
3. Diagnostic and Statistical Manual of Mental Disorders, 5th edition. Washington, DC: American Psychiatric Association; 2013. pp. 311-27.
4. Dutta S, Mehta M, Verma IC. Recurrent abdominal pain in Indian children and its relation with school and family environment. Indian Pediatr. 1999;36:917-20.
5. Egger HL, Costello EJ, Erkanli A, Angold A. Somatic complaints and psychopathology in children and adolescents: stomach aches,

musculoskeletal pains, and headaches. J Am Acad Child Adolesc Psychiatry. 1999;38:852-60.
6. Engel GL. The clinical application of the biopsychosocial model. Am J Psychiatry. 1980;137:535-44.
7. Faust J, Soman TB. Psychogenic movement disorders in children: characteristics and predictors of outcome. J Child Neurol. 2012;27:610-4.
8. Gerber M, Pühse U. "Don't crack under pressure!"—do leisure time physical activity and self-esteem moderate the relationship between school-based stress and psychosomatic complaints? J Psychosom Res. 2008;65:363-9.
9. Griffin A, Christie D. Taking the psycho out of psychosomatic: using systemic approaches in a paediatric setting for the treatment of adolescents with unexplained physical symptoms. Clin Child Psychol Psychiatry. 2008;13:531-42.
10. Gupta V, Singh A, Upadhyay S, Bhatia B. Clinical profile of somatoform disorders in children. Indian J Pediatr. 2011;78:283-6.
11. Hjern A, Alfven G, Oestberg V. School stressors, psychological complaints and psychosomatic pain. Acta Pediatr. 2008;97:112-7.
12. Obeid M, Mikati MA. Expanding spectrum of paroxysmal events in children: potential mimickers of epilepsy. Pediatr Neurol. 2007;37(5):309-16.
13. Ramya SG, Kulkarni ML. Bullying among school children: prevalence and association with common symptoms in childhood. Indian J Pediatr. 2011;78:307-10.
14. Rickert VI, Jay MS. Psychosomatic disorders: the approach. Pediatr Rev. 1994;15:448-54.
15. Spender Q. A short guide to understanding behavioural difficulties. Arch Dis Child. 2013;98:625-8.
16. Starfield B, Gross E, Wood M, Pantell R, Allen C, Gordon IB, et al. Psychosocial and psychosomatic diagnoses in primary care of children. Pediatrics. 1980;66:159-67.

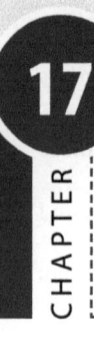

Psychological Effects of Chronic Illness

Jai Ranjan Ram

■ INTRODUCTION

Chronic pediatric illnesses have been shown to affect the course of early emotional development in a significant proportion of children in a negative way. The volume of scientific evidence on this points to increased affection and vulnerability in terms of psychological, emotional, and behavioral development of children suffering from chronic diseases. Most of the chronic diseases exert a detrimental impact on the development of all domains at multiple levels.

One of the key deficiencies of the research in this area is that the key focus is on the child who fails to manage effectively and exhibit emotional and behavioral problems. It is important to keep in mind that the majority of children show excellent resilience while growing up with chronic illness.

■ EPIDEMIOLOGY

Studying the prevalence of psychological maladjustment in children is complex. There are problems in defining the threshold for "maladjustment" and the issue of sample selection. Cross-sectional community-based studies are always preferable to clinic-based studies as they are more likely to be based on broad representative samples, and the data generated could be widely generalized. But it is obvious that clinic-based studies are easier to conduct and hence done more often.

The probability and risk for identifiable psychiatric illnesses in children having chronic pediatric illnesses are nearly double that of similar conditions found in healthy children. It is estimated that about 30–40% of children with severe or chronic illnesses have some associated psychiatric illness.

Neurological illnesses represent a special subset of chronic pediatric illnesses. Childhood epilepsy, cerebral tumors, and various other chronic neurological disorders have a greater chance of comorbidities with various psychiatric conditions when compared to pediatric illnesses that do not encompass cerebral dysfunction.

In one population-based study, Cadman, Boyle, Szatmari, and Offord (1987) conducted a survey of 1,869 families in Ontario, Canada. It included 3,294 children aged 4–16 years. The incidence of chronic disease detected was 14%, which included 3.7% children who also suffered from different physical disability. It was also observed that children with chronic disease and various physical disabilities were at greater than three times risk for different psychiatric disorders and were also at "considerable" risk for social maladjustment compared with otherwise physically normal children. It was also noted that those children with chronic diseases (but without physical disability) were at lower risk, a twofold increase in psychiatric disorder.

In a recent study in the UK (2020), children with various chronic health problems had higher rates of mental illnesses at 10 years. These health problems persisted to be associated with poor mental health conditions at the ages of 13 and 15 years.

Clinical researchers reviewed a large sample of approximately 7,000 children in this study to assess the occurrence of various mental health disorders, which included anxiety or depression, and chronic illness. The measure of chronic illness was based on a mother's assessment of her child's health at 10 and 13 years. Chronic conditions are defined as those that cannot be cured effectively but can be controlled by medication and other therapies to some extent. Often, they may have little disease activity. This investigative measure included children presenting with minor health problems also.

The clinical researchers observed that children having chronic health conditions were approximately twice as likely at 10 and 13 years to present with some form of mental health disorder than the control group (children reported to be "healthy, no problems" by their mothers). Further at 15 years of age, children with chronic health problems were 60% more likely to present with mental disorders. They found that bullying and health-related school absenteeism emerged as the most significant additional factors for children with mental health issues. Health-related school absenteeism was identified as the most consistent factor predicting mental health problems over time.

FACTORS DECIDING ADAPTATION OF CHILDREN TO CHRONIC ILLNESS

The adaptability of children to persistent and chronic illness can be viewed as the product of the cumulative interactions of both risk and protective factors. An emotionally spontaneous child with a supportive family who has experienced a series of early successes can be expected to cope well with the early onset of a severe pediatric illness.

Age of Child at Time of Onset of Illness

Disfiguring illnesses at adolescence have more of an adverse outcome than the same in childhood. Illnesses that necessitate prolonged separation from primary caregivers are more damaging in early childhood than adolescence.

Parental Responsibility

Parental approach and responsibility for the management of pediatric illness are important factors related to the adaptability of a child to a serious or chronic pediatric illness.

Diagnosis of the Chronic Illness

Another important determining factor is initiation, timeliness, and accuracy of the process and establishment of diagnosis.

Process of Establishment of Diagnosis of the Chronic Illness

The steps and whole process by which the clinical diagnosis is established can also play a significant role in the ability of the child and also the parents to accept and adapt to the illness. A number of factors are involved:

- The duration of the process and the time required to come to conclusion on the nature of the condition
- The certainty with which the diagnosis can be made
- The empathy with which the diagnosis and its implications are explained and conveyed to the child and the family.

Interference with Function

Maintenance of body functions is an important factor for the ultimate outcome. School absenteeism is an important intermediary for psychological outcome.

Impact on Physical Appearance

Alteration in physical appearance has a lasting impact on the adaptability of the child.

Persistence of Symptoms

Prolonged illness has more lasting effect on the psychological reaction of the child.

Hope for Recovery

Any negativism is detrimental to psychological adaptability. Children who do not feel that there is a chance of recovery are more prone to having marked psychological impact.

CHILDREN WITH VARIOUS AILMENTS

There are many research articles on psychological effects of children suffering from cancer. Despite the fact that children suffer more frequently from other diseases than cancer, there are newer modalities of treatment and significant improvement in prognosis, and children with cancer continue to receive considerable attention.

Psychological problems in children, such as learning disabilities, academic failure, behavior, and adjustment problems, have all been reported in children suffering from cancer.

New research findings point to a positive psychological outcome, especially in childhood cancers. Post-traumatic growth (PTG) is one such. It is a frequently reported positive outcome of childhood cancer survivors and their family. It has been observed that childhood cancer survivors often express positive outcomes related to their cancer experience (meaning-making), better appreciation of life, enhanced self-knowledge, positive attitudes toward the family, and also motivation to give back to society. In childhood cancer warriors, PTG seems to be more associated with older age at diagnosis and initiation of measurement. It is imperative that a certain developmental stage (and as a result cognitive capacity) is necessary to experience PTG. Along with all these, a better social support and higher optimism among survivors have been shown to be associated with higher levels of PTG.

Survivors of childhood cancer due to their disease process and treatment are always at risk for developing neurocognitive impairments. Prevalence estimates vary across various studies. About 35% of survivors may experience neurocognitive effects at later stages. Children at the greatest risk of developing neurocognitive impairments are the survivors of central nervous system (CNS) tumors. Gross deficits in general intelligence are the most prominent feature. Besides this, impairments are often observed in other domains such as speed of processing, various executive functions such as verbal fluency and cognitive flexibility. Memory and attention are also likely to be affected. A high dose of cranial radiation therapy (CRT), larger brain volume irradiated, and younger age at diagnosis are the most profound risk factors for general neurocognitive impairments in CNS tumor survivors.

The plethora of psychological health problems in survivors of childhood cancer encompasses a variety of manifestations. These include depression, anxiety, various externalizing behavioral problems, and post-traumatic stress symptoms (PTSS).

Children suffering from diabetes often manifest adjustment problems. This is more prevalent in children with poorer health and children from dysfunctional families. It has also been debated that children with "better" diabetic control show improved adjustment scores over those with "poor" control.

But this view also has been challenged. Research suggests that the vigorous efforts to achieve and maintain good diabetic control may have countereffects. It may be so demanding that children find it difficult to adjust; they get more depressed. Parents and also doctors should be careful in this regard. Children are not expected to achieve unrealistic levels of glycemic control at the expense of quality of life.

Juvenile arthritis is another challenging condition. The extent of affection is dependent on the disease severity and age of the child. Increased incidence of maladjustment and social isolation was observed among older children and adolescents.

GENERAL INTERVENTION STRATEGIES

A careful attempt at increasing children's disease-specific knowledge has been partially successful. The access to knowledge has further complicated the issue. But increased knowledge is not the sole predictor for adaptation. Knowledge is principally important in enabling children with chronic diseases to become responsible for their self-care. Some interventions have focused on improving self-care skills.

Various other approaches have attempted to develop the social skills necessary to manage chronic disease and treatment process. Children are guided to understand the process and realize the difficulties they have in complying with treatment in different situations. Guidance is needed to manage certain challenging situations, as for example, diabetic children feeling embarrassed to handle their diet protocol at school. These "social skills" approaches enable in educating well children about health issues and are likely to have considerable potential with chronically sick children.

All the interventions and efforts of the professionals are to foster more independence and competence in dealing with stress situations by acquisition of relevant coping skills. At the same time, the potential for psychosocial maladjustment and need for continuous professional involvement is reduced.

GUIDELINES FOR PARENTS

- Children are often confused about their disease and outcome.
- They should be given some information about their disease.
- Positive attitudes from the family members help them cope with the stress of prolonged illness.
- Company of close family members and sympathetic attitude from the hospital staff give them comfort and courage.

BIBLIOGRAPHY

1. Barlow JH, Ellard DR. The psychosocial well-being of children with chronic disease, their parents and siblings: an overview of the research evidence base. Child Care Health Dev. 2006;32:19-31.
2. Brady AM, Deighton J, Stansfeld S. Chronic illness in childhood and early adolescence: a longitudinal exploration of co-occurring mental illness. Dev Psychopathol. 2021;33:885-98.
3. Cousens P, Ungerer JA, Crawford JA, Stevens MM. Cognitive effects of childhood leukemia therapy: a case for four specific deficits. J Pediatr Psychol. 1991;16:475-88.
4. Eiser C. Communicating with sick and hospitalised children. J Child Psychol Psychiatry. 1984;25:181-9.
5. Eiser C. Psychological effects of chronic disease. J Child Psychol Psychiatry. 1990;31:85-98.
6. Michel G, Brinkman TM, Wakefield CE, Grootenhuis M. Psychological outcomes, health-related quality of life, and neurocognitive functioning in survivors of childhood cancer and their parents. Pediatr Clin North Am. 2020;67(6):1103-34.

CHAPTER 18

Study Skills

Preeti M Galagali

■ INTRODUCTION

Learning is a tool for acquiring and developing abilities and capacities. Skill is the ability to perform a learned activity effectively and efficiently. A skill is developed through repeated practice and reflection. There are many skills that can be nurtured and developed, namely life skills, study skills, creative writing skills, mathematical skills, dancing skills, language skills, drawing skills, athletic skills, and so on. This chapter will focus on study skills and will cover its definition, research in Indian settings, essentials for learning, early foundations of learning, details of different evidence-based study strategies, and guidelines for parents.

■ DEFINITION

Study skills are defined as the conscious and intentional use of the processes of organizing and retaining new information to make learning more effective. These encompass a range of coordinated cognitive skills and processes that include acquiring, recording, organizing, synthesizing, remembering, and using information. Research has proved that inculcating study skills in students is critical for academic competence, excellence, and employability opportunities as adults. Success in school enhances the self-esteem of the child. In the current techno-savvy world, it is essential for school children to develop e-skills that train them to use electronic gadgets such as computers and tablets to enhance learning. Soft skill training that determines employability also forms an important part of study skills in school. These include skills in communication (verbal, nonverbal, and written), negotiation, networking, interpersonal relationships, teamwork, organization, and mentoring.

IMPORTANCE OF STUDY SKILLS IN AN INDIAN SCENARIO

Research from India in community settings has delineated poor study habits as a major cause for poor school performance in >50% of children. Hence, it is important to inculcate good study habits in students. In hospital-based referral centers, unrecognized specific learning disorder is a major reason for poor school performance. Children with specific learning disorder and intellectual disability are known to benefit from remedial teaching, individualized education plan, and acquiring study skills. Latest studies from India have also demonstrated the adverse effect of low birth weight, anemia, undernutrition, micronutrient deficiency, zinc deficiency, and poor aerobic fitness on the children's cognitive and intellectual functioning. It is a well-known fact that school performance is affected by a child's physical, emotional, and social health as well as by the environment at school and at home. Most parents and teachers are concerned and worried if children do not perform well in academics. Poor school performance may result in suicide, school refusal, drug addiction, anxiety, depression, psychosomatic disorders, stress in the adolescent and parents, school absenteeism and dropout, sexual promiscuity, aggressive behavior, and even runaway behavior. In a study from Maharashtra, 80% of the school dropouts cited poor school performance as the main reason for opting out of school.

ESSENTIALS FOR LEARNING

Motivation to learn, a nurturing home and school environment, balanced diet, adequate sleep and physical activity, stress management techniques, and effective study skills enable children to reach their academic potential.

Motivation is the fuel that drives the engine of life. A child with high motivation to study learns study skills much more easily than a child with low motivation. To develop a high intrinsic motivation to study, the child has to love and enjoy the process of learning and imbibe the importance of education. Parents and teachers play a major role in laying a firm foundation for life-long learning. At a very tender age, parents should nurture the feeling of "joy in learning" and teachers should further strengthen it in school.

A nurturing home environment is motivating, inspiring, encouraging, stable, and supportive. Marital harmony and respect for each family member characterize a stable home environment. In a "nurturing" home, the parents love unconditionally and follow an authoritative parenting style with assertive communication skills. They have realistic expectations from their children. They avoid comparisons with other children. They build up the self-esteem of their children by acknowledging their success and help them to overcome failure. They appreciate effort and do not focus only on the end result in terms of marks scored. Above all, they are good role models and teach life skills to their children to meet the challenges of life. Parents should provide a learning atmosphere at home with plenty of interesting books and educational toys that should satisfy the child's innate hunger for knowledge. They should try to link lessons with application in daily life. They should encourage the child to use all three learning modalities—visual, auditory, and kinesthetic.

The essential skills needed for schooling are the three Rs—reading, writing, and arithmetic. Children should be allowed to learn activities at their own pace; some may learn to recite rhymes at 15 months and some at 2 years. Parents and teachers should keep themselves updated about normal child development and should not pressurize the children to learn at a quick pace. In the early years, most of the learning takes place at home through the medium of play. At a later age, classroom teaching supports learning.

Multiple Intelligences

All children are not hardwired to excel in academics. Some are good in drawing while some in sports and dramatics. Educationists and parents should understand the concept of multiple intelligences proposed by Howard Gardner. He stated that there are different kinds of intelligence, namely linguistic, logical–mathematical, musical, spatial, bodily kinesthetic, intrapersonal, interpersonal, naturalist, and spiritual. Only linguistic and logical intelligence are tested by routine examinations in school. Parents and teachers should identify the interest of the children and accordingly encourage them in that particular field. Mastery in their field of interest will build up confidence and will have a "spillover" positive impact on the academic performance. For most people, the left cerebral hemisphere is associated with logical and analytical thinking and the right with creative thinking. To stimulate both hemispheres of the brain, caretakers and teachers should encourage both academic pursuits and creative arts and hobbies. Parents should help children to set up *smart* goals, i.e., specific, measurable, achievable, realistic, and time-bound goals. Career counseling for adolescents should be done on the basis of their interest and passion for a particular field.

Other Factors Affecting Learning

A balanced diet with appropriate quantities of macro- and micronutrients in the form of carbohydrates, proteins, vitamins, iron, zinc, iodine, calcium, and omega-3 fatty acids is essential for synaptogenesis, myelination, and neuronal growth. Apart from ensuring fitness, physical activity also promotes neuronal growth and synaptogenesis. Sixty minutes of moderate to vigorous physical activity is recommended for all children. Sleep is the elixir for good health and memory. Each child should sleep for an adequate time according to age.

Reasons for poor school performance could also include difficulty in the medium of instruction, procrastination, and poorly controlled chronic physical health disorder such as diabetes mellitus. Stress management techniques can be taught and modeled by teachers and parents. The children should be encouraged to follow a healthy lifestyle, pursue hobbies, and learn study skills, relaxation exercises such as *pranayam* and deep breathing, coping skills, and problem-solving skills. Children should accept the fact that they cannot completely eliminate stress from their lives but can keep it under control to allow optimum functioning.

■ EARLY FOUNDATIONS OF LEARNING

Can children learn in utero? Mythology mentions that Dhruva learnt Vedic *shlokas* in the womb and so did Abhimanyu who learned about the *Chakravyuh* in utero, but medical literature has yet to report such a miracle! It has been scientifically proven that a baby can hear and feel in utero. Immediately after birth, the baby has an innate tendency to bond with his parents. Parents should lovingly respond to all the needs of the baby and reinforce bonding. After birth until the first few months of life, the baby uses five senses of touch, smell, hear, sight, and taste to learn about the world. Parents should stimulate these senses appropriately by talking, singing, rocking, and cuddling their little ones. They should also show colorful toys preferably of different textures, rattles, and chimes to stimulate their sense organs.

Exposing the baby to the wonders of nature is another fine way of stimulating the young one. Walks in or out of the pram, gazing at greenery, listening to chirping of birds, sounds of splashing waves, and bathing in sunlight for a few minutes allow the baby to appreciate and love nature at a young age. Parents should do these activities with their infants in a quiet alert state and not when they are cranky or hungry or wet. They should guard against overstimulation of the infant.

In the early years, parents should form a scaffold for learning. They should teach, guide, and help the children in learning new tasks with a lot of patience and love until they can do them independently. This new learning could be making a house from blocks or completing a jigsaw puzzle or even cleaning a bicycle.

Language Development

Language development opens the gateway to the treasure of knowledge as it is an essential prerequisite for reading, writing, and even arithmetic. Reading out stories; showing picture books; reciting animated rhymes; *shlokas*, and *bhajans*; acting out action words such as "jump" and "run;" and speaking slowly with emphasis on phonetics can help in language acquisition and instill a love for reading. Five-year-old children can be asked to tell a story in their own words with actions and sound effects. This is usually an enjoyable activity for the children and it tests their comprehension and understanding.

Writing

Writing can be encouraged at a young age. Around 1.5 years of age, a child is able to grip a fat colorful crayon or a chalk piece. Parents should allow the child to scribble on paper or the blackboard and appreciate the efforts of the young writer in making. Drawing strokes and alphabets in the sand is another way of encouraging writing skills in a 2- or 3-year-old child. Children between 3 and 5 years enjoy paper tracing, making letters from clay dough, and joining dot to dot. It is only around 5–6 years that a child is able to grip a pencil firmly between the thumb and index finger. Painting with fingers, stamping pictures of various objects, stringing beads, making a collage by pasting pictures, and clay molding improve the dexterity of fingers. Parents and teachers should always remember to make these activities fun filled with a lot of mirth, laughter, and encouragement.

Arithmetic

Arithmetic is best learned by its application in daily life. Babies learn their first concept of shape, texture, and size by handling their dresses and toys. Stacking and nesting toys help infants to understand sizes. A 2-year-old can be told about various shapes by pointing to a full moon as a circle, a box as a rectangle, and an egg as an oval. At around 3 years, the child begins counting and by 5 years may be able to recite numbers 1–10. A 3-year-old can be given a simple task of counting mangoes or oranges or bananas in a fruit basket. Children also enjoy learning rhymes with numbers in them like "one, two buckle my shoe…." Parents can take a 4-year-old along for shopping to introduce the concept of money, weights, and sizes.

Creative Thinking

The seeds of creative thinking can be sown in a child's mind at an early age. Children are "natural" creative thinkers as they have free-thinking minds that are always bubbling with innovative ideas. They have not yet developed the ability of censoring their thoughts with notions of "possible" or "impossible" or "correct" or "wrong'" Parents should encourage this creative ability and allow active but safe exploration of the world. They can encourage their 3-year-old child to create a new story or dramatize a story or give a different ending to classics or folk tales. They can ask their child to discover new uses of simple things, like a pencil can become a rocket in a story or an empty bowl can become a hat for a doll or a ball can become earth and a smaller ball, the moon. Pretend play between the ages of 2 and 4 years also enhances creativity and social skills. Parents should allow the child to play "house" or "kitchen" or "doctor" and even join in the play when asked to. Parents and teachers should try to give simple and lucid answers to their constant barrage of questions such as "why does it rain?" or "why does the sun rise?"

Memory and Reasoning

Memory and reasoning should also be nurtured. A child responds to his name by 6–7 months. By 12–18 months, the child understands and can be taught the names of simple objects such as car, fan, table, and chair. For 2-year-old stacking toys and for 3-year-old building blocks stimulate creativity, reasoning, and memory. The child is able to identify colors at 3–4 years and can be given the task of matching colors. A 3-year-old child can fit pieces of a 4–10-piece jigsaw puzzle and can move to complex ones at a later age. The ability to follow and remember simple instructions indicates the memorizing and comprehension ability of the child. A 2-year-old can be taught to carry out a simple task of keeping a book in the rack after use, while a 3-year-old can be taught a little complex task of keeping all toys in the closet after playing. A child can be taught to self-feed at 18 months and to undress and dress by 3 years of age.

A preschool is not required if parents can spend adequate time with their children in appropriately stimulating them. The children can then begin regular schooling at 4–5 years of age. If parents are professionally engaged and unavailable, then a caretaker or a teacher in a play home can undertake the role of a parent and keep the child purposefully occupied with stimulating activities.

■ EVIDENCE-BASED STUDY STRATEGIES

Study skills are learning strategies that help the child to study in an organized manner and perform to his potential in school and college. These strategies have to be implemented right in the beginning of the academic session and should be diligently followed to ensure stress-free learning. A practical method to classify study skills is to

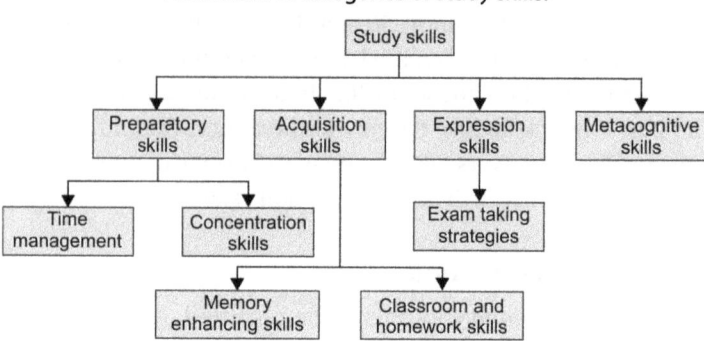

Flowchart 1: Categories of study skills.

divide them into four categories, namely preparatory, acquisition, expression, and metacognitive study skills, as shown in **Flowchart 1**.

CLASSIFICATION OF STUDY SKILLS

Preparatory Study Skills

Preparatory skills are essential prerequisites for academic success. They enable the student to prepare for acquiring knowledge. These include the following.

Time Management

Time management improves efficiency and avoids last-minute anxiety. Parents and teachers can help the children to make a daily timetable by asking them to list time spent every day in sleeping, grooming, meals, errands, school, television, meeting with friends, play, and hobbies. The remaining time can be planned for studies. Children can also be asked a few daily activities which they feel are a waste of time. Reducing time on these activities would give them more time to study. While making a timetable, it is important to leave some unscheduled time that can be used in case of an emergency. The study time can be split into time slots for revising each subject, doing homework, and for extra reading. A separate timetable should be made for the weekends. The schedule should be reviewed weekly and changes could be made according to the schedule of exams or extracurricular or sports activities. Parents should allow the children to make their "own" timetable and not dictate it to them. This will increase the likelihood of children following the time schedule. *ABC approach* can be used to categorize tasks into *a*bsolutely urgent (high importance), *b*etter do it soon (medium importance), and *c*an wait (low importance) for optimal utilization of time.

Concentration Skills

Parents can help their children to concentrate better by arranging for a "study niche" for them. It could be a separate room or even a corner of a room. It should preferably have a table and chair. Studying on a sofa or bed should be discouraged as that puts the mind in a state of relaxation and drowsiness. The study area should be free from distractions such as television, computer, radio, fridge, and phone. It should be well lit and ventilated. During the study time, the parents should make sure that the children are not disturbed by siblings or other relatives.

It is preferable to study at the same time everyday so that studying becomes an effortless enduring habit like taking a bath or brushing the teeth. It is essential to define goals before a study period. Setting specific goals such as planning to study one Physics chapter in 40 minutes will foster concentration and focus. It has been researched that an individual remembers best what he has read in the beginning and at the end of the study period. Hence, taking breaks after 40–50 minutes helps to sustain concentration and improves memory while continuous reading causes fatigue. Parents should insist on daily revision of lessons at home. They should also ask the children to clarify doubts rather than leaving the clarification to just before exams. This will help the children to be thorough with their learning.

Acquisition Study Skills

Acquisition skills develop expertise in gathering and retaining information and knowledge. These include the following.

Memory Enhancing Skills

There are three types of memory, namely sensory, short-term, and long-term. Sensory memory lasts only for a few minutes and consists of what one imbibes by senses of hearing, visualizing, and touch. Short-term memory lasts for 1–2 days. If a student pays keen attention to the teacher or to the reading material, the learned information gets stored in the brain for a couple of days. Most children who study for a few days to hours before the exam use this type of memory for answering the exam questions. No wonder all the knowledge is lost or deleted after exams are over! Long-term memory lasts for weeks to months and even a lifetime. All students should make efforts to maximize their long-term memory.

Strategies to enhance long-term memory include the following:
- Children should *understand and learn* the study material taught in the classroom on a daily basis. They should *revise* it at regular intervals, preferably weekly, fortnightly, and monthly to stamp it in memory. Preclass reading also helps in understanding the study material.
- They should use the method of association to form a *mind map* of the learned material.
- Colored pens can be used to *highlight* important facts.
- *Flash cards* can be used to record facts like formulae in physics and mathematics, number of bones in the body, smallest bone in the body, kings of Mughal dynasty, their date of accession, death, etc. Flash cards are useful for a quick revision of facts, especially prior to exams with multiple choice questions.
- Another useful technique is the use of *mnemonics*. For example, to remember the eight planets, students can form the mnemonic— "My Very Elegant Mother Just Showed Us Nine," the first alphabet of each word stands for a name of the planet—Mercury, Venus, Earth, Mars, Jupiter, Saturn, Uranus, and Neptune.
- SQ3R method can be used to improve textbook comprehension. SQ3R is an acronym that stands for Survey, Questions, Read, Recall, and Review. First, all the key points and diagrams of a particular chapter are *surveyed*. Then each bold heading in the chapter is converted to a *question*. Answers are *read* and then written in the student's language. Then the student *recalls* the answer. In the end, the entire chapter is *reviewed*. Portions that are not mastered are reread. The SQ3R method does not hold good for English and mathematics.

- *Multisensory learning* is the best mode of learning in which a combination of all senses is used to transmit information to the brain by the learner. The various senses used for learning include visual, auditory, kinesthetic, olfactory, and gustatory. It is estimated that students would remember 90% of what they study if they use the multisensory modality, that is, saying, seeing, hearing, and doing what has been taught, immediately after a learning session.
- *Group revision* may be helpful for some students in memorizing and understanding facts in a lucid manner.

Classroom and Homework Skills

Parents and teachers can teach children to actively listen in class. They should encourage preclass reading and ask them to correlate the newly acquired knowledge with the previous knowledge to improve understanding of the subject. The children should avoid chatting in class and listen attentively to the teacher. Teachers can guide children regarding the methodology of taking good notes in class. Children should revise notes after the class and update the notes using textbooks and reference books. Teachers and parents should stress on the importance of regular studying and procrastination should be avoided at all costs. Children should give top priority to completion of homework. While doing homework, emphasis should be laid upon understanding and memorizing the study material.

Expression Study Skills

Expression skills enable students to demonstrate their knowledge in tests and include exam-taking strategies.

Parents should ensure that children get enough sleep and healthy nutrition, especially during exam time. All the things needed for the exams such as pencils, erasers, pencil sharpeners, rulers, and pens should be kept ready a day before the exam. On the day of the exam, children should have a light nutritious breakfast. They should think and verbalize positive self-motivating statements such as "I have studied regularly throughout the year and I shall do well in the exams." Last-minute discussions with friends should be avoided. They should "time" the question paper and leave a few minutes at the end of the paper for revision. They should write legibly and neatly. They should first attempt those questions that they know the best. Students must be taught about the nuances of answering different types of questions such as multiple choice, short answer, and essay type. For example, while answering essay-type questions, the students should focus on structuring the answer in a way that demonstrates their detailed understanding of concepts and issues in comparison to answering short answer questions where only discrete facts need to be written.

After the exam, the parents should refrain from discussing the answers and mistakes and should allow the children to prepare calmly for the next exam. Mistakes could be discussed after completion of all the exams. Students should avoid stress building beliefs such as "I should always stand first" or "I should always score 100%." Students should believe that putting in their best effort would ensure the best results! Students should enjoy the process of learning and should not feel burdened by exams. They should consider exams as a "celebration of learning"—a time where they can showcase what they have learned and not simply a time of "groans" and "moans." This would enable children to treat exams as just another milestone, albeit an important one, that they can achieve easily without any stress!

Metacognitive Skills

Metacognitive skills help the students to assess the need, plan, implement, monitor, and evaluate each study strategy and use it efficiently. Students with good metacognitive skills are able to select, monitor, and use different strategies for different subjects. For example, the SQ3R strategy cannot be used for learning mathematics and languages but is effective for social studies and science. Students with good metacognitive skills can flexibly use interrelated study strategies.

Study skills should be personalized and adapted for individual learning as each student has a unique learning style. A study strategy that might work out for one student may not benefit the other. Teachers and parents can use the technique of social cognitive structuring to teach study skills to students. They can first model the strategy and then coach the students to use it under supervision and finally allow them to implement it on their own with flexibility.

Objective Assessment of Study Skills

Parents and students should not hesitate to seek counseling for improving study skills. LASSI (Learning and Study Strategies Inventory), ASSIST (Approaches and Study Skills Inventory for Students), DCSSI (Denver Congos Study Scale Inventory), and SSI (Study Skill Inventory) are few validated tools for objective assessment of study skills and identify areas of strengths and weaknesses. Each tool has subscales to assess reading skills, concentration, memory, time, and emotional management. Specific counseling can be provided in the areas of deficit to strengthen the overall learning capability. Anxiety, depression, and neurodevelopmental and mental disorders can be also screened for and managed by health professionals during these counseling sessions.

Conclusion

Goal-directed use of learning strategies is one of the important characteristics of a high achiever apart from self-efficacy, high prior achievement, intelligence, and conscientiousness. Research has clearly proved that students who have learned different study skills have a better academic performance compared to those who have not. Academic performance builds up a student's self-esteem and lays the foundation for future learning, career, and employment opportunities. Hence, effective study skills should be taught to all students by parents, teachers, and counselors.

GUIDELINES FOR PARENTS

- Parents should provide a nurturing, stimulating, and inspiring home environment for children. Such an environment is conducive for learning.
- The feeling of "joy in learning" has to be inculcated at a very young age.
- From younger years onward, children should be engaged in creative and enjoyable learning pursuits.
- Parents should ensure adequate nutrition, physical activity, and sleep for an optimum learning experience.
- Parents should model and teach stress management techniques.

Contd...

Contd...

- Parents should teach the children effective study strategies, e-learning skills, and soft skills. The study skills may have to be individualized and modified according to the learning style of each child.
- Children should not be put under pressure to perform.
- Parents should offer unconditional love and support to their children.
- Parents should not hesitate to seek professional help for improving learning strategies.

BIBLIOGRAPHY

1. AlFaris E, Irfan F, AlSayyari S, AlDahlawi W, Almuhaideb S, Almehaidib A, et al. Validation of a new study skills scale to provide an explanation for depressive symptoms among medical students. PLoS One. 2018;13(6):e0199037.
2. Alloway TP, Alloway RG. Investigating the predictive roles of working memory and IQ in academic attainment. J Exp Child Psychol. 2010;106:20-9.
3. Chandrashekhar CR. Improve Learning and Memory. Bangalore: Navakarnataka; 2001.
4. Chaudhari S, Otiv M, Chitale A, Pandit A, Hoge M. Pune low birth weight study—cognitive abilities and educational performance at twelve years. Indian Pediatr. 2004;41:121-8.
5. Chowarghde SW. How to handle stress of examinations in adolescents. In: Bhave SY (Ed). Course Manual for Adolescent Health Part 2. Mumbai: IAP ITPAH; 2002.
6. Cottrell S. The Study Skills Handbook, 2nd edition. New York: Palgrave Macmillan; 2003.
7. Eilander A, Muthayya S, van der Knaap H, Srinivasan K, Thomas T, Kok FJ, et al. Undernutrition, fatty acid and micronutrient status in relation to cognitive performance in Indian school children: a cross-sectional study. Br J Nutr. 2010;103(7):1056-64.
8. Galagali P, Bhave SY. Motivation. In: Bhave SY (Chief Ed). Bhave's Textbook of Adolescent Medicine. New Delhi: Jaypee Brothers Medical Publishers (P) Ltd; 2006. pp. 897-907.
9. Galagali P. Scholastic skills. In: Ugra D, Yamuna S, Galagali P, Prasad C (Eds). Stepping Stones. India. IAP Action Plan, 2010. Mumbai: Indian Academy of Pediatrics. pp. 67-83.
10. Galagali P. Study skills. In: Unni J (Ed). Poor Scholastic Performance Module. India. IAP Action Plan, 2011. Mumbai: Indian Academy of Pediatrics. pp. 21-8.

11. Gettinger M, Seibert JK. Contributions of study skills to academic competence. School Psychol Rev. 2002;31:350-65.
12. Guerrasio J, Nogar C, Rustici M, Lay C, Corral J. Study skills and test taking strategies for coaching medical learners based on identified areas of struggle. MedEdPORTAL. 2017;13:10593.
13. Jacob A, D'Souza CD, Sumithra S, Avadhani S, Subramanya CM, Srinivasan K. Aerobic fitness and cognitive functions in economically underprivileged children aged 7-9 years: a preliminary study from South India. Int J Biomed Sci. 2011;7(1):51-4.
14. John P, George SK, Mampilly AB. Handbook on Poor School Performance. New Delhi: CBSE; 2001.
15. Karande S, Doshi B, Thadhani A, Sholapurwala R. Profile of children with poor school performance in Mumbai. Indian Pediatr. 2013;50:427.
16. Karande S, Kulkarni M. Poor school performance. Indian J Pediatr. 2005;72:961-7.
17. Kawade R. Zinc status and its association with the health of adolescents: a review of studies in India. Glob Health Action. 2012;5:7353.
18. Kelly PD. Learning disorders in adolescence: the role of the primary care physician. Adolesc Med. 2008;19:229-41.
19. Khwaja A. Study Skills—How to Learn Better and Enjoy the Learning Process. Bangalore: Banjara Academy; 2005.
20. Moffat G. The Parenting Journey: From Conception through the Teen Years. Westport, CT: Praeger; 2004.
21. Mundkur N, Sankar C. Early diagnosis and management of learning disabilities. Indian J Pract Pediatr. 2010;12(1):71-8.
22. Nair MK, Paul MK, Padmamaohan J. Scholastic performance of adolescents. Indian J Pediatr. 2003;70:629-31.
23. Nair MKC, Sumaraj L, Swapna S, Sajitha JJR. Academic success—student support and guidance. Ind J Pract Pediatr. 2020;22(1):100-4.
24. Orpinas P, Raczynski K, Hsieh HL, Nahapetyan L, Horne AM. Longitudinal examination of aggression and study skills from middle to high school: implications for dropout prevention. J Sch Health. 2018;88(3):246-52.
25. Pratinidhi AK, Kurulkar PV, Garad SG, Dalal M. Epidemiological aspects of school dropouts in children between 7-15 years in rural Maharashtra. Indian J Pediatr. 1992;59:423-7.
26. Ramaprasad D. The Art and Science of Studying. Bangalore: Intellect Publishing House; 2006.
27. Schneider M, Preckel F. Variables associated with achievement in higher education: a systematic review of meta-analyses. Psychol Bull. 2017;143(6):565-600.

28. Seshadri S, Saksena S, Saldanha S. On Track a Series on Life Skills and Personal Safety. Parents Manual 1-3. New Delhi: MacMillan; 2008.
29. Shashidhar S, Rao C, Hegde R. Factors affecting scholastic problems. Indian J Pediatr. 2009;76:495-9.
30. Thacker N. Poor scholastic performance in children and adolescents. Indian Pediatr. 2007;44:411-2.
31. Veena SR, Krishnaveni GV, Srinivasan K, Wills AK, Hill JC, Kurpad AV, et al. Infant feeding practice and childhood cognitive performance in South India. Arch Dis Child. 2010;95:347-54.
32. Williams M, Burden RL. How does the learner deal with the process of learning? In: Williams M, Burden RL (Eds). Psychology for Language Teachers—A Social Constructivist Approach. Cambridge: Cambridge University Press; 1997. pp. 143-66.
33. Wingate U. Doing away with 'study skills'. Teach High Educ. 2006;11:457-69.

CHAPTER 19

School Problems

Ketan Bharadva

▪ INTRODUCTION

School-going children can face many types of behavioral problems either due to their ailments such as learning disability, attention-deficit hyperactivity disorder (ADHD), conduct disorder, or due to specific conditions in the school environment. The most common end result can be school refusal. Most of the primary diagnoses are dealt with in other chapters; here, school refusal and bullying are discussed.

▪ SCHOOL REFUSAL

School refusal, earlier termed as school phobia, is a serious emotional upset of the child at prospect of attending school with antipathic parental awareness, and there is no significant antisocial behavior. This particular behavior refers to those school-age children who miss the entire or partial school days, sometimes skip classes, or reach late to school for unjustified reasons. This behavior is differentiated from parents who decide to withdraw their child from school deliberately and older children who are runaway or homeless that prevent regular school attendance. It is considered an emergency. School refusal affects 1–2% of school-aged children and about 5% of clinic-referred children.

"School refusal" as "school phobia" was associated with anxiety disorders only. School refusal is now known to be multifactorial with increasingly complex patient and family situations. It includes other underlying disorders such as antisocial disorders and behaviors such as school truancy.

There is not much breakthrough in knowledge and treatment modalities in practice as found in review of literature from

1999 to 2019. There is lack of rigorous randomized controlled trial (RCT) studies, mechanisms behind the issue, and interventional effects on long term.

Etiology

School refusal mainly affects 11–13-year-old children but may be observed at any age from 5 to 15 years without socioeconomic or gender bias. School refusal can be because of school phobia directed toward school or its environment or separation anxiety of separation with closely attached relatives, the mother being common. Various contextual risk factors are street children, homelessness and poverty, school violence, bully and victimization, school environment and connectedness, parental education and concern, family variables, teenage pregnancy, etc.

Clinical Features

School refusal often builds up gradually, after a holiday or illness, stressful event with peers or at home or other places. It can present somatic manifestations such as autonomic symptoms (dizziness, palpitation, sweating, headache, trembling, or chest discomfort), gastrointestinal complaints (abdomen pain, nausea, vomiting, or diarrhea), or musculoskeletal pain. They can also present as emotional features of fearfulness, panic symptoms, crying episodes, temper tantrums, threats of self-harm. Symptoms peak before school-going time and improve when child stays away from school. Returning to school becomes more difficult if the child is allowed to remain away from school for a longer time. Separation anxiety is always as default in every such child.

It has been observed that psychiatric morbidity may be as high as 88.2% in a population of youngsters with school refusal. It is usually associated with various temperamental, familial, and other environmental factors. Studies have revealed that 87.9% had a psychiatric disorder at baseline. Depressive disorder (63.6%) was the most common. Anxiety disorders were second most common (57.6%), encompassing separation anxiety, specific phobias, obsessive–compulsive disorder, generalized anxiety disorder, adjustment disorder, and mood disorders. Anxiety has many faces, offshoots like depression, and may be masked by aggression. Different psychosocial factors influenced school refusal in many children. Younger age, last-birth order, no or a single diagnosis, and good baseline functioning predicted a favorable outcome.

School refusal is a multifactorial entity. School avoidance may fulfill various purposes depending on the individual child. These may include avoidance due to specific fears provoked by the school environment (e.g., exams or performance in sports, bathrooms, and teachers), as a means to escape from certain aversive social situations (e.g., problems with classmates or teachers), separation anxiety, or attention-seeking behaviors (e.g., functional somatic complaints, prolonged crying spells) that worsen over time if the child is allowed to stay home.

Short-term sequelae of school refusal include poor academic performance, family disharmony, and disturbed peer relationships. Long-term consequences are academic underachievement, employment difficulties in adult life, and increased risk for various psychiatric illnesses. The long-term outcome of school phobia after age 30 years was studied. School phobia cases had more psychiatric consultations, lived with their parents more often than the general population group, and had fewer children than comparison groups. There is a higher rate of depressive and anxiety disorders, panic disorder, and agoraphobia in first-degree relatives of children with school phobia. Parents of children with school phobia have more disturbances in family functioning in the areas of role performance, communication, affective expression, and control.

Anxious school refusal and truancy: These are distinct but not mutually exclusive and are significantly associated with psychopathology, as well as adverse experiences at home and school. Truancy is reported in 11–16% school-going children, with risk factors identified as parental education, having large amounts of unsupervised time after school, school disengagement variables (e.g., poor grades and low educational aspirations), and drug use. Children with mixed school refusals co-existing (anxious school refusal and truancy) had a psychiatric disorder or emotional and behavior disorders in 88.2% of cases. Fear from specific factors, sleep difficulties, various somatic complaints,

TABLE 1: School refusal versus truancy.	
School refusal	**Truancy**
Significant emotional disturbances (such as anxiety/fear, temper tantrums, misery, depression, or somatic symptoms)	No significant anxiety about going to school. May have oppositional defiant disorder, conduct disorder, or depression
Parents aware of the issue; child attempts influencing parents to allow him or her to stay home	Child often attempts to hide school absence from parents
No significant antisocial behaviors	Often antisocial delinquent and disruptive behavior and antisocial company
During school hours, child prefers to stay in safe and secure environment such as home	During routine school hours, child regularly does not stay home
Child willing to do schoolwork and homework	Uninterested in schoolwork and do not conform to academic and behavior expectations

difficulties in peer relationships, and adverse psychosocial conditions had different associations with the three types of school refusal. Unsupervised and unmonitored time spent with peers may be a factor for substance abusers to be a truant. The differences between school refusal and truancy are presented in **Table 1**.

Evaluation

The evaluation should be comprehensive and include interviews with close family members and also separate individual interviews with the child and parents. Assessment should include a complete medical history and thorough physical examination. History of the onset and progress of school refusal symptoms, associated stress factors, school attendance history, peer relationships, family functioning, psychiatric history, substance abuse history, and a mental status examination should be done. Identification of factors responsible for school avoidance behaviors is important. Collaboration with school teachers and staff with regards to assessment and treatment is necessary for initiation of successful management. School personnel can provide additional information to aid in assessment. It includes review of attendance records, report cards, and psychoeducational evaluations. More specific assessment scales to measure symptoms of school refusal have been developed recently.

Management

Early recognition and intervention are the determining factors for the prognosis. Many approaches are tried for the management.

Individualized treatment focusing on function rather than symptoms seems to be working the best.

Behavioral management: It includes systematic desensitization (i.e., gradual graded exposure and adjustment to the school environment), relaxation training, social skills training, and cognitive behavior therapy.

Parental involvement and caregiver training: These are crucial factors in enhancing the effectiveness of behavior treatment. The high rates of psychopathology in parents of children with school phobia suggest that treatment of children diagnosed as anxiety disorder should include the treatment of parents as well.

Interventions to help children develop skills to master their academic/ social or other difficulties: This is employed to prevent a recurrence of symptoms after medication is discontinued. Hospital management and/or medication may be necessary in severe forms.

Spending regular time at school also helps truants to prevent substance abuse.

There are rare studies on comparison of impact of child training or combine child with teacher/parent training.

Pharmacologic treatment: Drug therapy should not be the sole intervention but used in addition to behavioral or psychotherapeutic interventions. Tricyclic antidepressants and selective serotonin reuptake inhibitor (SSRI) group of drugs have been usually helpful. Hospital management may be needed in severe cases.

■ BULLYING IN SCHOOL

Bullying in school is a universal and serious problem of specific type of aggression. There is pervasive systematic abuse of power between peers, which is *intentional* to harm or disturb, *repetitive* over time, and has a power *imbalance* with relatively stronger person or group attacking the weaker one. Various observations indicate that as many as half of all children are bullied at some time in one or more situations during their school years, and at least 10% are bullied on a regular basis. Boys usually use physical intimidation, assault, or threats, regardless of the gender of their victims. Bullying by girls is more often verbal, more commonly with another girl as the victim by defamation, ostracizing, etc. Most bullying occurs during break time, on playgrounds, in lunchrooms, sometimes washrooms, on school buses, or in unsupervised halls. Bullies are less likely to pick on a child in a group. Bullying is hurtful and can happen in many ways in academics, social, and emotional health, with long-term consequences also, including self-harm and committing suicide by victims.

Though there is no characteristic profile of a victim or a bully, there are some who seem to be more prone. But then while describing for purpose of understanding, there should not be any labeling or profiling of either. *Victims* are more often typically passive, weaker personality, easily intimidated, or have few friends. Victims may also be smaller in physical structure or younger, with lower self-esteem, depression or anxiety, and have difficulty in defending themselves. A *bully* may have been a victim of physical abuse or bullying. Bullies may also be depressed, angry, or upset about certain situations at school or at home. Usually, they are impulsive, short tempered, and dominant; many are physically strong, with inflated self-esteem, and feel little responsibility for their actions and are unable to empathize with others. They have acceptance toward violence. They may be facing academic difficulties or have difficulty conforming to rules. Psychiatric illness or substance abuse may be aggressor in the background.

Resilience to bullying is rendered by involvement of caring adults, development of cognitive and social skills, and presence of strong social support systems, which includes close family relationships, attachment to school personnel, and involvement in positive peer groups such as sports teams and community service groups.

Types of Bullying

- *Physical:* It may be hit or punch, kick or tripping up the victims, and take or spoil their belongings, etc.
- *Psychological/verbal:* The various forms are calling by names, teasing, giving nasty looks, threatening, making racist remarks, spreading nasty rumors or stories about victim, hindering them from joining in play or games, or avoiding talking to them.
- *Relational:* It is a less common and more subtle form of aggression. It intends to harm by damaging the victim's relationships with others or impairing the victim's ability to maintain a social reputation and usual relationships among peers.
- *Cyberbullying:* It is a relatively new form of bullying that uses electronic communication technology. Cell phones and various social networking sites are used to spread rumors, intimidate directly, or damage the cyber-visual reputation of the victim. Characteristics of traditional bullying (intent, repetition, and power imbalance—technological power in cyberbullying) may not be always seen here. In the absence of definitive evidence, it is said that cyberbullying is worse than traditional bullying. Adolescents experiencing social and emotional difficulties were more likely to be cyberbullied and traditionally bullied than traditionally bullied only. Those targeted in both ways experienced more harm and stayed away from school more often than those traditionally bullied only. It was observed that about 16% bully via the internet and text messages, and 23% were victims of cyberbullying. Cyberbullying is more often anonymous, personal activity, usually committed from home. Victims often respond by pretending to ignore it, often by really ignoring it, or sometimes by retaliating. Some parents set rules for their children about the way they should use the internet but are not really conscious of the harassments that may be the outcome of internet use. They often misjudge their own children's bullying behavior and have improper idea of their

children as victims of bullying. Gender differences are not very prominent. Victims of cyberbullying usually chose to tell their friends or sometimes to no one at all. Victims may feel unable to escape the cruelty, whereas traditional bullying does not typically carry over into the home setting.

Evaluation

- As bullying is a common issue, doctors dealing with children are likely to see some who are victimized at school. Bullying may be a vital factor in the development and maintenance of interpersonal, psychological, and somatic symptoms, and this should be considered in their management. Victims may be reluctant to attend school. They may present to doctors with various stress symptoms such as fits, faints, vomiting, limb pains, pseudoparalysis, hyperventilation, visual symptoms, headaches, stomachaches, fugue states, and also hysteria. Bullied children are less likely to disclose it on their own due to shame, embarrassment, and fear of retaliation. Over time, they feel that they are at fault and deserve the bullying.
- There are rare obvious signs of bullying; hence, doctors should therefore ask directly about bullying. They should identify at-risk children and families, ask status of peer relations, screen for psychiatric morbidities, substance abuse, self-harm tendencies, and advocate for antibullying steps in schools.
- Bullies also deserve proper attention. They themselves are vulnerable to many negative outcomes affecting their well-being and social functioning throughout childhood, adolescence, and into adulthood. They are learning to achieve and exercise their dominance over others through misuse of power. Bullying may even be a component of antisocial and defiant behavior. As adults, they are more likely to have criminal behavior and be involved in serious, habitual crime.

Management

Appropriate intervention of bullying in childhood could not only reduce children's and adolescents' immediate mental health issues but also prevent psychiatric and socioeconomic difficulties in future

up to adulthood and reduce considerable burden and costs for society:
- Affected children should be provided plenty of opportunities to talk with dependable adults in a positive, open, and honest way. The victim should be conveyed that it is not a fault of him or her. If a child says that he or she is being bullied, they should be believed and reassured that they have done the right thing by disclosing to dependable adults.
- Parents should be informed and advised to inform the matter to the school teachers directly.
- Children should be taught simple measures to protect themselves, for example, ignoring name calling, making friends with a peer or group which is not involved. They may convey it to someone such as a teacher or playground supervisor. They should be advised not to fight back and escalate the issue. The child should be prepared to face similar situations.
- The child should be helped to practice being assertive. The simple act of insisting that the bully should leave the victim alone may have a surprising effect. The child should be explained that the bully's true goal is to get a response.
- Encourage the child to be always with close friends when traveling back and forth from school or on other outings.
- Strong antibullying policies in schools and college help to prevent the issue. School initiatives for prevention of bullying should include training in peer mediation, prompt conflict resolution, anger management training, and proper adult supervision. Whole-school interventions such as promoting overall attitudes against bullying and prosocial behaviors using short videotapes, interactive lectures and discussions around the topic of bullying, training teachers in handling bullying effectively, conflict resolution strategies, and counseling obtained the best results. Broader interventions are more efficacious in fighting bullying, perhaps because they consider it to be a complex phenomenon that goes beyond the dyadic relationship between bully and victim. They effectively reduced all forms of bullying, including exclusion, cyber and threats, between 21% up to 63% in older pupils and younger as well.

Parent training, improved playground supervision, disciplinary methods, school conferences, videos, information for parents, work with peers, classroom rules, and management play an important role in antibullying strategies.

GUIDELINES FOR PARENTS

- The child should be encouraged to attend schools as per routine. School avoidance should be discouraged. The longer the child is allowed out of school, the more difficult it is to return.
- Most of the time teachers are the best person to handle school phobia, and parental support is important.
- Active involvement and training of parents and caregivers are critical factors in enhancing the effectiveness of behavior treatment.
- Early recognition and intervention are determining factors for the prognosis.
- Like other forms of abuse, children are unlikely to voluntarily disclose being bullied as they feel ashamed, embarrassed, and fear countercharge accusation.
- If children convey that they are being bullied, they should be believed and reassured that they have done the right by telling. Parents should be informed and advised to take the matter up with the teachers and school directly.
- Children can be trained in simple measures to protect themselves.

BIBLIOGRAPHY

1. Bernstein GA, Massie ED, Thuras PD, Perwien AR, Borchardt CM, Crosby RD. Somatic symptoms in anxious-depressed school refusers. J Am Acad Child Adolesc Psychiatry. 1997;36(5):661-8.
2. Cross D, Lester L, Barnes A. A longitudinal study of the social and emotional predictors and consequences of cyber and traditional bullying victimisation. Int J Public Health. 2015;60(2):207-17.
3. da Silva JL, de Oliveira WA, de Mello FCM, de Andrade LS, Bazon MR, Silva MAI. Anti-bullying interventions in schools: a systematic literature review. Cien Saude Colet. 2017;22(7):2329-40.
4. Dehue F, Bolman C, Völlink T. Cyberbullying: youngsters' experiences and parental perception. Cyberpsychol Behav. 2008;11(2):217-23.
5. Desombre H, Fourneret P, Revol O, De Villard R. School phobia: diagnosis and management. Arch Pediatr. 1999;6(1):97-101.
6. Egger HL, Costello EJ, Angold A. School refusal and psychiatric disorders: a community study. J Am Acad Child Adolesc Psychiatry. 2003;42(7):797-807.

7. Elliott JG, Place M. Practitioner review: School refusal: developments in conceptualisation and treatment since 2000. J Child Psychol Psychiatry. 2019;60:4-15.
8. Elliott JG. School refusal: issues of conceptualisation, assessment, and treatment. J Child Psychol Psychiatry. 1999;40(7):1001-12.
9. Englander E, Donnerstein E, Kowalski R, Lin CA, Parti K. Defining cyberbullying. Pediatrics. 2017;140(Suppl. 2):S148-51.
10. Flakierska-Praquin N, Lindström M, Gillberg C. School phobia with separation anxiety disorder: a comparative 20- to 29-year follow-up study of 35 school refusers. Compr Psychiatry. 1997;38(1):17-22.
11. Fremont WP. School refusal in children and adolescents. Am Fam Physician. 2003;68(8):1555-60.
12. Heyne D, King NJ, Tonge BJ, Cooper H. School refusal: epidemiology and management. Paediatr Drugs. 2001;3:719-32.
13. Kearney CA. School absenteeism and school refusal behavior in youth: a contemporary review. Clin Psychol Rev. 2008;28:451-71.
14. King NJ, Tonge BJ, Heyne D, Pritchard M, Rollings S, Young D, et al. Cognitive-behavioral treatment of school-refusing children: a controlled evaluation. J Am Acad Child Adolesc Psychiatry. 1998;37(4):395-403.
15. Lyznicki JM, McCaffree MA, Robinowitz CB. Childhood bullying: implications for physicians. Am Fam Physician. 2004;70(9):1723-8.
16. Mouren MC, Delorme R. School phobia or school refusal: controversial concepts. Bull Acad Natl Med. 2006;190(8):1629-39.
17. Martin C, Cabrol S, Bouvard MP, Lepine JP, Mouren-Siméoni MC. Anxiety and depressive disorders in fathers and mothers of anxious school-refusing children. J Am Acad Child Adolesc Psychiatry. 1999;38(7):916-22.
18. Menesini E, Salmivalli C. Bullying in schools: the state of knowledge and effective interventions. Psychol Health Med. 2017;22(Sup1):240-53.
19. Nissen G. Separation anxiety, school anxiety, depression... pediatric anxiety disorders have many faces. MMW Fortschr Med. 2001;143(5):26-8.
20. Prabhuswamy M, Srinath S, Girimaji S, Seshadri S. Outcome of children with school refusal. Indian J Pediatr. 2007;74(4):375-9.
21. Salmivalli C, Kärnä A, Poskiparta E. Counteracting bullying in Finland: the KiVa program and its effects on different forms of being bullied. Int J Behav Dev. 2011;35(5):405-11.
22. Slonje R, Smith PK. Cyberbullying: another main type of bullying? Scand J Psychol. 2008;49(2):147-54.
23. Ttofi MM, Farrington DP. What works in preventing bullying: effective elements of anti-bullying programmes. J Aggression Conflict Peace Res. 2009;1:13-24.

CHAPTER 20

Fussy Child

Piyali Bhattacharya

▪ INTRODUCTION

The dictionary meaning of "fussy" is "easily upset." When given to bouts of ill temper, it is a "fussy baby." One in five babies has parent-reported cry–fuss problems. Parents continue to receive conflicting advice about caring for their unsettled baby from the primary, secondary, and tertiary sectors. Organic disturbance is implicated in only 5% of cases, while it may be normal for children to get fussy or irritable most of the times. Young children, who cannot talk, will let others know something is wrong by acting fussy or irritable.

Normally, children get fussy because of hunger, frustration, fight with a sibling, being too hot or too cold, poor sleep patterns, diaper rash, thrush, overtiredness, overstimulation, loneliness, discomfort, food sensitivities, etc.

To Distinguish Between "Normal" and a Problem

Normal fuss usually occurs around the same time of day, with approximately the same intensity; it responds to some of the same things each time, such as passing stools, holding the baby, or frequent breastfeeding. It occurs in a baby who has at other time of the day been contentedly awake or asleep.

Looking after the child's basic needs, for example, nursing baby to the breast, burping the baby, changing his wet diaper, and checking to make sure that no clothing is irritating him and creating discomfort, helps in soothing a fussy child. Sometimes, a comforting touch or rhythmic rocking motion may be all that the baby needs. Reduced stimulation, for example, dimming overhead lights and playing soft music, is a useful strategy in such children.

A serious thought about an underlying cause should be given if the child is:
- Getting worse or not gradually getting better
- Awakening frequently with painful cries
- Inconsolable crying
- Not thriving/poor weight gain
- Having frequent respiratory or intestinal illnesses.

A child's fussiness may be an early sign of a problem such as:
- Anemia, asthma, or other health problems
- Unwitnessed head injury
- Hearing or speech problems
- Autism or abnormal brain development
- Depression or other mental health problems.

COMMON CHILDHOOD ILLNESSES WHICH MAKE A CHILD FUSSY

Upper Respiratory Infection with Nasal Block

Infants younger than 3 months are usually protected by maternal antibodies. However, by 3-6 months, upper respiratory infection rates increase. In toddlers and preschool ages, there is an increased rate of infections once they start going to crèche or play school. Viral infections, for example, respiratory syncytial virus, adenovirus, rhinovirus, influenza, and parainfluenza, and other infections due to organisms such as group A beta-hemolytic streptococci, staphylococci, pneumococci or *Hemophilus influenzae*, can give rise to considerable discomfort in children.

Children have relatively small airways, and mucous or edematous swelling during an infection would change the diameter and increase the resistance, giving rise to difficulty in respiration, irritability, and fussiness.

Clinical manifestations:
- Fever (temperature varies with the age of the child)
- Irritability, restlessness
- Decreased appetite and fluid intake
- Nasal congestion, runny nose, mild cough
- Vomiting and diarrhea.

Ear Infection

Diameter and distances of airways play a significant role in respiratory illnesses in children. The Eustachian tubes are horizontal and not diagonal, and the distance between structures is shorter in children. This allows organisms to rapidly move up or down the respiratory tract. Acute otitis media occurs when the child's Eustachian tube becomes swollen or blocked and traps fluid in the middle ear. Once fluid accumulates, the stasis may be associated with infection.

Infants and children may have one or more of the following symptoms:
- Crying, irritability
- Sleeplessness
- Pulling on the ears
- Ear pain, fullness in the ear
- Drainage from the ear
- Headache
- Fever
- Vomiting
- Diarrhea

The risk factors for acute otitis media are magnified manyfold with factors such as the use of pacifier, bottle feeding, or having had a recent cold, sinus, or ear infection.

Urinary Tract Infection

Normally, girls are more likely to get urinary tract infections (UTIs) than boys because their urethra is shorter. However, in children <1 year of age, there is a male preponderance. Stasis of urine, as in vesicoureteral reflux (VUR) where urine backflows into the ureters and kidneys, is one of the prominent disorders that need investigation in early childhood to prevent ongoing damage.

The main symptoms are pain and burning in the lower abdomen, back, or side with frequent urination. Children who are already toilet trained may lose control and start bed-wetting. There may be drops of blood in the urine or pink urine. Younger children may have general symptoms, such as fussiness, little interest in food, or nausea, vomiting, and/or fever.

Constipation

Bowel patterns vary from child to child. Children with constipation may have stools that are hard, dry, and difficult or painful to pass. A short history will reveal the diet and physical activity patterns of the child. The abdomen is generally soft, nontender on palpation, and a simple per rectal examination will be mostly sufficient to ascertain the presence of impacted stool in the rectum.

Adding dietary fiber and adequate fluids work well. Glycerine suppositories can be used to soften the stools in younger children.

Worm Infestation

Worm infestation is endemic in India. According to the World Health Organization, out of the total 836 million children at risk worldwide, 241 million children between the ages of 1 and 14 years are at risk of parasitic intestinal worms in India. The infestation is acquired through the fecal-oral route by unwashed hands, drinking contaminated water, eating unwashed or undercooked food, using contaminated utensils, handling of infected pets, and sometimes by direct entry through the skin while walking barefoot.

Children with a worm infestation may show a lack of concentration in school, loss of appetite, loss of weight, abdominal pain, and diarrhea.

Teething or a Toothache

Some babies breeze through teething while others suffer from a good deal of pain due to the inflammation of the gums. Teething babies may be edgy or hard to settle at naptime and bedtime. They become more fussy and clingy and drool saliva most of the time. They have an urge to bite to try to ease the pain and chew almost anything they can get hold of.

■ SOME SERIOUS CONDITIONS

Gastroesophageal Reflux

Gastroesophageal reflux maybe suspected if the child experiences the following:
- Painful bursts of night waking
- Cries painfully after eating

- Draws up his legs, knees to his chest, and arches his back as if writhing in pain.

Food Sensitivities

When a child has a food allergy, their immune system overreacts, producing antibodies to the food. Common suspects include peanuts and tree nuts (walnuts, almonds, cashews, pistachios), dairy products, eggs, fish and shellfish (shrimp, lobster), soy, wheat, caffeine-containing foods and beverages (soft drinks, chocolate, coffee, tea), and certain vegetables.

The child may present with a runny/congested nose, stomach pain, vomiting, diarrhea, nausea, itching around the mouth or ears, red, itchy rashes on the skin (hives), swelling of the lips, tongue, and/or face, or shortness of breath.

The Colic: Cow's Milk Protein Allergy

It deserves a special mention. One possible cause of a fussy baby could be an allergy to cow's milk protein, and it is important to distinguish cow's milk protein allergy (CMPA) from other food allergies. Information about this disease from India is scanty, and only one study has highlighted a prevalence of 13% among children <2 years of age with malabsorption.

Signs and symptoms consist of frequent spitting up or vomiting, abdominal pain or colic-like symptoms (excessive crying and irritability, especially after feedings), diarrhea, blood in stool, hives, scaly skin rash, and coughing or wheezing. The presence of aphthous ulcers and abnormal rectal biopsy are clues to initial diagnosis.

Diagnosis can be confirmed by a positive milk challenge test 2-3 months after cow's milk-free diet.

Transient Lactase Deficiency

Babies may acquire transient secondary lactose intolerance due to damage of the intestinal villi commonly due to gastroenteritis or CMPA. Research has shown that 38% infant colic cases can be attributed to a temporary insufficiency of lactase enzyme that digests the lactose sugar in milk. Colic comes in many shapes and sizes, from the evening-only screamer to the all-day fusser. Symptoms usually improve when babies start producing the enzyme around 4 months of age. Weaning is not indicated in breastfed babies with secondary lactose intolerance, although probiotics and CMPA maternal elimination diet may have a role.

> **GUIDELINES FOR PARENTS**
> - Caring for a fussy baby can be quite stressful.
> - Do not be alarmed or feel guilty all the time.
> - When you stay with your baby, provide comfort so that he feels connected and loved.
> - Be positive and affirm to yourself that you are doing a great job.
> - A little *me* time always helps.
> - Mothers must surround themselves with supportive people and de-stress in other areas, such as time spent in the kitchen and listening to music.

BIBLIOGRAPHY

1. Freedman SB, Al-Harthy N, Thull-Freedman J. The crying infant: diagnostic testing and frequency of serious underlying disease. Pediatrics. 2009;123:841-8.
2. Poddar U, Yachha SK, Krishnani N, Srivastava A. Cow's milk protein allergy: an entity for recognition in developing countries. J Gastroenterol Hepatol. 2010;25:178-82.
3. Savino F, Cordisco L, Tarasco V, Palumeri E, Calabrese R, Oggero R, et al. *Lactobacillus reuteri* DSM 17938 in infantile colic: a randomized, double-blind, placebo-controlled trial. Pediatrics. 2010;126:e526-33.
4. Wake M, Morton-Allen E, Poulakis Z, Hiscock H, Gallagher S, Oberklaid F. Prevalence, stability, and outcomes of cry-fuss and sleep problems in the first 2 years of life: prospective community-based study. Pediatrics. 2006;117:836-42.
5. Yachha SK, Misra S, Malik AK, Nagi B, Mehta S. Spectrum of malabsorption syndrome in North Indian children. Indian J Gastroenterol. 1993;12:120-5.

CHAPTER 21

Behavioral Problems in Adolescents

Suchit Tamboli

EATING DISORDERS

■ INTRODUCTION

Eating disorders are classic examples of illness with biopsychosocial determinants. Anorexia nervosa involves a distorted body image and self-imposed severe dietary limitation that results in malnutrition. Bulimia nervosa is binge eating with inappropriate measures taken to avoid weight gain. Cyclic vomiting manifests itself as repeated severe episodes of vomiting in the absence of the usual causes. Rumination disorder is repeated significant regurgitation.

■ RISK FACTORS OF EATING DISORDERS

Social, family environment and media are the most prominent risk factors for eating disorders. The influence of the media and social environment has been related to the worship of thinness. As to the family environment, mealtimes appeared to be fundamental in shaping eating behavior and the development of disorders. Eating disorders were associated with nutritional problems (growing impairment and weight gain), oral health (cheilitis, dental erosion, periodontitis, and hypertrophy of salivary glands), and social prejudice.

The chapter on feeding and eating disorders in the fifth edition of the Diagnostic and Statistical Manual of Mental Disorders (DSM 5) includes several changes to better represent the symptoms and behaviors of patients dealing with these conditions across the life span. Among the most substantial changes are the recognition of binge eating disorder, revisions to the diagnostic criteria for anorexia nervosa and bulimia nervosa, and the inclusion of pica, rumination, and avoidant/restrictive food intake disorder.

BARRIERS INFLUENCING EATING BEHAVIORS

Inadequate nutrient intake because of dieting or concern for weight gain, eating patterns, and food selection directly or indirectly influence eating behaviors.

Interventions must be appropriate and sustainable to halt the growing number of obese, overweight, and malnourished adolescents. It is important to assess nutritional status and needs during adolescence.

"Adolescent nutritional status must be assessed individually using information from clinical, biochemical, anthropometric, dietary, and psychosocial assessments."

ANOREXIA NERVOSA

The patient has an obsessive desire to lose weight. They are usually physically hyperactive and often experience sleep disturbances and are characterized by distorted body image and excessive dieting that leads to severe weight loss with a pathological fear of becoming fat. The criteria have several minor but important changes as per DSM 5.

DSM 5 Diagnostic Criteria

- *Restriction of energy intake relative to requirements:* It leads to a significantly low body weight in the context of age, sex, developmental trajectory, and physical health. Significantly low weight is defined as a weight that is less than minimally normal or for children and adolescents less than minimally expected. The word "refusal" was omitted because this was viewed as possibly pejorative and difficult to assess, as it implies intention. Rewording of the criterion to focus on behaviors was recommended.
- *Intense fear of gaining weight or becoming fat:* It means persistent behavior that interferes with weight gain, even though at a significantly low weight. Clarification with regard to "fear of weight gain" took place. A significant minority of individuals with the syndrome explicitly deny such fear. Therefore, the addition of a clause to focus on behavior was recommended.
- *Disturbance in the way in which one's body weight or shape is experienced:* This means undue influence of body weight or shape on self-evaluation or persistent lack of recognition of the seriousness of the current low body weight.

The criterion D of DSM-IV was removed in DSM 5, which is a substantial change. In criterion D, amenorrhea was required to meet an eating disorder diagnosis. However, individuals have been clearly described who exhibit all other symptoms and signs of anorexia nervosa but who report at least some menstrual activity. In addition, this criterion cannot be applied to premenarche females, to females taking oral contraceptives, to postmenopausal females, or to males. However, there are some data that women who endorse amenorrhea have poorer bone health than women who fail to meet this criterion.

Specific Current Type: Restricting Type

During the last 3 months, the person has not engaged in recurrent episodes of binge eating or purging behavior (i.e., self-induced vomiting or the misuse of laxatives, diuretics, or enemas).

Binge Eating/Purging Type

During the last 3 months, the person has engaged in recurrent episodes of binge eating or purging behavior (i.e., self-induced vomiting or the misuse of laxatives, diuretics, or enemas). DSM-IV requires that the subtype (binge eating/purging or restricting) be specified for the current episode. While there are data that such subtyping is useful clinically and for research purposes, there is significant crossover between subtypes, and resultant difficulty in specifying the subtype for the "current episode" of illness. Therefore, it was recommended that the subtyping be specified for the last 3 months. The 3-month timeframe was used for bulimia nervosa and proposed for binge eating disorder.

Clinical Features

Physical Symptoms

- Loss of weight
- Amenorrhea, absence of cyclic symptoms or physical changes of menstruation (anovulatory)
- Hyperactivity (psychological and motor)
- Aberrant behavior, such as irritability, isolation-withdrawal, and sleep disturbances

- Hyperacusis or optic hyperesthesia
- These children may present with depressed mood, feelings of ineffectiveness, and low self-esteem.

Physical Signs

These children may present with typical features such as cachexia, emaciation, debilitation, or dehydration. There may be possible signs of shock or impending shock. Coexisting infections (pneumonia or sepsis; immunologic problems) may be present.

- Typical skin changes (dryness, pale yellowish palms and soles, desquamation)
- Loss of scalp and pubic hair. Presence of lanugo hair or increased pigmented body hair
- Hypothermia (rectal temperature below 96.6°F/36.2°C)
- Decreased respiratory rate
- Bradycardia, "quiet" heart (decreased basal metabolic rate)—pulse below 60 beats/min, usually as low as 25 beats/min
- Hypotension as per age, often below 70/50 mm Hg
- Sometimes heart murmur
- Pedal edema
- Various signs of estrogen deficiency—dry skin, osteoporosis, small uterus-cervix, vaginal mucosa pink and dry
- Signs of decreased androgen—absence of acne, nonoily skin

Laboratory Findings

Biochemical

- Most laboratory tests are normal initially.
- Elevated blood urea nitrogen (BUN) levels—as a consequence of dehydration
- Hypercarotenemia
- High serum cholesterol levels in the early stage, which may decrease later
- Decreased transferrin, normal protein and albumin to globulin ratio, low complement C, fibrinogen, and prealbumin
- Elevated serum lactate dehydrogenase and alkaline phosphatase—possibly related to growth

- Decreased phosphorus level is a late and ominous sign, magnesium level is decreased. Calcium levels may be low or high.
- Sometimes depression of plasma zinc, urinary zinc, and urinary copper levels.

Endocrine

- Low normal thyroxine (T4), reduced tri-iodothyronine (T3), elevated reverse T3, and normal thyroid-stimulating hormone (TSH)
- Low normal fasting glucose
- Low luteinizing hormone (LH), low or pseudonormal follicle-stimulating hormone (FSH), deficiency of gonadotropin-releasing hormone (GnRH), normal prolactin, low testosterone in males, and low estradiol in females
- Elevated circulating cortisol
- Sometimes elevation of parathyroid hormone (PTH) secondary to hypomagnesemia with resultant hypercalcemia
- Raised resting growth hormone levels.

Hematological

- Leukopenia with relative lymphocytosis due to bone marrow hypoplasia, sometimes absolute lymphopenia
- Thrombocytopenia
- Very low erythrocyte sedimentation rate (ESR)
- Anemia in the late phase, especially after rehydration.

BULIMIA NERVOSA

DSM 5 Proposed Diagnostic Criteria

- *Recurrent episodes of binge eating:* An episode of binge eating is characterized by both of the following:
  1. Eating, in a discrete period of time—for example, within any 2-hour period, an amount of food that is definitely larger than most people would eat during a similar period of time and under similar circumstances
  2. A sense of lack of control over eating during the episode—for example, a feeling that one cannot stop eating or control what or how much one is eating.

- *Recurrent inappropriate compensatory behavior in order to prevent weight gain:* Such as self-induced vomiting; misuse of laxatives, diuretics, or other medications, fasting; or excessive exercise.
- *Binge eating and inappropriate compensatory behaviors:* Both occur, on average, at least once a week for 3 months.

    Criterion C is a modest change in DSM 5. Previously, DSM-IV required that episodes of both binge eating and inappropriate compensatory behaviors occur on average twice/week over the last 3 months. A literature review found that the clinical characteristics of individuals reporting a lower frequency of once/week were similar to those meeting the current criterion. Therefore, it was recommended that the required minimum frequency be reduced to once/week over the last 3 months.
- Self-evaluation is unduly influenced by body shape and weight.
- The disturbance does not occur exclusively during episodes of anorexia nervosa.

Subtypes have been deleted, which also resulted in some rewording of criterion B. DSM-IV required that the subtype (purging or nonpurging) be specified. A literature review indicated that the nonpurging subtype had received relatively little attention, and the available data suggested that individuals with this subtype more closely resembled individuals with binge eating disorder. In addition, how to precisely define nonpurging inappropriate behaviors (e.g., fasting or excessive exercise) was considered to be unclear.

Clinical Features

Physical Examination

- Weight is variable. It may be normal, overweight, or underweight.
- Occasional complaints of bloating, diarrhea, and swelling
- Usually hyperactive (mental and motor), but exceptions common
- Constant or extreme thirst and increased urination (hypokalemic nephropathy, hypovolemia)
- May present with depression, anxiety, despair, and suicidal ideation.

Physical Signs

- These children are usually well groomed and maintain proper hygiene. There may be definite exceptions, especially in patients with severe character disorders or chronic addictive conditions.
- Weight is usually normal or mild to moderate obesity. Exceptions are food restrictors or anorexia nervosa patients with associated bulimia-vomiting-purging.
- Generalized or localized edema of lower extremities may be present due to compensatory renal retention of sodium and water that is hypovolemia with secondary hyperaldosteronism or pseudo-Bartter syndrome.
- Physical examination findings of extreme weight loss due to self-starvation of bulimia-vomiting-purging are complications of anorexia nervosa or food restriction. There may be loss of scalp hair and skin changes in anorexia.
- Parotid and other salivary glands may be swollen.
- Dental enamel dysplasia and discoloration due to gastric secretions as a result of vomiting.
- Bruises and lacerations of the palate and posterior pharynx, lesions of fingernails, fingers, and dorsum of the hand as a result of trauma due to self-induced vomiting.
- Pyorrhea and other gum disorders
- Diminished deep tendon reflexes, generalized muscle weakness, paralysis, and rarely, peripheral neuropathy with muscle weakness and paralysis
- Muscle cramps may be elicited by induced hypoxia or positive Trousseau sign.
- Signs of hypokalemia, cardiac dysrhythmias, hypotension, decreased cardiac output, weak peripheral pulse and feeble heart sounds, abdominal distention, ileus, acute gastric dilatation, and myopathy. Shortness of breath, depression, and mental clouding.

Laboratory Findings

Bulimia Alone

Usually, no abnormalities are reported. There may be possible alterations in glucose metabolism.

Bulimia with Vomiting
- Metabolic alkalosis with hypochloremia, elevated serum bicarbonate levels
- Hypokalemia, secondary to the above condition
- Hypovolemia with secondary hyperaldosteronism also contributes to hypokalemia (pseudo-Bartter syndrome).

Bulimia with Vomiting and Laxative-diuretic Abuse
- All findings as mentioned above
- Decreased body potassium level due to small bowel diarrhea and renal losses
- Metabolic acidosis with spurious normal serum potassium levels
- Hypokalemic nephropathy with a urine-concentrating deficit
- Hypokalemic myopathy
- Hypocalcemia or hypercalcemia, hypomagnesemia, hypophosphatemia.

BINGE EATING DISORDER

Binge eating disorder is defined as recurring episodes of eating significantly more food in a short period of time than most people would eat under similar circumstances, with episodes marked by feeling of lack of control. Someone with binge eating disorder may eat too quickly, even when he or she is not hungry. The person may have feelings of guilt, embarrassment, or disgust and may binge eat alone to hide the behavior. This disorder is associated with marked distress and occurs, on average, at least once a week over 3 months.

This change is intended to increase awareness of the substantial differences between binge eating disorder and the common phenomenon of overeating. While overeating is common and recurrent, binge eating is much less common, far more severe, and associated with significant physical and psychological problems.

DSM 5 Proposed Diagnostic Criteria
This is a new diagnostic criterion; therefore, no changes are noted in DSM 5.

- *Recurrent episodes of binge eating:* An episode of binge eating is characterized by both of the following:
  1. Eating, in a discrete period of time (e.g., within any 2-hour period, an amount of food that is definitely larger than most people would eat in a similar period of time under similar circumstances)
  2. A sense of lack of control over eating during the episode (e.g., a feeling that one cannot stop eating or control what or how much one is eating).
- The binge eating episodes are associated with three (or more) of the following:
  - Eating much more rapidly than normal
  - Eating until feeling uncomfortably full
  - Eating large amounts of food when not feeling physically hungry
  - Eating alone because of feeling embarrassed by how much one is eating
- Feeling disgusted with oneself, depressed, or very guilty afterward.
- Marked distress regarding binge eating is present.
- Binge eating occurs, on average, at least once a week for 3 months.
- Binge eating is not associated with the recurrent use of inappropriate compensatory behavior (e.g., purging) and does not occur exclusively during the course of bulimia nervosa or anorexia nervosa.

EATING DISORDER NOT OTHERWISE SPECIFIED
DSM 5 Proposed Diagnostic Criteria

It is noted that there is a considerable change to DSM-IV, which specified fairly vague criteria and did not suggest any clusters of illnesses that this was based on. The Work Group has recommended that the category Eating Disorder Not Otherwise Specified be replaced by a section termed Feeding and Eating Conditions Not Elsewhere Classified. Brief descriptions of several conditions that may be listed in the DSM 5, should sufficient data be available to justify them as designated disorders, have been included in the proposal.

Atypical Anorexia Nervosa

All of the criteria for anorexia nervosa are met, except that, despite significant weight loss, the individual's weight is within or above the normal range.

Subthreshold Bulimia Nervosa

It is of low frequency or limited duration. All of the criteria for bulimia nervosa are met, except that the binge eating and inappropriate compensatory behaviors occur, on average, less than once a week and/or for <3 months.

■ PURGING DISORDER

Purging disorder is recurrent purging behavior to influence weight or shape, such as self-induced vomiting, misuse of laxatives, diuretics, or other medications in the absence of binge eating. Self-evaluation is unduly influenced by body shape or weight or there is an intense fear of gaining weight or becoming fat.

■ NIGHT EATING SYNDROME

Night eating syndrome is characterized by recurrent episodes of night eating, as manifested by eating after awakening from sleep or excessive food consumption after the evening meal. There is awareness and recall of the eating. Night eating is not better accounted for by external influences such as changes in the individual's sleep/wake cycle or by local social norms. Night eating is associated with significant distress and/or impairment in functioning. The disordered pattern of eating is not better accounted for by binge eating disorder, another psychiatric disorder, substance abuse or dependence, a general medical disorder, or an effect of medication.

■ OTHER FEEDING OR EATING CONDITION NOT ELSEWHERE CLASSIFIED

This is a residual category for clinically significant problems meeting the definition of a feeding or eating disorder but not satisfying the criteria for any other disorder or condition.

MEDICAL COMPLICATIONS OF EATING DISORDERS

- *Fluid and electrolyte imbalance:*
  - Hypokalemia
  - Hyponatremia
  - Hypochloremic alkalosis
  - Elevated BUN
  - Inability to concentrate urine
  - Decreased glomerular filtration rate (GFR)
  - Ketonuria
- *Cardiovascular:*
  - Bradycardia
  - Orthostatic hypotension
  - Dysrhythmias
  - Electrocardiographic abnormalities
    - Prolonged QT interval
    - T-wave abnormalities
    - Low voltage
    - Conduction defects
  - Ipecac cardiomyopathy
  - Mitral valve prolapsed
  - Congestive cardiac failure
  - Pericardial effusion
- *Gastrointestinal:*
  - Parotid hypertrophy
  - Perimolysis and increased incidence of dental caries
  - Constipation
  - Bloody diarrhea
  - Delayed gastric emptying
  - Intestinal atony
  - Esophagitis
  - Mallory-Weiss tears
  - Esophageal or gastric rupture
  - Perforation/rupture of the stomach
  - Barrett's esophagus
  - Fatty infiltration and focal necrosis of liver
  - Acute pancreatitis

- Superior mesenteric artery syndrome
- Gallstones
- *Dermatologic:*
  - Acrocyanosis
  - Yellow dry skin (hypercarotenemia)
  - Brittle hair and nails
  - Lanugo
  - Hair loss
  - Russell sign (calluses over the knuckles)
  - Pitting edema
- *Endocrine:*
  - Growth retardation and short stature
  - Delayed puberty
  - Amenorrhea
  - Low T syndrome
  - Partial diabetes insipidus
  - Hypercortisolism
- *Skeletal:*
  - Osteopenia
  - Fractures
- *Hematologic:*
  - Bone marrow suppression
    - Mild anemia
    - Leukopenia
    - Thrombocytopenia
  - Low sedimentation rate
  - Impaired cell-mediated immunity
- *Neurologic:*
  - Seizures
  - Myopathy
  - Peripheral neuropathy
  - Cortical atrophy.

Inpatient Medical Hospitalization

Inpatient medical hospitalization is indicated in many cases with dehydration and electrolyte disturbances.

Day Treatment

Day treatment is indicated if the patient is medically stable but needs structure to gain weight and avoid compulsive exercising and purging.

Intensive Outpatient Psychiatric Treatment

Intensive outpatient psychiatric treatment can be done if the patient can be self-sufficient in eating, is able to avoid compulsive exercising, accepts support from other individuals, and is highly motivated to recover. Because anorexia nervosa is a complex, serious, chronic, and potentially fatal condition, multiple treatment modalities are used at different stages of illness and recovery.

- *Attending physician:* He is the team leader who oversees evaluation, general care, and the development of the overall treatment plan. He also anticipates common problems so that those may be prevented or recognized and treated early. Ultimately, he is responsible for the care that the patient receives.
- *House staff member:* The in-house physician makes day-to-day treatment decisions in conjunction with the nursing staff. He also ensures that orders are written so that treatment plan can be implemented, facilitates communication among team members, monitors patient's progress, and learns about the subtleties of working with behavioral patients and their families.
- *Nurse:* They are consistent caretakers who act as a healthy role model for patients, give emotional support, suggest strategies for patients to resolve conflicts, and make decisions. They help patients take increasing control over eating behaviors and monitor compliance with the program.
- *Psychiatrist/psychologist:* They help patients resolve conflicts from food and eating to larger concerns about identity, trust, control, and conflict resolution. These specialists confirm psychiatric diagnoses and recommend and oversee psycho-pharmacologic issues.
- *Nutritionist:* A nutritional consultant guides in healthy food choices by focusing on food groups and not specifically on energy value. They monitor nutrient and energy intake and

body composition. Thus, they help patients plan increase or decrease in food intake. They gradually transfer decision-making to the patient so that by the end of the hospital stay, the patient is choosing and eating appropriate meals without input from anyone.
- *Activities therapist:* They encourage socialization and social competence through peer-related activities, such as the production of a pediatric newsletter.
- *School teacher:* They provide continuity in education.
- *Parents and family:* Parental participation is vital in management.

Medications

Drugs have a limited role in the integrated treatment of anorexia nervosa. If the patient has comorbid depression or obsessive-compulsive disorder, initiation of a selective serotonin reuptake inhibitor (SSRI) is indicated.

MANAGEMENT

Four general principles of care that should be followed are:
1. Establishment of rapport and trust
2. Restoration of nutritional and metabolic state to normal
3. Involvement of the family
4. Implementation of a team approach

The primary goal is to save life by restoration of body weight and physiologic homeostasis. The secondary goal is the development of trust by the patient in the physician and other members of the eating disorder team.

Bulimia Nervosa

Treatment goals include restoring the patient to a healthy weight, treating the physical complications, increasing the patient's motivation to change, educating the patient about healthy nutrition and eating patterns, modifying dysfunctional thoughts and feelings associated with the eating disorders, addressing co-occurring psychologic symptoms (mood disturbance, self-esteem), engaging the family and providing family therapy where appropriate, and developing relapse prevention skills. Bulimia nervosa has been treated with a variety of psychotherapeutic approaches, including cognitive-behavioral therapy (CBT), behavioral therapy, psychodynamic therapy, family therapy, experimental therapy, and an addiction model.

Hospitalization

- It is indicated when the patient has severe symptoms that do not respond to outpatient treatment.
- General medical problems (metabolic abnormalities, hematemesis, vital sign changes, uncontrolled vomiting)
- Need for intravenous fluids to correct electrolyte abnormality
- Refeeding for severe malnutrition
- Suicide tendency
- Assessment and management of self-harm
- Psychiatric disturbances independent of the eating disorder that require hospitalization
- Severe co-occurring substance abuse
- Management of uncontrolled compensatory behaviors (excessive exercise, vomiting)
- Initiation or trial of medication
- Most patients with uncomplicated bulimia nervosa may be seen in intensive outpatient psychiatric treatment.

Psychodynamic Therapy

It may be helpful once binge eating and purging behaviors are improved, and family therapy may be considered for adolescents who are still living at home or for older patients who are still struggling with family conflicts. Behavioral strategies include stimulus control procedures and exposure with response prevention. The most widely used and empirically supported treatment for bulimia nervosa is CBT. Remission rates and long-term outcomes are also favorable after therapy. CBT also appears to affect both the specific and the general psychopathology associated with bulimia nervosa, such as depression, self-esteem, social functioning, and personality disturbance.

Interpersonal Therapy

It focuses on relationship stressors that contribute to the eating disorder and is another empirically supported therapy for bulimia nervosa that is relatively equal in effectiveness to CBT at long-term follow-up.

Nutritional Counseling

Nutritional counseling in bulimia nervosa is also warranted to decrease the behaviors associated with the eating disorder, such as decreasing food restriction, increasing the variety of foods eaten (especially high-protein foods), and encouraging healthy exercise behaviors.

Pharmacologic Therapy

The primary drugs are antidepressants. They have also been used to correct hypothesized serotonin deficits that may be linked to bulimia nervosa. Both tricyclic antidepressants and fluoxetine have been reported to be significantly more effective than placebo. Treatments that integrate both CBT and antidepressants are more effective than either treatment individually. Antidepressant medications can also reduce binge eating and purging behavior and may assist in preventing relapse. A combination of psychotherapy and medication may improve remission rates.

Prevention

Eating disorders are complex biopsychosocial conditions; hence, the cause is indefinite and multifactorial. Risk factors are difficult to know; therefore, preventive measures are uncertain. Parents should provide a nurturing environment without being overprotective or overinvolved. They should be alert to the needs of the child and avoid putting their own vicarious pleasure from the child's accomplishments over the inner joy felt by the child. They should encourage autonomy and independence, but not as a justification for neglect or preoccupation. Parents should make the child feel wanted, loved, and valued but not possessed, overprized, or indulged. Mealtimes should be regular and relaxed; it does not mean that we should not totally avoid conflict; they can express differing opinions. Fat restriction, avoidance of obesity, and the need for exercise must be explained. The role of media is too effective. We should be alert to inappropriate media messages that generate anxiety about body shape, appearance, and physical fitness. Exercise should be reasonable and appropriate.

Social Skills: A Factor of Protection Against Eating Disorders in Adolescents

Social skills begin to be formed in infancy. A child's first formative environment is the family and, subsequently, environments such as school, place of sports and games, and club. These abilities relate to a group of behaviors practiced by the individual in a given context, expressing her/his feelings, attitudes, desires, opinions, and rights in a way that is appropriate to the situation while respecting the behavior of others.

The occurrence and sustaining of eating disorders can be influenced by the current society's standards of beauty, by messages and values transmitted by the media, by the influence of peers, and by emotions which, when not properly administered, exacerbate the situation, creating a predisposition to the disorder.

Individuals who receive training for social skills since their early days as children, whether in school, at home, or in club, are able to deal with situations that are stressful or those that could have emotional influence in a more appropriate way compared to those who have not received this training. It is possible to infer that the greater the repertoire of the adolescent's social skills, the greater the protection against behaviors of risk for eating disorders. Thus, it is postulated that all those involved in dealing with children and adolescents, especially professionals in health and education, should be trained, aware, and qualified to work on the development of such skills among the people under their care, helping in the formation of healthy individuals and, thus, individuals who are able to integrate effectively into society and into the culture to which they belong. These professionals would thus be helping with the children's and adolescents' development.

Outcomes and Continuity into Adult Life

Around 50% of adolescents with anorexia nervosa respond to treatment within 12 months, and 75-80% achieve full or partial remission, regardless of treatment type. This means, however, that 20-25% will still meet diagnostic criteria for anorexia nervosa after 2 years of treatment. Factors that have been associated with poorer outcomes include admission to a psychiatric hospital, eating-related obsessionality, and eating disorder-specific.

For bulimia nervosa, around 40% abstain from bingeing/purging after treatment, but relapse is common even by 6 months. Those with less severe eating concerns at baseline, lower baseline depression, fewer binge/purge episodes at presentation, and receiving family based rather than individual treatment are more likely to be in remission at follow-up.

Previous studies have suggested that the outcome for childhood-onset eating disorders might be worse than for those with onset in adolescence.

PROGNOSIS

Anorexia Nervosa

Mortality is a substantial risk in individuals with anorexia nervosa, and it results from suicide or the physical complications of the chronic eating disorder. The mortality risk has declined over the last 25 years with improved identification and treatment of anorexia nervosa. The majority of patients with anorexia nervosa recover from their initial illness. Approximately 25% of patients remain symptomatic. The recovery process usually occurs within 2 years of the onset of anorexia nervosa and is atypical beyond 5 years after onset in some cases. A strong risk factor for the development of bulimia nervosa is recovery from anorexia nervosa.

Bulimia Nervosa

Spontaneous improvement is seen in bulimia nervosa with reduction of symptoms over 1-2 years. Patients who received psychological treatment or medications report a short-term success rate of 50-70%. Relapse rates for patients with bulimia nervosa after 6 months to 6 years range from 30 to 50%, although slow improvement has been reported as follow-up studies extend to 10–15 years. Patients who are functioning well and have milder symptoms at the beginning of treatment have a more favorable prognosis, as do outpatients compared with hospitalized in-patients with severe symptoms. Some studies have reported that a higher frequency of pretreatment vomiting is predictive of poorer outcomes.

GUIDELINES FOR PARENTS

- Parents should not blame themselves for the condition.
- Their creative resources and strengths should be drawn to move their child toward a healthy state.
- Recovery is best achieved when it is treated at an early stage.
- Parents should avoid criticizing their child during their resistance to eating.
- Parents need to give considerable time and energy.
- Sympathetic sibling plays a role in refeeding and restoration of health.
- Make sure to keep healthy boundaries in your marriage and build a positive relationship with your child.
- Be patient, careful, and focus on refeeding and physical health indicators.
- Take professional help whenever necessary.

SEXUALITY AND DEVIANT SEXUAL BEHAVIOR

INTRODUCTION

Sexuality is the sum total of one's thinking, behavior, and attitude. Sexuality is becoming comfortable with one's own body, emotions, and feelings. To develop a positive sexuality concept, one has to free the mind from all fears, misconceptions, myths, and complexes.

Different types of sexual behaviors in children are common, occurring in 42–73% of children by the time they reach 13 years of age. There may be various factors of parental concern about their child's sexual behavior like anxiety, the extent to which the behavior is disruptive at home or in school, the origin of the behavior, and effective management of the behavior.

Sexual behaviors are influenced or modified by several factors:
- Normal development
- Parent's reaction to the behavior
- Changes in family stressors
- Access to sexual material. For example, recent technology, such as the internet, chat rooms, and texting, has opened new ways through which children are exposed to sexually explicit information. Contemporary television and music provide more frequent exposure to sexual material.

Sexual behavior that is developmentally inappropriate requires an evaluation of other factors, such as conduct and behavior disorders in the child, violence, abuse, and neglect in the home. Age-appropriate sexual behaviors in children are given in **Table 1**. While assessing the sexual behaviors in children, the questions that caretakers should be asked are given in **Table 2**.

TABLE 1: Age-appropriate sexual behaviors in children.		
Age (years)	**Gender**	**Behaviors**
2–5	Boys	*More common (observed in 25–60% of children):* Touch genitals, breasts, stand too close to other persons, try to look at persons when they are nude, touch genitals in public
		Less common (15–20%): Very interested in opposite sex, masturbates with hand, hug adults he does not know well, display the anogenital area to adults
	Girls	*More common (25–44%):* Touch the anogenital area and breasts, try to look at persons when they are nude, stand too close to other persons
		Less common (10–16%): Masturbate with hand, very interested in the opposite sex, touch the anogenital area in public, display the anogenital area to adults, hug adults she does not know well, get upset when adults kiss, dress like the opposite sex
6–9	Boys	*More common (14–40%):* Touch genitals, try to look at persons when they are nude, stand too close to other persons, touch breasts, touch genitals in public

Contd...

Contd...

Age (years)	Gender	Behaviors
		Less common (8.5–13%): Very interested in the opposite sex, know more about sex, masturbate with hand, try to look at pictures of nude persons, talk about sexual acts
	Girls	*More common (15–21%):* Touch the anogenital area, try to look at persons when they are nude, stand too close to other persons, touch breasts, knows more about sex
		Less common (8–14%): Very interested in the opposite sex, try to look at pictures of nude persons, dress like the opposite sex, want to watch nudity on media
10–12	Boys	*More common (9–24%):* Interested in the opposite sex, want to watch nudity on media, know more about sex, try to look at pictures of nude persons, touch the anogenital area
		Less common (6–8%): Stand too close to other persons, try to look at persons when they are nude
	Girls	*More common (15–29%):* Interested in the opposite sex, knows more about sex, stand too close to other persons, want to watch nudity on media, touch the anogenital area at home
		Less common (5–9%): Talk about sexual acts, dress like the opposite sex, masturbate with hand, get upset when adults kiss, try to look at persons when they are nude, talk flirtatiously

TABLE 2: Questions for caretakers regarding sexual behaviors in children.

Question	Comments
When the concerned behavior was first noticed? Have there been any recent changes or stressors in the family?	The behavior may be related to a recent stressor, such as a new sibling, disharmony, or parent separation
Does the behavior involve other persons?	Most sexual behavior problems involve responses from other persons

Contd...

Contd...

Question	Comments
How often have you noticed the behavior? Is the frequency or nature of the behavior changing?	Recent escalation in the frequency of behaviors may indicate increased anxiety or stressors contributing to the behavior
Can the child be easily distracted from the behavior? How do you (the caretaker) respond to the behavior?	Normative behavior is usually easy to divert; caretaker distress may escalate the behavior
Does the behavior occur at home, school/daycare, or both?	If the typical behavior occurs only at home, the behavior may be related to stressors or changes at home, or the behavior may be related to differences in observer perception
If the concerned behavior involves another person, how old is the person?	Behaviors involving persons of 4 or more years' difference in age are age inappropriate
Is the typical activity disruptive, instructive, coercive, or forceful?	These are abnormal situations
Does the child become overtly anxious or fearful during the behavior? Has the child been diagnosed with emotional or behavioral problems?	Sexual behavior problems in children have often been associated with conduct and other behavior disorders
Is there any disharmony or violence in the home?	Intimate partner violence has been associated with sexual behaviors in children
Does the child have or had access to sexual material, acts, or inappropriate information, including pornographic movies or images, nudity, internet chat rooms, and texting that includes sexual language?	Children may imitate what they see or hear
Has anyone ever spoken to the child about possible abuse?	Sexual behaviors in children are associated with physical or sexual abuse and neglect

SEXUALIZED BEHAVIOR

The sexuality dilemma in adolescents is because of the fact that they do not understand their body image. They fail to realize that they are not comfortable with their emotions and feelings. The characteristic features of adolescent sexuality are the 3 Es: *E*xperimenting, *E*xperiencing, and *E*xpanding.

ISSUES BOTHERING GIRLS

- *Breast size and shape:* The size and shape of the breast vary from individual to individual. Even the enlargement of breast is not similar in two girls. But adolescent girls are more often than not bothered by the variation when they compare themselves with their peers.
- *Masturbation:* It is a harmless, normal physiological outlet for sexual tension in both sexes.
- *Lesbianism:* Attraction toward another girl may just be a passing phase, but if it is persistent and associated with lack of interest in boys, then it is deviation.
- *Privacy:* In a sense, it is a way of establishing individual identity. Parents often misinterpret it as an attempt to hide.
- *Peer pressure:* Adolescents trust their peers more than anybody else. It is a phase when the individual can be molded in any form by peer influences.

ISSUES BOTHERING BOYS

- *Onset of puberty:* Boys undergo a lot of stress because they lag behind in physical growth and size. They think that they cannot establish a normal healthy relationship with girls. This may result in shyness, withdrawal, anger, and aggression. Even a delay in the appearance of facial hair may cause inferiority complex.
- *Gynecomastia:* It is a normal phenomenon in adolescence, but often, it causes great concern. It disappears within a few years.
- *Nocturnal emission:* It is also a normal phenomenon in adolescent boys just like menarche in girls.
- *Masturbation:* It is a harmless practice among boys. Keeping oneself busy is one way to curb too much of masturbation.

- *Homosexuality:* It may be a passing phenomenon in boys.

Sexuality is defined as the "condition of being characterized and distinguished by sex, concern with or interest in sexual activity, sexual character, or potency." Hence, sexuality does not exclusively mean sex, but it is one aspect of it. Sex, which is sexual behavior or act, is part of our sexuality. Sexuality is an instinct. The facts that sexuality involves thinking, emotions, and behavior about getting attracted, coming together, performing sexual acts, and staying together and that each person requires to go through all of the above to perform satisfactorily during the sexual act show that there is much more than mere sexual act. Sexual acts and relationships are considered as two different things. Sexual act is part of sexuality, which it consumes a comparatively small portion of the day; the rest of the day is consumed by the relationship. The richest relationship thus would be one where there is sexual attraction as well as intellectual and emotional compatibility.

Sexuality is a complex phenomenon that involves interaction between one's (1) biological sex, (2) core gender identity (sense of maleness and femaleness), (3) gender identity (sense of masculinity and femininity), and (4) gender role behavior (nonsexual as well as sexual).

Therefore, it is necessary that both husband and wife are comfortable at the time of intercourse. It acknowledges the fact that even females have the right to experience pleasure. Thus, sex is not just equal to intercourse. It is much more than that. In fact, it is the most intimate form of communication, where one can express one's liking, love, appreciation, comfort, and care through thoughts. A key component to the healthy development of the teenager is how he/she proceeds with their stages of adolescent sexuality. During this time, the individual must develop healthy self-esteem and also sexual comfort, learning to deal with those in his/her "sexual" universe.

■ GENDER IDENTITY DISORDER

Gender identity refers to a person's sexual self-concept, the feeling of being male or female. In gender identity disorder of childhood, children who have not yet reached puberty express extreme distress at their gender and intense desire to be of the opposite sex.

Sigmund Freud felt that individuals began human life with biopotentiality; that is, they could become homosexual or heterosexual. Usually, the heterosexual aspect dominates. Freud did not consider homosexuality a mental illness. "Homosexuality assuredly is no advantage, but nothing to be ashamed of, no vice, no degradation; it cannot be classified as an illness; we consider it to be a variation of sexual functioning produced by a certain arrest of sexual development." Homosexual behavior refers to sexual behavior with members of one's own sex. Kinsey's scale of sexual orientation is used for the detection of homosexuality.

Troiden's Model of Sexual Identity Development and School Needs of LGBTQ Youth (1989) has outlined four stages in the development of homosexual identity:

1. *Sensitization:* Gains homosexual experiences in childhood and adolescence while learning about the general society's negative views on homosexuality.
2. *Dissociation and signification:* Struggles to reject the concept that society's negative views on homosexuality, applies to one's self.
3. *Coming out:* Identifies oneself as "gay" and reaches out to become involved in some aspect of gay society culture; begins to consider homosexuality as a viable lifestyle option.
4. *Acceptance:* Fuses one's concepts of sexuality and emotionality as an adult; some are "arrested" at stage 3, while others will eventually arrive at stage 4.

Adolescent crossdressing or, more specifically, boys dressing in female clothing, however, signifies the existence of transsexualism, transvestism, or effeminate homosexuality; the differences are given in **Table 3**.

ETIOLOGY OF DEVIANT SEXUAL BEHAVIOR

Theories outlined to explain the inherent causes of deviant sexual behavior in adolescents are primarily based on adult models. The most frequently offered explanations include reconstituted and combined versions of (1) social learning theory, (2) developmental theory, (3) cognitive-behavior theory,

TABLE 3: Categorization of male gender identity variants.

	Transsexuals	Effeminate homosexuals	Transvestites
Core gender identity	Female	Male	Male
Crossdressing	To fulfill feminine role	To attract partner	Fetishistic
Desired sex partner	Heterosexual male	Homosexual male	Heterosexual female
View of penis	Abhorrent	Source of gratification	Source of gratification

(4) attachment theory, (5) psychosis theory, (6) addictions theory, and (7) biological theory.

There are mainly three viewpoints of deviant sexual behavior. It may be learned behavior caused by biological factors or caused by a combination of learning and biological factors. Unfortunately, most concepts do not relate the basic cause of deviant sexual behavior to other factors that may impair treatment, such as financial, parental, community, or peer resources.

It is generally agreed that there are multiple factors (psychological, biological, and sociological) that interact in complex and generally poorly understood ways. A history of prior physical or sexual abuse, impaired family dynamics, alcohol and substance abuse, exposure to pornography, neurobiological factors, and psychiatric comorbidities have been found to be associated with a higher prevalence of abnormal adolescent sexual behavior.

In the DSM, paraphilic disorders are often misunderstood as an encompassing definition for any unusual sexual behavior. In DSM 5, the Sexual and Gender Identity Disorders Work Group has sought to draw a line between atypical human behavior and behavior that causes mental distress to a person or makes the person a serious threat to the psychological and physical well-being of other individuals. While legal implications of paraphilic disorders were considered seriously in revising diagnostic criteria, the goal was to update the disorders in this category based on the latest science and effective clinical practice.

■ CHARACTERISTICS OF PARAPHILIC DISORDERS

Several important changes have been made to the criteria of paraphilic disorders or paraphilias as they have been called in previous editions of the DSM manual. Most people with atypical sexual interests do not have a mental disorder. To be diagnosed with a paraphilic disorder, DSM 5 requires that people with these interests:

- Feel personal distress about their interest, not merely distress resulting from society's disapproval, or have a sexual desire or behavior that involves another person's psychological distress, injury, or death.
- A desire for sexual behaviors involving unwilling persons or persons unable to give legal consent.

To further define the line between an atypical sexual interest and disorder, the work group revised the names of these disorders to differentiate between the behavior itself and the disorder stemming from that behavior; that is, sexual masochism in DSM-IV will be titled sexual masochism disorder in DSM 5.

It is a subtle but crucial difference that makes it possible for an individual to engage in consensual atypical sexual behavior without inappropriately being labeled with a mental disorder. With this revision, DSM 5 clearly distinguishes between atypical sexual interests and mental disorders involving these desires or behaviors.

Additional Changes to Paraphilic Disorders

Other changes to the diagnostic criteria for two DSM 5 paraphilic disorders should also be noted. The first concern is transvestic disorder, which identifies people who are sexually aroused by dressing as the opposite sex but who experience significant distress or impairment in their lives, socially or occupationally, because of their behavior. DSM-IV limited this behavior to heterosexual males. DSM 5 has no such restriction, opening the diagnosis to women or gay men who have this sexual interest. The change in paraphilic disorders could increase the number of people diagnosed with transvestic disorder. The requirement remains that individuals must experience significant distress or impairment because of their behavior.

In the case of pedophilic disorder, the notable detail is what was not revised in the new manual. Although proposals were discussed throughout the DSM 5 development process, diagnostic criteria ultimately remained the same as in DSM-IV-TR. Only the disorder name is changed from pedophilia to pedophilic disorder to maintain consistency with the chapter's other listings.

DSM-IV-TR describes three general classes of paraphilia (the name means attraction to the deviant):
1. Preference for the use of a nonhuman object for sexual arousal
2. Repetitive sexual activity with humans that involves real or simulated suffering or humiliation
3. Repetitive sexual activity with nonconsenting partners

DSM-IV-TR classification of the paraphilias takes into account the duration of the fantasies, urges, or behavior, which must be present for at least 6 months, and the level of distress or impairment of function that they cause. In a mild condition, the individual may be distressed by the imagery but not have ever acted on it; in a moderate condition, imagery may have been transformed into action leading to impairment of social or occupational functioning; and in a severe condition, the urges may have been repeatedly acted upon and have come to occupy a central role in the person's life.

Clinical Features of Major Paraphilias

Paraphilic disorders include eight conditions—exhibitionistic disorder, fetishistic disorder, frotteuristic disorder, pedophilic disorder, sexual masochism disorder, sexual sadism disorder, transvestic disorder, and voyeuristic disorder.

The clinical features must be present for at least 6 months and cause significant distress or impairment in social, occupational, or other important areas of functioning.

Fetishistic Disorder

Recurrent, intense, sexually arousing fantasies, sexual urges, or behaviors involving the use of nonliving objects (such as female undergarments) are characteristics of fetishistic disorder.

Transvestic Disorder

Recurrent, intense, sexually arousing fantasies, sexual urges, or behaviors in heterosexual crossdressing men are characteristics of transvestic disorder.

Sexual Masochism Disorder

Recurrent, intense, sexually arousing fantasies, sexual urges, or behaviors involving, in masochism, real or simulated humiliation, beating and suffering are characteristics of sexual masochism disorder; in sadism, it actually causes psychological or physical suffering (including humiliation) to the victim. The essential feature of sexual masochism is the feeling of sexual arousal or excitement resulting from receiving pain, suffering, or humiliation. The pain, suffering, or humiliation is real and not imagined and can be physical or psychological in nature. The comparison of sexual masochism in DSM-IV-4-TR and the proposed DSM 5 diagnostic criteria is given in **Table 4**.

TABLE 4: Comparison of DSM-IV-TR and proposed DSM 5 diagnostic criteria for sexual masochism.

DSM-IV-TR sexual masochism	DSM 5 sexual masochism
Over a period of at least 6 months, recurrent, intense sexually arousing fantasies, sexual urges, or behaviors involving the act (real, not simulated) of being humiliated, beaten, bound, or otherwise made to suffer	• Over a period of at least 6 months, recurrent, intense sexually arousing fantasies, sexual urges, or behaviors involving the act of being humiliated, beaten, bound, or otherwise made to suffer • It is to be noted that "real not stimulated" is deleted
The fantasies, sexual urges, or behaviors cause clinically significant distress or impairment in social, occupational, or other important areas of functioning	The fantasies, sexual urges, or behaviors cause clinically significant distress or impairment in social, occupational, or other important areas of functioning
No such mention	*Specify if:* With asphyxiophilia (sexually aroused by asphyxiation)

Sexual Sadism Disorder

The essential feature of sexual sadism is a feeling of sexual excitement resulting from administering pain, suffering, or humiliation to another person. The pain, suffering, or humiliation inflicted on the other is real; it is not imagined and may be either physical or psychological in nature. A person with a diagnosis of sexual sadism is sometimes called a sadist. The name of the disorder is derived from the proper name of the Marquis Donatien de Sade (1740–1814), a French aristocrat who became notorious for writing novels around the theme of inflicting pain as a source of sexual pleasure.

Voyeuristic Disorder

Recurrent, intense, sexually arousing fantasies, sexual urges, or behaviors involving the act of observing an unsuspecting person who is naked, in the process of disrobing, or engaging in sexual activity are characteristics of voyeuristic disorder.

Exhibitionistic Disorder

Recurrent, intense, sexually arousing fantasies, sexual urges, or behaviors involving the exposure of one's genitals to an unsuspecting stranger are characteristics of exhibitionistic disorder.

Pedophilic Disorder

Recurrent, intense, sexually arousing fantasies, sexual urges, or behaviors involving sexual activity with a child or children who have not yet gone through puberty (generally 13 years or younger) are characteristics of pedophilic disorder.

Frotteuristic Disorder

Frotteurism refers to a paraphilic interest in rubbing, usually one's pelvis or erect penis, against a nonconsenting person for sexual gratification. It may involve touching any part of the body, including the genital area. A person who practices frotteurism is known as a frotteur. The majority of frotteurs are male and the majority of victims are female, although female-on-male, female-on-female, and male-on-male frotteurs exist. This activity is often done in circumstances where the victim cannot easily respond, in a public place such as a crowded train or concert.

■ MANAGEMENT OF SEXUAL DYSFUNCTION

A persistent impairment of sexual interest or response is called a sexual dysfunction. Sexual dysfunction is often associated with anxiety about performance or cultural inhibitions.

■ TREATMENT OF SEXUAL DYSFUNCTION

When an adolescent is brought for therapy of sexual dysfunction or disorder, the clinician should get detailed medical history and social history. Sex therapy is often carried out by working with the couple involved rather than with one person. The therapist attempts to decrease the fear of failure and to focus on sensory pleasure rather than on the sexual act itself. The sexual retaining technique is developed by Masters and Johnson in their pioneering work on sex therapy. Behavioral and cognitive elements are widely used in current treatments of sexual dysfunction. Some therapists use an approach that combines these elements with a more traditional psychodynamic approach. Many therapists believe that aspects of the relationship between the members of the couple may be a major force in a negative therapeutic outcome.

Treatment of Paraphilias

Each of the perspectives has something to offer in understanding the paraphilias. Because many of the paraphilic behaviors are carried out in private, their causes are poorly understood. Conventional psychotherapy seems ineffective in treating paraphilias.

Biological Treatment

Therapy using hormones has been used, but long-term effects have not yet been evaluated.

Behavioral Therapy

Using aversion techniques has been tried but is found objectionable by many people. The interactional view of paraphilic sexual behavior maintains that biological and environmental factors as well as personality development may play a role. From this perspective, effective treatments must consider all of these aspects of paraphilic behavior rather than focusing on any single causal factor.

If the "sex play" is determined to be experimental or exploratory, the pediatrician should discuss normal childhood and adolescent sexual behavior with parents and outline measures to minimize inappropriate sexual stimulation in the home. Parents should be advised to provide closer supervision of the adolescent. Older adolescents can be instructed to stay away from compromising situations with younger children. If the sexual behavior is determined to be exploitation, in addition to the preceding suggestions, medical examination and documentation should be performed, and as required by state child abuse laws, the family should be referred to the appropriate agency for further evaluation. If the adolescent has access to other children, especially very young ones, the pediatrician should assess the level of risk posed to those children. If it is determined that the child or adolescent is at high risk for sexually assaulting children, the pediatrician should inform the family. Furthermore, the family should be advised to stop all babysitting and childcare activities to limit the adolescent offender's opportunity to reoffend. A more definitive treatment may not be within the purview of all pediatricians, and generally, adolescent offenders will be referred to professionals and programs specializing in such treatment.

DISTINGUISHING SEXUAL EXPLOITATION

- *What is the age difference between the participants?* Exploitation is likely if the children are not peers in terms of age or cognitive level.
- *Is the activity consistent with the developmental level of the participants?* Prepubertal exploratory behavior typically involves mutual genital display, touching, and fondling. Intercourse or attempted intercourse is unusual among preschoolers and is rare in the young school-aged child (6–9 years).
- *What is the motivation of the participants?* Curiosity about differences and similarities in anatomy and pleasurable feelings associated with masturbation are the main motivating factors.

- *Is the activity consensual or coercive?* Mutual consent is usually present in exploratory behaviors. Abusive behavior often involves elements of pressure, force, threat, secrecy, or other forms of coercion. Although some of the threats or coercion are obvious and violent, there may be subtle emotional pressure or the use of implied authority by an older child or adolescent in some cases.
- *Is there an outside influence involved?* Two children or adolescents may be involved in age-appropriate exploratory behavior, but if the activity has been arranged for the pleasure of another older individual, it is exploitative.
- *What is the response of the child to the contact?* Mutual exploratory behavior may result in some guilt feelings in children. Exploitation is more often viewed negatively by the child; however, some abused children may appear to have a neutral or positive emotional response to abuse. The victims' denial may mask the negative responses in some cases.

Adolescent Sexual Offenders

The treatment of adolescent sexual offenders is controversial. Many of the management interventions have not been scientifically evaluated on adolescents. Most treatment programs focus on the rehabilitation of adolescent offenders and on the prevention of reoffending. Each intervention program is designed for use with adolescents by adding components to address developmental issues. These programs typically include several treatment modalities, such as individual, family and group formats, biological therapy, substance abuse interventions, cultural sensitivity training, victim empathy training and protection, cognitive restructuring, values clarification, consideration of victimization issues, anger management, social skills training, assertiveness training, problem-solving skills training, grief counseling, stress management, peer counseling, sex education, and covert sensitization. Unfortunately, there remains little empirical evidence of the long-term effects of different interventions with adolescent sexual offenders.

Evidence suggests short-term benefits of some treatment modalities with adolescents, but long-term recurrence rates remain high.

> **GUIDELINES FOR PARENTS**
> - Understand what is sexuality and sexual deviant behavior. All professionals who work with children or families need practical guidelines as to which child sexual behaviors are natural and healthy and which behaviors indicate a need for specialized assessment.
> - Parents should not blame themselves for the condition.
> - Parents should minimize criticizing their child. One important aspect of deviant behavior is the development of self-image; hence, labeling the child should be avoided.
> - Supervise the child without hurting them.
> - Explain what is normal and the effects of deviant behavior. Accurate information and a forum in which to ask questions about sexuality are essential for these children.
> - Professional help may be taken so that a child can understand changes in their body, mind, and sexuality.
> - Parents need to give considerable time and energy.
> - Make sure to keep healthy boundaries in your marriage and build a positive relationship with your child.
> - Be patient, careful, and focus on cognitive and physical health. Keep them engaged in creative activities.
> - Children should be aware that no other person (whether that person is an adult or another child) has the right to force or pressure them into unwanted sexual behaviors.
> - Use of behavioral, psychotherapy, counseling, and, if required, medicines will recover the adolescent from their problems.

SUICIDE

INTRODUCTION

Suicidal behavior is often an unpremeditated, impulsive act used by individuals who do not have psychiatric morbidity in the face of predominantly interpersonal crisis with significant others in their lives. As such, it is an inappropriate problem-solving skill to deal with distress. Suicides among young people nationwide have increased dramatically in recent years. Suicide is the second most common cause of death among 10-24-year-old. Suicide rates among 10-19-year-old increased by 56% between 2007 and 2016. 13.6% made a suicide plan, and 7.4% made one or more suicide attempts. Males are more likely to die by suicide; however, incident rate

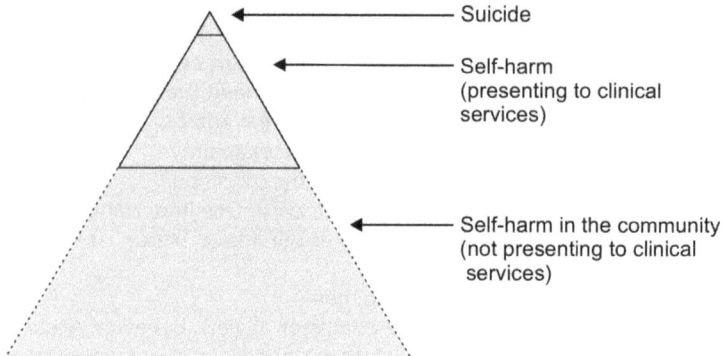

Fig. 1: Prevalence of self-harm and suicide.

ratios comparing deaths by suicide between adolescent males and females have been decreasing since 2007. Young adults experience strong feelings of stress in various situations, confusion, self-doubt, pressure to succeed, financial insecurity, and various other concerns while growing up.

Most of the time, depression and suicidal ideas are treatable mental disorders. Psychiatric examination may be very helpful if there is doubt. Many of the symptoms of suicidal feelings are similar to those of depression.

The American Psychiatric Association's (APA) proposed diagnostic criteria for DSM 5 include a new suicide assessment tool developed to help clinicians better identify individuals at risk for suicide. The prevalence of self-harm and suicide is depicted in **Figure 1**.

ASSESSMENT FOR SUICIDE RISK

The proposed DSM 5 revisions include two new scales for assessing individuals' risk factors for committing suicide, one for adolescents and one for adults. While the current version of *DSM* includes thoughts of suicide as a symptom of some mental disorders, such as major depression, the proposed suicide risk techniques have been designed to be applied to anyone receiving an evaluation for a mental disorder, regardless of diagnosis, to help clinicians identify those at risk for suicide.

NEW RISK SYNDROMES CATEGORY

The APA is also considering the inclusion of a new category in DSM 5 for risk syndromes, in which symptoms are identified that place a person at higher risk of later developing a mental disorder. The first risk conditions proposed for inclusion are psychosis risk syndrome and minor neurocognitive disorder, also known as mild cognitive impairment.

Psychosis Risk Syndrome

Psychosis risk syndromes are mild versions of the symptoms found in psychotic disorders, such as unusual suspicion, delusions, and disorganized speech or behavior. It is anticipated that 25–30% of people with these symptoms will go on to develop a psychotic disorder. Interestingly, many of these symptoms, in their milder forms, can also be found in the normal population.

Definitions of Self-injurious Behaviors

Suicidal attempts (SAs) and nonsuicidal self-injury (NSSI) can be grouped into the category of self-harm. SAs are potentially self-injurious behaviors attempted with some intent to die (i.e., to cause one's own death) as a result of the behaviors. Self-injurious behaviors are performed without any intent to die and include behaviors such as scratching the skin, cutting, burning, headbanging, hitting oneself, and so forth. The purposes, or functions, of NSSI are typically to reduce or distract from negative emotions, punish oneself, and/or reduce feelings of numbness or dissociation. The key risk factors in adolescents for self-harm and suicide are shown in **Figure 2**.

Parents should be aware of the following signs in adolescents:
- Change in eating and sleeping habits
- Withdrawal from friends, family, and regular activities
- Violent actions, rebellious behavior, or running away
- Drug and alcohol use
- Unusual neglect of personal appearance
- Marked personality change

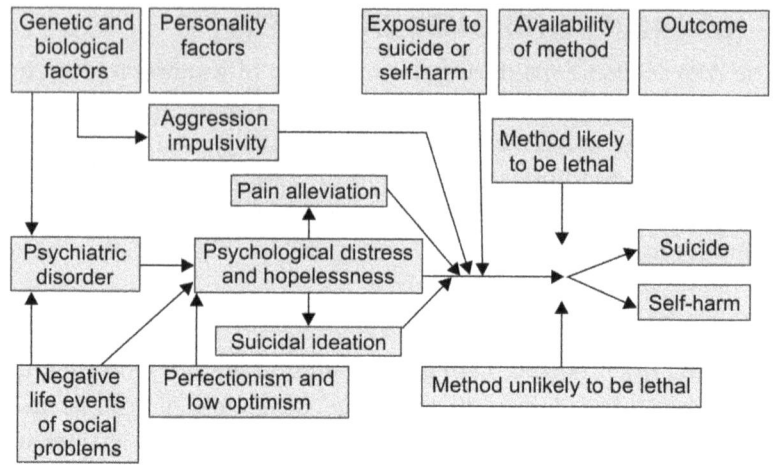

Fig. 2: Key risk factors in adolescents for self-harm and suicide.

- Persistent boredom, difficulty concentrating, or a decline in the quality of schoolwork
- Frequent complaints about physical symptoms, often related to emotions, such as stomachaches, headaches, and fatigue
- Loss of interest in pleasurable activities; history of running away from school
- Not tolerating praise or rewards
- History of suicide by friend or death wish.

An adolescent who is planning to commit suicide may have the following features:
- Complain of being "bad" or feeling rotten inside.
- Give subtle verbal hints with statements such as I will not be a problem for you much longer, nothing matters, its no use, and I will not see you again.
- Put his or her possessions in order; for example, give away favorite possessions, clean his or her room, throw away important belongings.
- Become suddenly cheerful after a period of depression.
- Have signs of psychosis (hallucinations or bizarre thoughts).

If a child or an adolescent says "I want to kill myself" or "I am going to commit suicide," always take the statement seriously and immediately seek assistance from a psychiatrist. If one or more of these signs occurs, parents need to talk to their child about their concerns and seek professional help when the concerns persist. With support from family and professional treatment, adolescents and young adults who are suicidal can heal and return to a healthier path of development.

RISK FACTORS FOR SUICIDE

- Previous suicide attempts
- Close family member who has committed suicide.
- History of psychiatric illness
- *Social isolation:* The individual does not have social alternatives or skills to find alternatives to suicide.
- Physical abuse by parents and feeling neglected by parents.
- *Drug or alcohol abuse:* Drugs decrease impulse control, making impulsive suicide more likely. Additionally, some individuals try to self-medicate their depression with drugs or alcohol.
- *Exposure to violence in the home or the social environment:* The individual sees violent behavior as a viable solution to life problems.
- *Talking about dying:* Any mention of dying, disappearing, hanging, jumping, shooting oneself, or other types of self-harm
- *Recent loss:* Death, divorce, separation, broken relationship, self-confidence, self-esteem, loss of interest in friends, hobbies, and activities previously enjoyed
- *Change in personality:* Sad, withdrawn, irritable, anxious, tired, indecisive, and apathetic
- *Change in behavior:* Cannot concentrate on studies, at school, work, and routine tasks
- *Change in sleep patterns:* Insomnia, often with early waking or oversleeping, and nightmares
- *Change in eating habits:* Loss of appetite and weight or overeating
- *Low self-esteem:* Feeling worthless, shame, overwhelming guilt, self-hatred, everyone would be better off without me
- *No hope for the future:* Believing things will never get better, that nothing will ever change.

Characteristics of the Index Event

The following four characteristics of the index episodes are of particular importance: Suicidal intent, motivation, lethality, and method.

Motivation

Adolescents may have a range of motives for self-harm: To die, to escape thoughts and feelings, to feel better, to get help, or to replace emotional pain with physical pain.

Lethality

Clinicians should distinguish between objective lethality, which is the actual degree of danger to life, and subjective lethality, the youth's anticipated consequences of self-harm.

Method

This refers to the way or the process that is used by the youth to self-harm. Method is closely linked with objective lethality, ranging from highly lethal behaviors such as shooting and hanging at one extreme to cutting and burning on the opposite side of the spectrum. One of the key questions in assessing risk is whether the youth has access to lethal agents such as dangerous drugs or firearms.

Prevention of Self-harm and Suicide

Activities to prevent suicide and self-harm should take into account the particular characteristics of adolescent suicide and self-harm. For example, they should target issues around the social transmission of suicide and self-harm, address concerns about sexual orientation and bullying in young people, promote help-seeking behavior, and foster self-esteem and resilience. School-based suicide-prevention strategies are growing and include screening at-risk young people, gatekeeper training, skills training, and whole-school programs although there is some evidence that screening programs can identify at-risk young people not recognized by school professionals and increase the uptake of mental health services in untreated at-risk young people.

Approaches to Prevent Self-harm and Suicide in Adolescents

Population Measures
- School-based psychological well-being and skill training programs
- Training of schoolteachers and peers
- Screening to identify those who might be at risk
- Restriction of all access to means used for self-harm and suicide
- Improved media reporting and portrayal of suicidal behavior
- Encouragement of help-seeking behavior
- Public awareness campaigns
- Child and adolescent helplines
- Internet sources of help
- Reduction of stigma associated with mental health problems and help-seeking.

Management

Therapeutic assessment is based on the Cognitive Analytic Therapy Model and is as follows:
- Standard psychosocial history and risk assessment (approximately 1 hour)
- A 10-minute break to review the information gathered and to prepare for the rest of the session, followed by a 30-minute intervention covering the next four steps
- Joint construction of a diagram aiming to capture the vicious cycles that maintain self-harm
- Identifying a target problem
- Considering and enhancing motivation for change
- Exploring potential "exits" (i.e., ways of breaking the vicious cycles identified)
- Describing the diagram and the exits in an "understanding letter," which the clinician is required to prepare on the basis of the initial assessment.

A successful treatment regimen includes assessment and treatment by a multidisciplinary team that integrates psychotherapy (both individual and family), behavior modification techniques, pharmacologic therapy, group therapy, and moral treatment. Treatment is given for those who have suicide potential and to those who have already attempted suicide. A supportive environment, family, and group therapy are the mainstay of treatment.

Dialectical Behavior Therapy

Dialectical behavior therapy (DBT) is the first and only "well-established" treatment for suicidal and self-harm adolescents. DBT targets both SA and NSSI by identifying the function of the behavior (e.g., reducing emotional distress) for the given individual and finding ways to obtain that function safely using DBT-based coping skills. Components of standard DBT are the same for adolescents and adults **(Table 5)**, with the exception of there being parenting and family sessions with the individual therapist as needed and the skills class including both teens and parents.

Multisystemic Therapy

Multisystemic Therapy (MST) is a treatment package that takes into account multiple systems that the family and the adolescents interact with. The main target of the therapy is effective parenting skills and enhanced community supports (school, peers, and other community supports), primarily targeted at engaging adolescents with prosocial activities and disengaging with antisocial one, removing potential methods of suicide, and monitoring and support of the youths by responsible adults. The therapy is intensive (contact could be daily) and time-limited (3–6 months). Contacts are made in adolescents' homes, and the average caseload of the therapists is low (four to six families).

Metallization-based Therapy

Metallization could be defined as implicitly and explicitly interpreting the actions of oneself and others as meaningful on the basis of intentional mental states, in other words, having the awareness that all people have their own feelings and thoughts (mental states) that determine their actions while, by their very nature, mental states are opaque and cannot be "read" directly.

TABLE 5: Components of stage I standard dialectical behavior therapy for adolescents.

Component	Function	Structure
Individual psychotherapy (at least 1 session per week)	• Enhance capacities related to skills development • Skills application to patient's unique circumstances • Improve motivation and reduce dysfunctional behavior • Structure the environment to reinforce effective behavior and positive change	Treatment hierarchy: • Life-threatening behavior • Therapy-interfering behavior (TIB) • Quality of life-interfering behavior
Multifamily group skills training (1 session per week)	Teach skills: • Mindfulness • Distress tolerance • Emotion regulation • Interpersonal effectiveness • Middle path skills	• Mindfulness exercise • Homework review • Teaching of new skill
Telephone coaching (available 24/7 for youth and parents)	• Help with skills application in context (e.g., in a crisis) • Unavailable for 24 hours after the patient engages in self-injurious behavior	Brief, focused calls for: • Skill use in a crisis • Addressing therapist–patient rupture • Reporting good news
Therapist consultation team (1 session per week)	Support therapist's motivation, adherence, and effectiveness	• Mindfulness exercise • Clinical concerns, including therapist's TIB

Cognitive Behavioral Therapy

- CBT has been shown to reduce self-harm repetition in independent trials.
- CBT showed significant reductions in self-harm behavior, depression symptoms, and trait anxiety.

- Person's awareness of internal positive and negative self-talk patterns and behavioral habits
- To develop effective problem-solving strategies
- Self-directed development of positive coping strategy
- Perception of self-efficacy
- Encourage them to identify problems and respond with acceptable adaptive behavior.
- Impulse-control problems, anxiety, acute and chronic pain
- Rational emotive therapy, stress inoculation training.

Three Steps Parents can take
1. Help the child (medical or mental health professional).
2. Support the child (listen, avoid undue criticism, remain connected).
3. Become informed (library, local support group, internet).

Three Steps Friends can take
1. The friend's actions seriously.
2. Encourage friends to seek professional help and accompany them if necessary.
3. Talk to a trustworthy adult.

Prevention of Suicide
- *Primary prevention:* Strong family life and religion integrate the person within the social group. It is concerned with eradicating the causes leading to self-destruction.
- *Secondary prevention:* It relates to reducing the association disability and preventing recurrence.

Suicide Crisis and Intervention
There are four phases of any suicide plan:
1. An intention to end one's life
2. Decision about the lethality of the means
3. Making it available
4. Execution of the plan of suicide

Intervention can be done at any stage stated above.

Postvention

Postvention is concerned with the alleviation of the effects of stress in the survivor victims of suicidal deaths. Survivor victims develop unhealthy emotions such as shame, guilt, hatred, and perplexity. Postvention process emphasizes looking after the survivor victims and helps them overcome their negative emotions. Adolescents may be referred to suicide prevention clinics run by a team of psychiatrist, psychologist, and pediatrician.

KEY POINTS

- Suicide among children and adolescents is related to a morbid process of neurobiological etiopathology, rather than the desires of the individuals themselves.
- 10% of adolescents will have self-harmed by the time they finish secondary school, and 10% of the adolescents who engage in self-harm will repeat self-harm within a year.
- Therapeutic Assessment and the Family Intervention for Suicide Prevention may lead to improved engagement; MST may reduce self-harm repetition in comparison with hospitalization.
- DBT and CBT have the best evidence in adults with self-harm, while DBT and CBT with adolescents require rigorous evaluation in randomized clinical trials (RCTs).
- Pharmacological agents require evaluation in adolescents with self-harm.
- Positive findings of the Signs of Suicide (SOS) programs need to be independently replicated, and MST needs to be studied in adolescents presenting with self-harm.
- SSRIs can trigger suicidal thoughts in children and adolescents.
- International consensus regarding definitions and measurements of self-harm is required.
- The more we limit children and adolescents access to toxic substances, firearms, railway lines, bridges, etc., the greater number of suicides we can prevent.
- The main objective is to be able to draw up reliable protocols for early diagnosis and to develop effective primary, secondary, and tertiary prevention methods.

> **GUIDELINES FOR PARENTS**
> - Keep abreast with the activities and friends of the child, particularly the adolescents.
> - Do not be too intrusive, but enquire about the latest development in the adolescent's life.
> - Be careful if there is a drastic change in behavior, particularly the risk factors as stated above.
> - Take nihilistic comments seriously.
> - If in doubt, take the help of a psychiatrist.

BIBLIOGRAPHY

1. Abraham A, Stafford B. Eating disorders. In: Jenson HB, Behrman RE, Kliegman R (Eds). Nelson Textbook of Pediatrics, 18th edition. Philadelphia: WB Saunders; 2008. pp. 127-30.
2. American Psychiatric Association. Diagnostic and Statistical Manual of Mental Disorders, DSM-IV, 4th edition. Washington, DC: American Psychiatric Association; 1994. pp. 544-5.
3. American Psychiatric Association. Diagnostic and Statistical Manual of Mental Disorders, DSM-IV, 4th edition. Washington, DC: American Psychiatric Association; 1994. pp. 549-50.
4. Brown JD, Witherspoon EM. The mass media and American adolescents' health. J Adolesc Health. 2002;31(6 Suppl):153-70.
5. Center for Disease Control and Prevention. 10 leading causes of death by age group, United States. [online] Available from https://www.cdc.gov/injury/wisqars/pdf/leading_causes_of_death_by_age_group_2017-508.pdf.
6. Chambless DL, Hollon SD. Defining empirically supported therapies. J Consult Clin Psychol. 1998;66(1):7-18.
7. Comerci GD, Greydanus D. Eating disorders: anorexia nervosa, bulimia. In: Hormann AD, Greydanus D (Eds). Adolescent Medicine, 3rd edition. Norwalk, CT: Appleton and Lange; 1997.
8. Deshpande CG. Suicide and Attempted Suicide, 1st edition. Pune: Uma Publication; 1999. pp. 115-29.
9. Eisler I, Dare C, Russell G, Szmukler G, Le Grange D, Dodge E. Five-year follow-up of a controlled trial of family therapy in severe eating disorders. Arch Gen Psychiatry. 1997;54:1025-30.
10. Field AE, Sonneville KR, Micali N, Crosby RD, Swanson SA, Laird NM, et al. Prospective association of common eating disorders and adverse outcomes. Pediatrics. 2012;130:e289-95.

11. Friedrich WN, Fisher J, Broughton D, Houston M, Shafran CR. Normative sexual behavior in children: a contemporary sample. Pediatrics. 1998;101(4):E9.
12. Goerge DC. Disordered eating behaviors: anorexia nervosa, bulimia nervosa, cyclic vomiting syndrome, and rumination disorder. In: Levine MD, Carey WB, Crocker AC (Eds). Developmental-Behavioral Pediatrics, 3rd edition. Philadelphia: WB Saunders Co.; 1999. pp. 380-91.
13. Gould MS, Marrocco FA, Hoagwood K, Kleinman M, Amakawa L, Altschuler E. Service use by at-risk youths after school-based suicide screening. J Am Acad Child Adolesc Psychiatry. 2009;48:1193-201.
14. Gowers SG, Clark A, Roberts C, Griffiths A, Edwards V, Bryan C, et al. Clinical effectiveness of treatments for anorexia nervosa in adolescents: randomized controlled trial. Br J Psychiatry. 2007;191:427-35.
15. Greydanus DE. Adolescent Sexuality: American Perspective. Course Manual for Adolescent Health, Part-I US Perspective. IAP-ITPAH; 2004. pp. 271-80.
16. Haugaard JJ, Tilly C. Characteristics predicting children's responses to sexual encounters with other children. Child Abuse Negl. 1988;12(2):209-18.
17. Herpertz-Dahlmann B, Muller B, Herpertz S, Heussen N, Hebebrand J, Remschmidt H. Prospective 10-year follow-up in adolescent anorexia nervosa—course, outcome, psychiatric comorbidity, and psychosocial adaptation. J Child Psychol Psychiatry. 2001;42:603-12.
18. Kann L, McManus T, Harris WA, Shanklin SL, Flint KH, Queen B, et al. Youth Risk Behavior Surveillance—United States, 2017. MMWR Surveill Summ. 2018;67(8):1-114.
19. Keel PK, Brown TA. Update on course and outcome in eating disorders. Int J Eat Disord. 2010;43:195-204.
20. Klonsky ED. The functions of deliberate self-injury: a review of the evidence. Clin Psychol Rev. 2007;27(2):226-39.
21. Kotler LA, Cohen P, Davies M, Pine DS, Walsh BT. Longitudinal relationships between childhood, adolescent, and adult eating disorders. J Am Acad Child Adolesc Psychiatry. 2001;40:1434-40.
22. Kreipe RE, Uphoff M. Treatment and outcome of adolescents with anorexia nervosa. Adolesc Med. 1992;3:519-40.
23. Lake AM, Gould MS. School-based strategies for youth suicide prevention. In: O'Connor RC, Platt S, Gordon J (Eds.). International Handbook of Suicide Prevention. Hoboken: Wiley-Blackwell; 2011.
24. Lamb S, Coakley M. "Normal" childhood sexual play and games: differentiating play from abuse. Child Abuse Negl. 1993;17(4):515-26.
25. Larsson I, Svedin CG. Sexual experiences in childhood: young adults' recollections. Arch Sex Behav. 2002;31(3):263-73.

26. Le Grange D, Crosby RD, Lock J. Predictors and moderators of outcome in family-based treatment for adolescent bulimia nervosa. J Am Acad Child Adolesc Psychiatry. 2008;47:464-70.
27. Le Grange D, Lock J, Agras WS, Moye A, Bryson SW, Jo B, et al. Moderators and mediators of remission in family-based treatment and adolescent focused therapy for anorexia nervosa. Behav Res Ther. 2012;50:85-92.
28. Linehan MM. Cognitive Behavioral Treatment of Borderline Personality Disorder. New York: Guilford Press; 1993.
29. Litt IF, Martin JA. Development of sexuality and its problems. In: Levine MD, Carey WB, Crocker AC (Eds.). Developmental-Behavioral Pediatrics, 3rd edition. Philadelphia: WB Saunders Co.; 1999. pp. 466-8.
30. Lock J, Le Grange D, Agras WS, Dare C. Treatment Manual for Anorexia Nervosa: A Family-Based Approach. New York: The Guilford Press; 2001.
31. Lock J, Le Grange D, Agras WS, Moye A, Bryson SW, Jo B. Randomized clinical trial comparing family-based treatment with adolescent-focused individual therapy for adolescents with anorexia nervosa. Arch Gen Psychiatry. 2010;67:1025-32.
32. Miller AL, Rathus JH, Linehan MM. Dialectical Behavior Therapy with Suicidal Adolescents. New York, NY: Guilford Press; 2007.
33. Miller AL, Rathus JH, Linehan MN, Wetzler S, Leigh E. Dialectical behavior therapy adapted for suicidal adolescents. J Psychiatry Pract. 1997;3(2):78-86.
34. Nadkarni A. Sexuality. Family Health Guide. Maharashtra: Institute for Psychological Health; 2002. pp. 47-8.
35. Nair MKC, Chacko DS, Paul MK. TEENS: Mental health in family life education module for young adults. Child Development Centre, Thiruvananthapuram. 2004;3(15-16):108-10.
36. Nair MKC. Introducing sex and sexuality to adolescents. Course Manual for Adolescent Health, Part-II Indian Perspective. IAP-ITPAH; 2004. pp. 206-7.
37. Nicholls DE, Lynn R, Viner RM. Childhood eating disorders: British national surveillance study. Br J Psychiatry. 2011;198:295-301.
38. Nock MK. Self-injury. Annu Rev Clin Psychol. 2010;6:339-63.
39. Patel DR. Eating disorder. Course Manual for Adolescent Health, Part-I US Perspective. IAP-ITPAH; 2004. pp. 406-10.
40. Russell GFM, Szmukler GI, Dare C, Eisler I. An evaluation of family therapy in anorexia nervosa and bulimia nervosa. Arch Gen Psychiatry. 1987;44:1047-56.

41. Sarason IG, Sarason BR. Abnormal Psychology, 11th edition, New Delhi: Prentice Hall of India; 2005. pp. 270-300, 362-8.
42. Scott MA, Wilcox HC, Schonfeld IS, Davies M, Hicks RC, Turner JB, et al. School-based screening to identify at-risk students not already known to school professionals: the Columbia suicide screen. Am J Public Health. 2009;99:334-9.
43. Sidhartha T, Jena S. Suicidal behaviors in adolescents. Indian J Pediatr. 2006;73:783-7.
44. Spear B. Adolescent growth and development. J Am Diet Assoc. 2002;102(Suppl. 3):23-9.
45. Vawda N. Suicidal behaviour among Black South African children and adolescents. In: Malhotra S (Ed.). Mental Disorders in Children and Adolescents, 1st edition. New Delhi: CBS Publishers; 2005. pp. 94-9.

CHAPTER 22

Adolescent Parenting

Sukanta Chatterjee

■ INTRODUCTION

The period of adolescence is 10-19 years. Parenting of adolescents is a different than that of children. Why it is such is the point of discussion in this chapter. Adolescents undergo transformation of mind to mature into adulthood, characterized by autonomy. The parents find it difficult to change from an all-control child–parent relation to an autonomy-acceptance adolescent–parent relation. There is a well assessed gradual and mutual decision-making in each and every sphere of life of an adolescent, which will make them a confident adult. This is the basis of good parenting of the adolescent. The series of biological, emotional, social, and cognitive changes that they come across demands independent decision-making, which parents are not ready to accept. This leads to conflict between parents and the adolescent, reflected in their behavior. Due to lack of adequate development of the frontal lobe, the seat of judgment, the adolescent may take an amygdala-dominant emotional decision having a harmful outcome. Ideal adolescent parenting is to recognize that this conflict is natural yet transient and to guide the adolescent with love and affection, guarding them from the harmful effects of emotional decisions through discipline and discussion.

■ ACTIONS THAT SHOULD MAKE PARENTS CAUTIOUS

- Sudden deterioration in school performance
- Drastic changes in behavior and mood swings
- Isolation from family and friends; prefers to remain alone most of the time

- Separation from long-time friends, changes in peer group, or frequenting strange friends
- Unusual requirements and demands for money
- Lack of interest in hobbies or usual social and recreational activities

Any of these features does not mean that the adolescent is in a grave situation. Some change in friends, change in hobbies, or spending time alone is normal in adolescence. But alert and caring parents often can make out if the adolescent is deviating from normalcy beyond 6 weeks; in such cases, parents should intervene early before the situation goes beyond control.

ROLE OF PARENTS

Adolescent years could be of great importance for parents in many aspects as they find the outcome of their parenting efforts through the childhood and adolescent years coming together and their offspring is maturing into an adult ready to face the challenges of life in modern society.

From the teenager's perspective, this is again a risky time since the protective parental guidance diminishes gradually when the adolescents are increasingly attracted to the opportunities of society but unaware of the accompanied risk. This modern commercial society wants to make them clients and present the item in a luring manner, hiding the risk or bad effects. The teenagers being impulsive and emotional often make judgment errors and get trapped in the risk. Their decision is more influenced by peers and new members outside the family, and both may add to the risk exposure.

At this age, controlling the behavior of adolescents is a challenging task. The exploring instinct drives them to late-night parties and experiment with drinks and drugs. The development of sexuality involves them in sexual fantasies, desire for opposite-sex partner, and falling in love and romantic relations. The desire and attempt of romantic relation expose adolescents to significant mental stress. They need help and guidance at this stage from parents and seniors but not in a mood to accept it.

The hormonal changes make them liable to sudden mood change, emotional outbursts, defiance, defensiveness, and withdrawal in divergent situations. The identity crisis or sense of self is gets obstructed by society norms, putting them in a stage where they are neither a child nor an adult. This puts them in embarrassment and confusion toward independent decision-making, leading to timid personality or anger–defiance–violence chain of activities.

The civilized and modern society exposes adolescents to different useful and risky situations. They are often being attracted toward harmful activities. Good parenting principle is to take stock of their time spent outside and discuss the benefit–risk ratio of the activities. Respect their opinion. Try to convince them with logic and respect. Never say bad about their friends but point out the outcomes. Talk about media literacy. Let them learn from you about the commercial intent of many of the Google search sites attracting them. Encourage good relations and information search. Discuss, monitor, and counsel unwanted relation and risky Google search. Conflict between adolescent and the parent should be viewed as a difference in opinion of two persons, one maturing and the other mature. It needs to be dealt with calm, love, and quality time.

▪ DEALING WITH THE SITUATION

The most important step is to maintain good communication. But it should always be nonconfrontational. Adolescents may not communicate at all or behave rudely. But the parents approach with care. All adolescents need support and guidance. Parents should try to be good role models.

▪ DIFFERENT PARENTING STYLES

Classically, we describe four parenting styles: Authoritarian, permissive, neglectful, and authoritative. Each parenting style has got its own characteristics with different outcome on the adolescent. We shall now describe each of them to understand which pattern is the best. It also helps us to clinically evaluate the cause-and-effect relationship of the administered parenting style to an individual adolescent's symptoms.

Authoritarian Parenting

Parental directions and rules are binding to the adolescents. In case of noncompliance, they are punished. There is no discussion or flexibility on the enforced discipline. Moreover, the rules are changed according to the wish or mood of the parents. The adolescents are growing in a state of fear and find it difficult to choose an expected behavior.

The adolescents raised in this constant state of threatening atmosphere become poor in self-confidence and are often withdrawn from social situations. They might rebel and defy parents openly, leaving home and start taking drugs, alcohol, and other substances. They may become sexually active early and choose a partner whom their parents are unlikely to approve. Antisocial associations are more likely.

Permissive Parenting

Permissive parenting maintains a parent–child love and affectionate relation without standard expectations on lifestyle behavior. All the demands of the adolescent are fulfilled so that they are not disheartened. So, in other words, all demands are permitted without expectation of responsible behaviors.

These adolescents in their life exhibit immaturity, lack of decision-making, and emotional impulsivity. In society and family, they are unable to take the responsibility of any adverse outcome due to their activities and try to pass it on to others. They remain more dependent and prefer to remain in the childhood-protective environment. They avoid living away from home either for education or for job.

Neglectful Parenting

In this type of parenting, the love, affection, and attachment to the adolescent are missing, but the parents provide food, shelter, and other materialistic requirements as a responsibility to the child. They do not care for the friends, school, or how was the day for the adolescent. Neglectful parenting is therefore one step ahead of permissive parenting toward the worse side where love and care are missing.

Adolescents brought up with neglectful parenting get in trouble going out of the family due to lack of acceptable social behavior. Parents are not aware of it since they do not take stock of "how was the day" for the adolescent. There could be something serious or tragic only when parents come to know. Adolescents themselves gradually develop resentment against parents and blame the neglectful parenting for their fate.

Authoritative Parenting

In this type of parenting, there is love and care along with high expectations of the parents from their adolescent. Here, the adolescent is also allowed to discuss freely about their expectations, experiences, and difficulties. Finally, a happily acceptable compliance of discipline and behavior comes from both sides. Any change of rules, directions, or expectations from parents are intimated and discussed for acceptable compliance. Parents discuss the cause-and-effect relationship of the acts and behavior with their offspring. This is considered the ideal parenting style.

Adolescents raised in this style of parenting become self-sufficient, taking responsibility of their behavior. They are usually happy and generous to others. They respect their parents and get acceptance from society through their responsible involvement.

GUIDELINES FOR PARENTS

- Raise your adolescent in a balanced permissive parenting style.
- In case of a troubled parent–child relation during the preadolescent years, it is advised to take professional help.
- Investment of quality time in the early years of the child will help parents to prevent small problems of childhood from being carried forward as bigger problems into adolescence.
- Parents should start early to get best results for their child's adolescence.
- The home environment should be safe and caring with unconditional love.
- Maintain a relation with the adolescent based on mutual trust, honesty, and respect.
- Accept situation-appropriate assertiveness and independent decisions of the adolescent.
- Make them responsible for their belongings and the family as well as for household tasks.
- Let them understand the advantages of thinking before acting and also in accepting limitations.
- Remember that we often underestimate the impact of an affectionate touch, a smile, a listening ear, honest complimenting words, or the smallest act of caring; all of them have the potential to turn a life around.

BIBLIOGRAPHY

1. Brody GH, Yu T, Beach SR, Kogan SM, Windle M, Philibert RA. Harsh parenting and adolescent health: a longitudinal analysis with genetic moderation. Health Psychol. 2014;33:401-9.
2. Chatterjee S, Chatterjee R. Adolescent crisis. Indian J Pract Pediatr. 2007;9:65-9.
3. Fabrizio CS, Lam TH, Hirschmann MR, Stewart SM. A brief parenting intervention to enhance the parent-child relationship in Hong Kong. J Child Fam Stud. 2013;22:603-13.
4. Kao TS, Salerno J. Keeping adolescents busy with extracurricular activities. J Sch Nurs. 2014;30(1):57-67.
5. Kim SY, Wang Y, Orozco-Lapray D, Shen Y, Murtuza M. Does "tiger parenting" exist? Parenting profiles of Chinese Americans and adolescent developmental outcomes. Asian Am J Psychol. 2013;4:7-18.
6. Leemreis WH, Okkerse JM, de Laat PC, Madern GC, van Adrichem LN, Verhulst F, et al. Educational paper: parenting a child with a disfiguring condition-how (well) do parents adapt? Eur J Pediatr. 2014;173(6):699-709.
7. Moilanen KL, Shen YL. Mastery in middle adolescence: the contributions of socioeconomic status, maternal mastery and supportive-involved mothering. J Youth Adolesc. 2014;43(2):298-310.
8. Nair MKC. Parenting adolescents. Indian Pediatr. 2004;41:887-90.
9. Patalay P, Fitzsimons E. Development and predictors of mental ill-health and wellbeing from childhood to adolescence. Soc Psychiatry Psychiatr Epidemiol. 2018;53:1311-23.
10. Smetana JG, Rote WM. Adolescent-parent relationships: progress, processes, and prospects. Ann Rev Dev Psychol. 2019;1:41-68.
11. Yuwen W, Chen AC. Chinese American adolescents: perceived parenting styles and adolescents' psychosocial health. Int Nurs Rev. 2013;60:236-43.

CHAPTER 23

Digital Media and Children

Samir Hasan Dalwai

INTRODUCTION

Digital media has become a part of daily life for children and adolescents. Its use is growing even in infants and toddlers. Exposure to digital media is perceived to be beneficial without considering its negative impact. Besides, its contribution in keeping the baby engaged, distracted, or feeding well leads to misuse. Caregivers are often impressed with the child's expertise with gadgets. Consequently, their use is reported up to 7 hours of the day or more.

Infants learn social human behavior and language best by social interaction with other humans, and social feedback is important for the quantity and quality of infant social behavior and communication. Excessive digital time interferes with a child's language and social development because children spend less time interacting with caregivers and may internalize what is seen on the screen.

PATTERNS OF MEDIA USE IN CHILDREN AND ADOLESCENTS

Traditional media (TV) has physical and mental health concerns that correlate with the duration and content of viewing. Digital media, including interactive and social media, is a blend of technology and content on easily available electronic gadgets. Its use is fast replacing traditional media because it is more engaging, easy to use, and addictive.

Screen time is the time spent in viewing TV/video, computer, electronic games, hand-held devices, or other visual devices.

Addictive behaviors are defined by the person's progressive exclusion of other activities, causing physical, mental, and social harm while attempting to control one's dysphoric feelings. Addiction presents as abuse without control, alterations in mood, tolerance (the need for more), abstinence (ability to avoid), and personal harm or conflicts in the environment (family, peers, school), as well as a tendency to relapse.

Digital media (internet, video games, smartphones) and its applications (gaming, gambling, social media) constitute the highest form of behavioral addictions. Addiction may develop to the gadget itself, the search for information, interaction compulsions (chatting, online games, shopping), cybersexuality, and cybercontacts.

Thus, digital media addiction is one of the most pervasive addictions inspiring new terminologies, such as "FOMO" (Fear Of Missing Out) and "Textiety"—the anxiety of receiving and responding immediately to text messages.

CLINICAL FEATURES

Factors associated with high TV and mobile screen viewing:
- *Age:* Younger children watch more of TV, whereas older children are more likely to use mobile screen devices.
- *Devices:* Higher number of media gadgets at home; gadgets in the bedroom
- Higher parental use and poor parental control

Clinical features associated with digital media exposure:
- *Developmental delay:* Early exposure to screens and gadgets can lead to delay and/or deviance in the development of speech and language.
- *Sleep:* Exposure to light and stimulating content can disturb sleep. Teens with a high number of calls and messages and on social networks may develop anxiety and insomnia.
- *Obesity:* Decreased physical activity along with increased consumption of food leads to obesity.
- *Behavioral problems:* Irritability, inattention, emotional, and psychological issues including auditory and tactile illusions (heard a ring or felt a vibration)
- Poor academic performance
- *Physical problems:* Muscular rigidity and pain

- *Ophthalmological:* Dry eyes, fatigue, blurry vision, irritation, or ocular redness
- *Risk-taking behaviors:* Higher risk of addiction and earlier initiation of substance use, self-injury, or eating disorders. Sexting is sending nude or seminude images and sexually explicit text messages using a cell phone. Exploitation may lead to further behavioral emotional concerns. *Cyberbullying leads to* social, academic, and health issues.

Addiction and dependence may signify underlying emotional disturbances such as impulsivity and sensation seeking, poor conflict resolution, and low self-esteem.

MANAGEMENT

Healthcare workers need to guide caretakers about the potential of addiction and abuse with digital media and offer recommendations as part of routine consultation **(Box 1)**.

The way ahead:
- **Which is the best app for my child?** More than 80,000 apps are labeled as educational, but little research has demonstrated

BOX 1: American Academy of Pediatrics: Recommendations for children's media use (2016).

- For children younger than 18 months, avoid use of screen media other than video-chatting
- For children 18–24 months of age, parents who want to introduce digital media should choose high-quality programming and co-view it with their children
- For children aged 2–5 years, limit screen use to 1 hour per day of high-quality programs. Parents should co-view media with children to help them understand what they are seeing and apply it to the world around them
- For children aged 6 years and older, place consistent limits on the time spent using media, and the types of media, and make sure media does not take the place of adequate sleep, physical activity, and other behaviors essential to health
- Designate media-free times together, such as dinner or driving, as well as media-free spaces, such as bedrooms
- Have ongoing communication about online citizenship and safety, including treating others with respect online and offline

their actual quality. Some benefits of digital and social media may accrue provided they are of high quality and mandatorily involve parent co-play and supervision.
- In his clinical practice, the author has noted a tendency to expose children as young as 6 months to apps and nursery rhymes on devices with a belief that this would increase their cognitive and communication abilities, make them eat more, or soothe them. The author has counseled parents about the need to increase social interaction with their child and that "their lap is the best app for infants and toddlers." Infants and toddlers learn best through two-way communication. Children learn more by face-to-face back-and-forth conversation and playful animated interaction, rather than "passive" listening or one-way exposure to screens. In his service evaluation, the author recounts the significant number of children with social communication concerns whose parents had reported compelling amount of screen time and who reported significant improvement on eliminating screen time.
- Digital media will be a part of our life. Hence, parents need to choose digital products that are appropriately engaging and can be used as co-view and co-play by parent and child.

GUIDELINES FOR PARENTS

- *Eye care:* Follow the 20/20/20 rule—look away from the screen every 20 minutes and focus on an object at least 20 feet away for at least 20 seconds (American Optometric Association). *Take frequent breaks from the screen*—at least 10 minutes every hour. *Remember to blink.* Use moisturizing eye drops or a room humidifier if indicated. *Position the screen slightly below eye level.* Follow the 1/2/10 rule—mobile phones ideally at 1 foot, desktop devices and laptops at 2 feet, and TV screens at 10 feet. Increase the font size. Prevent *ambient lighting* from windows and overhead light fixtures shining directly on screens. Decrease the brightness of the screen to a comfortable level. *Get regular ophthalmological screening done.*
- *Make your own family media use plan—Set limits:* Designate time and place for media activities for everyone. Teach and role model good manners online. *Create tech-free zones* at home.
- *Encourage playtime:* Physical unstructured interactive play is essential on a daily basis.

Contd…

Contd...

- *Exercise:* Children aged 6 years and older need at least an hour of physical activity each day [American Academy of Pediatrics (AAP)].
- *Sleep:* No devices should be kept in the child's bedrooms, including TVs, computers, and smartphones. Avoid screen time 1 hour before going to bed.
- Counsel children about *privacy settings, predators, and sexting*. Caregivers are encouraged to know your children's friends, both online and offline, and what digital media they are using, what sites they visit, what they are doing online.
- *Co-view, co-play, and co-engage* with children when they are using screens.
- *Do not use technology as an emotional pacifier:* Let children learn how to manage their boredom with activities and to communicate their feelings or to self-soothe.

BIBLIOGRAPHY

1. Council on Communications and Media. Media and young minds. Pediatrics. 2016;138(5):e20162591.
2. De-Sola Gutiérrez J, Rodríguez de Fonseca F, Rubio G. Cell-phone addiction: a review. Front Psychiatry. 2016;7:175.
3. Madigan S, Browne D, Racine N, Mori C, Tough S. Association between screen time and children's performance on a developmental screening test. JAMA Pediatr. 2019;173(3):244-50.

CHAPTER 24

Street Children

Sunita Shanbhag, Jaydeep Choudhury

INTRODUCTION

The United Nations International Children's Emergency Fund (UNICEF) describes street children as:
- Those on the street to make a living for their families and/or themselves. For these children, the street is, above all, a workplace.
- Those that spend large amounts of time on the street frequently because of the low returns on their labor
- Those who make their way into the informal sector as petty hawkers, shoeshine boys, scavengers of raw materials, or even thieves and street prostitutes.
- Those by the nature of their work and life, who are normally on their own, largely unprotected by adults

The UNICEF definition concentrates on four major dimensions, namely:
1. The ones whose place of congregation or coming together is the street
2. The ones who spend a large amount of time on the street
3. The ones whose level of working and living conditions are low
4. The ones who lack adult protection

For these reasons above all others, they are vulnerable to many dangers and abuses, and they tend to receive very few services essential for their protection and development.

Thus, the children who live on the streets can be categorized as follows:
- Who work on the street but return to their families at night
- Who work on the street but whose family ties are dwindling

- Who live and work with their families on the street
- Who work and live on their own on the street

CATEGORIES

Based on the relationship of the child with his family, there are three categories of street children which are as follows:

1. *Children on the street:* This category comprises children working on the street but maintaining more or less regular ties with their families. Their focus is home to which they return at the end of the working day and have a sense of belonging to the local community.
2. *Children of the street:* Children in this category maintain only tenuous relations with their families, visiting them only occasionally. They see the street as their home where they seek shelter, food, and companionship.
3. *Abandoned children:* Children in this category are also children of the street. They have cut off all ties with their biological families and are completely on their own.

The sheer numbers, the characteristic features, and behavior make it necessary to handle this issue sensitively.

NUMBER

It is very difficult to state as to how many children are street children at any given point of time, the reason being that the population of street children is floating and transient in nature. Thus, the figures mentioned in literature are just estimates. While 18 million children work on the streets of India, it is estimated that only 5-20% of them are truly homeless and disconnected from their families. Children who decide to leave their homes do not want to be identified, so they make it a point to travel very far from their hometown and often to place themselves in big metropolitan areas. They tend to choose the metropolitan areas due to the glamour attached to such places and the fact that they can intermingle without being noticed in the large crowds. There are also many job opportunities in such large places, and lastly, no one goes hungry in large cities because there are many people who give alms.

The UNICEF's estimate of 11 million street children in India is considered to be a conservative figure. The Indian Embassy has estimated that there are 314,700 street children in metros such as Mumbai and Kolkata. It is difficult to count the number of street children living in India because of their floating (moving often) nature, but it is estimated that more than 400,000 street children in India exist in Mumbai, Chennai, Kanpur, Bengaluru, and Hyderabad and around 100,000 in Delhi alone.

AGE

A survey among 100 street children at the New Delhi Railway Station in India revealed that 86% of boys in the age group of 14-18 years were sexually active. Because it is difficult to obtain precise and accurate statistics about street children, information about their ages is approximate. Most of the street children in India are over 6 years old, and the majority are over 8 years old. The mean age of street children in a National Institute of Urban Affairs study in 1989 was 13 years. Another study in 1989 by UNICEF found that 72% of the street children studied were aged 6-12 years and 13% were under 6 years of age.

LOCATION

A study in 2007 in India found the following:
- 65.9% of the street children lived with their families on the streets.
- Out of these children, 51.84% slept on the footpaths, 17.48% slept in night shelters, and 30.67% slept in other places, including under flyovers and bridges, railway platforms, bus stops, parks, and market places.

GENDER

The majority of street children in India are boys with little or no education. While girls often work on the streets, they are much less likely to break family ties and live alone. A possible explanation for this is that girls are needed more in the household for day-to-day activities and thus never leave home for the streets. Another possible explanation is that boys may leave home more because of dominating nature and the conflict-filled dynamics that sometimes develop between a stepfather and male stepchildren that do not exist with female stepchildren.

REASONS WHY A CHILD CHOOSES STREET TO BE HIS HOME

There are different sets of factors that may prompt a child to leave home. These factors could be grouped into the following categories:

- *Economic factors*: Mainly poverty, a low standard of living, the child being forced to work at an early age
- *Familial factors*: Conflicts in the family, having a step-parent who is abusive, also lack of love and attention in the family
- *Social factors*: Pressure from peers to move away from home, freedom from familial bindings, attraction of city life as compared to the life of the smaller and rural areas
- *Psychological factors*: Need to assert one's independence, the need for more attention, and so on

Sociostructural Causes

The phenomenon of street children is also a repercussion of industrialization and urbanization. Migration of people from rural to urban places is the most crucial development-induced pattern. A large number of diverse opportunities in the developing urban areas and the additional lure of better life in towns and cities compared to villages have resulted in the allurement, particularly of young workforce toward the urban areas.

As people move from relatively backward places of the country to the developing regions, they often leave their families and homes back in their native places. But the city's development plans and programs do not give any importance or priority to their accommodation or housing. The migrated population has been uprooted from their native places, the only place they knew and could call their home. This population, men, women, and children alike, have no other option and take to the streets as their sole refuge. Only few lucky ones and with a great deal of difficulty, often at the mercy of various authorities these migrant families manage a roof over their heads in some slums.

Under the trying circumstances, the migrated parents can hardly do anything for their children. They are compelled to roam around in the streets, while their parents work until late hours to earn money. Some children are fortunate to have a "home" in a slum where they can retire to at the end of the day; many others have no other option but to seek shelter on the open pavements, bus stops, railway stations, in public places, and so on.

Economic Causes

It is not always lack of living space because of which the children are forced to be on the streets. Many parents are compelled to send their children for work to supplement the family's income as most of the times, the earnings of the working parent or parents are insufficient to secure even the family's very basic needs.

These young, uneducated, and unskilled children largely work in the unorganized sector and frequently end up in minor trades such as shoe-shining, rag-picking, and cleaning jobs. The economic compulsions of this new lifestyle are, however, more visible and apparent in them than others.

Quality of Education

Many street children are school dropouts, mostly by compulsion rather than by choice. The dropout rate in India is quite high (36-52%), the most common reasons for which are the poor quality of education, the irrelevance and monotony of the syllabi taught in schools, and child labor.

The curriculums of the free schools are most of the time uninteresting and monotonous. This is coupled with the fact that the teachers are most often inadequately trained to deal with children. This type of educational environment is detrimental in joining or continuing school. The teachers also follow traditional methods of disciplining and corporal punishment to discipline the children who in turn develop school phobia. As a consequence, the entire learning atmosphere is not stimulating or pleasurable but rather seems avoidable to many.

Some other children (mostly girls) are forced to leave school in order to join work with their parents or sometimes to look after their younger siblings while their parents are at work.

Subnormal intelligence quotient (IQ) levels sometimes lead to being stigmatized by family, friends, and society and act as the catalyst for running away from homes. In such situations, survival on the hostile streets is at the mercy of the street big brothers.

Natural Calamities

Natural calamities such as floods, droughts, earthquakes, and accidents often disrupt the family. As a consequence, they are displaced and torn apart (physically, socially, economically, and culturally). Relief operations are at the mercy of higher authorities. These not only arrive long after the disaster but are also woefully inadequate. Often, the relief efforts fail to address the most vital and demanding issue. Subsequently, the children orphaned by these disasters are compelled to move to the streets merely to survive.

Cruelty and Abuse

The stressed, overworked, frustrated parents, particularly from backward social background, still resort to traditional methods of disciplining children. They hit them with belts, canes, sticks, and hands or feet. These gruesome cruelties are more pronounced (such as the parent flinging the child against the wall, sexual abuse, etc.) in families where one or both the parents are alcoholic or drug addicted, and these children may sustain more severe injuries. The young, developing mind of a child is not adept in coping with such severe physical and psychological trauma and pain. When the situation becomes unbearable, the only escape the child knows is physical escape from home, which is the source of the pain and torture.

Broken Homes

Children who live with a single uncaring parent or a stepfather or stepmother or who are orphans are most prone to emotional trauma. They often suffer from feelings of helplessness, rejection, and insecurity. This feeling may drive them out in search of a safer place where they hope to be better accepted and loved. But unfortunately, they land up in a hostile environment.

Neglect

With both parents at work, the children go unattended for a major part of the day. In large or economically handicapped families, parents hardly get any opportunity to devote time, let alone quality time, to their children. In many situations, older siblings have to look after the younger ones. Children fail to understand this situation and feel that the parents do not love them adequately. In this state of neglect and rejection, they may turn desperate and hostile and in order to escape, run away from home in search of other places hoping to find solace.

Peer Group Influence

At tender ages and minds, peer influence plays a major role. Some children idolize their peers. They leave their homes for street life due to the influence of these peers. The peers encourage them to leave the conflict-ridden homes they live in because they had similar experience. The peers often glorify the idea of a better city life or an independent life out of restrictions and the confines of home.

Influence of Media

The media often plays a significant role in influencing the children and adolescents leaving home. Feature films largely dramatize, in a glossy exaggerated manner, the protagonist who leaves his home in the village, moves to the city, and makes a grand life for himself. Even the newspapers, television serials, and other audiovisual media glorify and overemphasize "city life" as being "lucrative," "exciting," "adventurous," and "filled with fun and entertainment." At the same time, they fail to realistically present the accompanying disadvantages of life in a strange place. As a result, children do not think deeply about leaving their homes for the cities because they presume they will definitely have no problems with city life as everything is available in abundance. Their illusions are shattered when they actually step into the cities. Then they are faced with the decision of realizing their mistake and returning home or struggling in the city in a desperate attempt to prove themselves right. Thus, the situation becomes more complicated and often beyond their control.

Street children live in an environment devoid of the affection, love, care, and comfort of a family life, which are vital in the development of a child. They are victims of their circumstances. They struggle to fulfill their most basic needs such as daily food and shelter at a very tender, impressionable age.

These children have to learn to make their own decisions at a very immature age. There is practically no one responsible to help them or guide them. Most of all, they are physically and emotionally worn down by the physical and mental pressure to fend for themselves and make a living at such a young age.

■ PHYSICAL PROBLEMS FACED BY A STREET CHILD
Lack of Adequate Nutrition
Street children usually get some amount of food to eat from various sources, but they do not have nutritious or balanced diets. This deficiency thus manifests in the form of anemia, malnutrition, and multiple vitamin deficiencies.

Homelessness
The most severe and demanding problems related to shelter are faced by those children who choose or are compelled to adopt the streets as their home. They are exposed and vulnerable to all types of weather conditions, be it hot summer, storms, rains, floods, or the extreme winter nights. These children have "nowhere to belong." They do not suffer merely from physical homelessness but also from a psychological homelessness and hopelessness. The homes they have left no longer remain their own; the streets are hostile and provide no comfort, and society keeps them at a distance.

Health Problems
Street children live in an environment of persistent physical and mental strain. Many of them rummage through the garbage

anywhere and anytime in a day to find food; others go hungry due to various factors and find solace in taking addictive drugs to diminish their pangs of hunger.

- *Nutrition:* Almost all street children suffer from various grades of malnutrition and many kinds of metabolic deficiencies.
- *Addiction:* The consumption of tobacco products, alcohol, or addictive drugs retards their growth at a growing age. All these addictive items are costly and that complicates the issue further.
- *Sexually transmitted diseases (STDs):* Most street children have no knowledge or have limited knowledge and awareness about hygiene or STDs. As a result, they encounter various sexual and reproductive health problems such as STDs and human immunodeficiency virus (HIV)/acquired immunodeficiency syndrome (AIDS).
- *Pregnancy:* Unwanted pregnancies, young age pregnancies, premature births, and unsafe abortions are common in street girls.
- *Medical care:* The lack of proper medical care, awareness about medical conditions, and opportunity to ever visit a hospital or doctor further compound all these health problems.
- *Dog bites:* When these children collect recyclable material from the garbage bins with gunny bags on their shoulder, they are met with hostile dogs. A large number of children are seen with some white powder on their legs. This is their way of managing dog bite, they apply lime over the wound.
- *Accidents:* These children, especially the adolescent ones, are always on the run either from the society or from the lawmakers. Being children at heart, they love to do stunts and be noticed by the onlookers. Travelling on train footboard and rooftops and doing other stunts in the moving trains are regular pictures seen, and this leads to accidents which are sometimes fatal and crippling.
- *Skin infections:* Most often, street children do not get an opportunity to bathe or bathe properly for many days at a time, and because of the unhygienic conditions in which they live and unclean water they use, they are prone to various skin diseases such as scabies, dermatitis, fungal infections, eczema, ulcers,

and other rashes. There is no proper place for these children, particularly girls, to take care of his or her personal needs such as bathing, maintaining personal hygiene, and toilet facilities. All these lead these children to staying unclean and defecating on either the railway track or open places. Once in a while, they take a bath in the local water bodies available. They have to do these under pressure of being driven out by the onlookers. Nonavailability of space to keep an extra pair of clothes makes them either wear the same clothes or wash them with or without soap; wearing them wet leads to skin infections, especially fungal infection.

- *Diarrhea:* It is common in these children because they do not have access to fresh food; they either beg or wait outside the wedding halls or outside restaurants where extra food is usually thrown off carelessly. Street children are found in flocks around these places. Personal hygiene is not maintained, adding to the risk of diarrhea. Lack of knowledge of oral rehydration solution (ORS) or not having access to public healthcare system due to their appearance and no money, as well as an insensitive attitude of the healthcare provider, keeps them away from early treatment, leading to severe complications later on.
- *Respiratory infections*: Sleeping in open or hidden and dingy places away from the police attention and having various types of addictions make them prone to having many episodes of respiratory infections and tuberculosis. Most of them go unnoticed till the later stages where some of the seniors of the street children dump him in the public hospital. Due to excessive exposure to automobile exhaust, smoke, dust, and other outdoor pollutants while they work near traffic junctions and other congested places, they suffer from respiratory disorders such as allergy, asthma, pneumonia, and even tuberculosis.

PSYCHOLOGICAL PROBLEMS FACED BY A STREET CHILD

A Stressful Past

There are many factors and successive events that ultimately compel some children to move to the streets. These factors often have a lasting and ongoing impact on their mental well-being. The effects of these events may deprive them of emotional, economic, and other kinds of support that are vital for any child for many years. The traumatic and often turbulent past also contributes a lot in predisposing street children to become more vulnerable to emotional, social, interpersonal, and psychological disorders in the future.

A Transitory Lifestyle

Street children often do not have a stable location. They frequently shift from one place to another. In majority of instances, it is by their choice, but at some other times, they are forced to keep moving. This is in order to hide from the police, sometimes welfare authorities, and also gangsters. This wandering and evasive lifestyle results in problems of social isolation and loneliness as they have not settled to a place or bonded with people. This leads to difficulties in developing bonding and emotional attachments to other human beings.

Substance Abuse

Many street children resort to using various addictive and high dependency substances (such as alcohol and drugs) by peer pressure, adolescent age risk-taking behavior, or as an attempt to escape from the overwhelming pressure of their traumatic past and their daily problems. This, in turn, can lead to various medical problems due to overdoses, infections, and an increase in the probability of accidents, violence, and also unprotected sex.

Unlearning of Learned Behavior

Universally, children learn a set of moral values and moral behavior from their close family members in their early formative years of family life. The children who leave home and begin to live on the hostile streets soon realize that the values their family taught them (such as honesty and integrity) are not helpful to their survival outside home on the streets. At times, they are forced to steal food and money because they have none of their own and no other option to meet their basic needs. Often, they have to unashamedly beg for food or money. They learn to live without a daily bath, in unhygienic and unsanitary conditions. They also ignore their shame when they have hardly any clothes to wear.

Depression

A large number of children go in for addictions due to mood changes and depression. These events are more common during the festive season when these children see all others enjoying with their families, and this is the time when they miss their families and near ones. They recollect the times when they have had good and happy moments, and this depression leads them to end up with easily available addictions such as glue sniffing, *ganja*, and others to forget the past.

Aggressiveness

Circumstance makes these children very violent at times. The feeling being cheated by the society makes them feel left out of the society. Sometimes they turn their anger on themselves by self-inflicting injuries.

SOCIAL PROBLEMS FACED BY A STREET CHILD

Deprivation of Needs and Lack of Resources and Opportunities

The daily and basic needs of street children are rarely met. Hunger, often fasting, and wearing torn, tattered, and dirty clothes or sometimes no clothes at all are frequent accompaniments of street children. They do not have a secure and definite place to stay, no educational facilities, no facilities for personal hygiene, and, in brief, no facilities at all for decent living. Psychologically, they are frequently deprived, exploited, and abused; thus, their basic needs of security and happiness are never met. Socioculturally, they lack opportunities for healthy recreation and lack social acceptance.

Exploitation

Children on the street have to work to survive and support themselves and sometimes their family. They have no skills with which to bargain for fair pay or to fight for their rights; they are vulnerable to employers who look to make a profit by using them. Often, they are forced to work for 10-12 hours a day for very meager payment or in exchange for just one square meal a day. In addition to this, exploitation, abuse, and harassment, either physical or sexual, by persons in authority, be they police personnel or others, are not uncommon. At times, they are paid a part of their payment in the form of addictive drugs so that the child gets hooked to the employer.

Children earn for their livelihood by doing petty jobs such as working as loaders and shoe-polish boys and collecting recyclable waste as ragpickers, and metal scrap from the streets and selling it in shops. It is difficult for them to keep the earned money safe at night when they sleep like logs after the day's hard work. The money so earned gets robbed, so either they spend it on food or finish it by seeing movies. Some of them keep the extra money in fixed shops with the hope of taking it with them when they would subsequently go home one day. These boys do not have mathematical skills and a lot of money is siphoned off from their total without thy being aware of it.

Security

These boys are found in groups and they are very loyal to the members of the group. This is the only social security they have on the streets. They hide mostly from police and the security agencies so that they are not spotted.

Besides the police, the street children are frequently taken advantage of by the underworld gangsters or by older street boys who bully them and use them to achieve their own ends. If the children do not oblige, they are threatened, beaten, and sometimes, in extreme cases, may even be killed.

Abuse

The overall incidence of physical abuse among street children, either by family members or by others or both, was 66.8% across the states. Out of this, 54.62% were boys and 45.38% were girls. A very low number of those boys who were sexually active were found to have adequate knowledge about safe sex, protection, and condom usage. No one reported having ever used a condom.

STIGMATIZATION

The image that is built up in our mind when we utter the word "street child" is that he is dirty, does not bathe for many days, wears tattered and dirty clothes, begs, is at the street corners selling some petty things, is polishing shoes on the streets or railway platforms, is a thief, is smoking, or is an addict, and many more such derogatory negative thoughts. This is the beginning of the society's indifferent and prejudiced outlook toward a street child.

Due to these general misconceptions about street children, people tend to be unsympathetic and indifferent to the actual plight. This lack of social acceptance pushes them further away from mainstream society and forces them to survive on the fringes of the social system.

IMMEDIATE MEASURES

- Providing facilities that the children need
  - Toilet, bathing, and personal hygiene
  - Nutritious food
  - Rest, recreation, and safe place for night rest
  - Safely storing their belongings
  - Secure place to keep the money earned
  - *Local shelters:* These can be taken on hire or built at strategic points. Facilities such as locker, small cupboards which can be locked, bathing, and resting facilities can be provided to these children here. The children can get adequate rest and nutritious food here. Their health ailments can be addressed early and proper treatment can be given. They can be educated on personal hygiene and other health care issues. They can learn a skill as per their interest and capabilities. A large number of agencies can come together to run such centers, and the overall directions can be given by experts and concerned government officials. Nongovernmental organizations in collaboration with the social welfare department of the state governments can be partners. It can also be taken up as a corporate social responsibility by some organizations.

- *Health care:* This can be looked after by the local or national medical bodies. These associations either have fixed day clinics providing curative services at the designated places or provide facilities free of cost/or reimbursed by the local governments or corporate bodies for the services provided to such homeless children.

LONG-TERM MEASURES

These need to be directed to reduce the chances of the child leaving and running away from home:
- Responsible parenting needs to be understood by each and every couple before marriage.
- Mass media, print media, and other educational measures to be used to create this awareness
- Each contact with the healthcare provider to be used to create understanding of this issue
- Every opportunity where youth and young adults come together can be used to build up strong family bonds.
- Help the society in early identification of the signs of psychological disturbance in a child
- Making services available for the child so that he is heard and to let him vent out his feelings and frustrations. This can be arranged at free counseling centers, especially for them.
- Giving a lot of publicity to this counseling center at every probable child contact area, so that each child on the street, whenever he needs a hearing ear, has someone available for him, and he is not strayed away further from the society which he considers is hostile to him.

GUIDELINES FOR PARENTS

- Based on the relationship with family, the categories of street children are children on the street, children of the street, and abandoned children.
- Majority of street children in India are boys with little or no education.
- Factors that may prompt a child to leave home are economic, familial, social, or psychological.
- A street child may face various physical, psychological, and social challenges.
- Exploitation, abuse, and stigmatization further complicate their life.

BIBLIOGRAPHY

1. Chempakathinal G. Social inclusion through education for children in street habitat. Salesian Journal of Humanities & Social Sciences. 2016: VII (1); 79-92.
2. Naga Seshamma S. Street Children of India: A Socio-legal Study. New Delhi: Anmol Publication Private Limited; 2010.
3. Nieuwenhuizen P. Street Children in Bangalore (India): Their Dreams and Their Future. New Jersey: Transaction Publishers; 2006. pp. 152.
4. Street Children: A Mapping and Gapping Review of the Literature 2000 to 2010 Consortium for Street Children.
5. Working with Street Children: A Training Package on Substance Use, Sexual and Reproductive Health Including HIV/AIDS. WHO http://www.who.int/substance_abuse/activities/street_children/en/ index.html.

CHAPTER 25

Substitute Care

Jaydeep Choudhury

■ INTRODUCTION

Substitute care, or foster care, is temporary or permanent out-of-home care provided to children and adolescents whose immediate families are unable to care for them due to various reasons. Children in substitute care are often unprepared for separations, which are usually abrupt and repeated in some situations. Early separation from the primary caregiver is a cause for major trauma for the child. Foster care children generally suffer from abandonment, neglect, rejection, emotional, physical, and sexual maltreatment.

■ REASONS FOR PLACEMENT IN SUBSTITUTE CARE

Children and adolescents in substitute care are "children in need of supervision" (CHINS), or sometimes they are juvenile delinquents (JD). These children are usually placed under foster care involuntarily. Abandonment remains the most common cause of substitute care. Most of these children are abandoned by their parents due to various reasons. Unwanted child, death of a parent, and unwed mother remain the leading causes. Other causes are neglect due to various factors, alcoholism and drug abuse of parent, domestic violence, inadequate housing, caregiver inability to cope, physical abuse, sexual abuse, child behavior problems, child alcohol or substance abuse, and child disability. Often, there are multiple and overlapping factors that necessitate foster care.

Few children and adolescents are voluntarily placed in foster care due to parent request. Some parents seek placement for children with serious mental or behavioral problems or children with complex chronic diseases.

TYPES OF SUBSTITUTE CARE

Ideally, the child should be placed in the least restrictive environment. But often the site of placement is determined by the child's needs and available facilities. The optimal placement for a child is within a well-supported family where the foster-care parents have received proper training related to child development, behavior, parenting, and the management of impact of childhood trauma.

The options include the following:
- *Foster care home:* Foster parenting is a voluntary program. It is generally guided by a personal need. Sometimes it is due to good intentions and abilities of people motivated by their love for children, religious conviction, or altruism.
- *Kinship care:* It encompasses the relatives who have become certified foster parents as well as relatives and friends who care for children placed with them by the legal authority. Placement in kinship care has many advantages. It maintains the child's sense of belonging to a family and is less likely to be a disruptive transition since children are likely to have had a preexisting relationship with the caregiver.
- *Residential or group homes:* Residential treatment facilities are intended to provide time-limited placement of the child. Sometimes care becomes extended for adolescents with major mental health issues.

CHALLENGES

Being removed from the real home and placed in substitute care is a difficult and stressful experience for any child. These children generally have enormous mental health needs. Some of them might have suffered some form of serious abuse or neglect previously. It is observed that about 30% of children in substitute care have severe behavioral, emotional, or developmental problems. Various physical health problems are also common. Most children, however, show remarkable adaptability, resiliency, and determination to go on with their lives. Children in substitute care often struggle with the following issues:
- Blaming themselves and feeling guilty about being removed from their birth parents

- Wishing to return to their birth parents even if they were previously abused by them
- Feeling unwanted when awaiting adoption for a long time
- Feeling helpless about multiple changes in substitute parents over time
- Having mixed emotions about accepting, adapting, and attaching to foster parents
- Feeling of insecurity and uncertainty about their future
- Having doubts about the positive feelings for foster parents.

On the other hand, foster parents also face some challenges from the situation, which include the following:
- Emotional attachment to the child
- Dealing with the complex needs, emotional factors, physical issues, etc., of children in their care
- Acceptance and influence of the relatives, friends, and society
- Financial issues related to child-rearing.

COMMON BEHAVIORAL PROBLEMS

A child's mental health, emotional issues, and ability to interact with others may be profoundly affected if the child is in substitute care or foster care. The frequency and severity of various emotional problems related to complex childhood trauma may be compounded by the child's lack of security and permanence in immediate foster care. Lack of stability in further placement exacerbates underlying emotional and behavioral problems. Foster parents or caregivers and others interacting with these children should be aware and oriented that the children's fluctuating emotions can also lead to changes in behavior in various circumstances such as home and in school. The more changes in substitute homes they experience over time, including changes in caregivers, the more likely these children are to develop various behavioral problems.

Behavioral manifestations may be precipitated by various factors, including:
- The stress of changes in the placement environment
- Unrealistic and demanding expectations of foster parents
- Poor quality visitation with birth parents, particularly if such interactions cause the child to relive the trauma of separation or rejection

- Changes in caregivers or therapists
- Court appearances
- Reminders of previous trauma, which may be subtle and escape the notice of the caregiver.

The various behavioral problems are as below.

Reactive Attachment Disorder

Reactive attachment disorder can occur due to disruptions in attachment relationships caused by substitute care. It can manifest in a variety of behaviors in relation to caregivers, including being withdrawn, not making eye contact, appearing sad, failing to smile, failing to reach out when picked up, and showing a lack of interest in interactive games or toys. Attachment issues are a cause of concern in these children because they did not get the opportunity to form secure attachments with consistent nurturing figures in early life. Children who shift from one foster home to another suffer from compromised enduring emotional attachments. Trusting somebody becomes a challenge for them.

Defying Authority

The whole process of being removed from their original home and being placed with strangers causes enormous emotional stress and insecurity among these children. They feel insecure and uncertain about their future. This insecurity frequently leads to children defying authority. The manifestations may be refusal to listen to authority figures or intentionally doing the opposite of what is asked.

Aggression

Substitute care children are at high risk for getting involved in aggression and violence with other children and siblings. This could mean initiating and participating in physical fights with friends, natural or foster care siblings. This aggressive behavior could originate from family separation or adversity between siblings in the child's biological family. Children who have experienced traumatic physical and sexual abuse often become mistrustful, sensitive, abusive, and aggressive.

Anger Outbursts

Anger outbursts are manifestations of frustration and helplessness. The outbursts are generally directed toward the foster parents, but they may also be directed toward other persons. During extremes of outbursts, they may be destructive and may even set fire. Sometimes they resort to self-destructive behavior.

Running Away

Problems in adjustment in a new home and a sense of insecurity may lead to running away.

Clinging and Crying

Constant crying and clinging behaviors are also sometimes observed in substitute care children, particularly young ones who have endured constant changes in caregivers and environments. They tend to get attached, depend upon, and cling to a particular caregiver whom they feel is dependable.

Stealing

Helplessness in children makes them seek some control and attempt to gain some measure of power by any means. Stealing is their attempt to assert their control and power. For some others stealing food, clothing, etc., may be a means of daily survival.

Lying

Telling lies at different situations by foster children may be the result of various underlying factors. These include the following:
- Fear of disappointing the adoptive parents
- Avoiding punishment, of which they are apprehensive
- Attention-seeking tactics
- Crying out for help
- The abnormal situations they grow up influence them to lie
- A means to avoid stressful situations
- Imitating the behavior of the adults around the child.

The pattern of lying must be looked into. It has to be assessed whether lying occurs only at specific times or in specific situations.

It has to be determined whether the child's unfulfilled needs drive him/her to lying.

Others

Children in substitute care may have various other behavioral problems such as feeding and eating disorders, sleep problems, enuresis, encopresis, and sexualized behaviors. The most prevalent psychiatric disorders among children in substitute care are attention deficit hyperactivity disorder (ADHD), oppositional defiant disorder, post-traumatic stress disorder, anxiety disorders, reactive attachment disorder, mood disorders such as depression or bipolar disorder, autism spectrum disorder, mental retardation, and obsessive–compulsive disorder. Adolescents in substitute care are at an increased risk of various risky situations such as substance abuse, teenage pregnancies, and sexually transmitted diseases.

> **GUIDELINES FOR PARENTS**
> - Children are usually placed under foster care involuntarily.
> - Abandonment remains the most common cause of substitute care.
> - Putting an orphan or abandoned child in foster care to avoid undesirable situations, injury, or even death is better than risking their lives and leaving them in a hostile environment.
> - How a child is able to cope with being placed in a new environment is contingent upon the support system that surrounds him/her.
> - Counseling and understanding, supportive foster parents are two main influences that determine the success of a healthy adjustment.
> - A foster child should be encouraged to talk about and express their needs.

BIBLIOGRAPHY

1. American Academy of Pediatrics. Fostering Health: Health Care for Children and Adolescents in Foster Care, 2nd edition. [online] Available from: www2.aap.org/fostercare/FosteringHealth.html. [Last accessed December, 2019].
2. Sadock BJ, Sadock VA. Kaplan and Sadock's Concise Textbook of Child and Adolescent Psychiatry. Philadelphia: Lippincott Williams and Wilkins; 2009.
3. Turney K, Wildeman C. Mental and physical health of children in foster care. Pediatrics. 2016;138:e20161118.

CHAPTER 26

Substance-related and Addictive Disorders

Mandira Roy

INTRODUCTION

Substance-related disorders are characterized by a cluster of cognitive, behavioral, and physiological symptoms indicating that the individual continues using the substance despite significant substance-related problems. These disorders encompass 10 separate classes of drugs out of which alcohol is the most common one to be used. Addiction is a distressing condition that is mainly characterized by compulsive drug-seeking behavior and consumption of drug despite experiencing severe adverse effects. Substance use and abuse is a major cause of morbidity and mortality for adolescents. The percentage varies in different countries. Lesser is the age of initiating substance abuse, greater is the risk of becoming addicted to it.

The Diagnostic and Statistical Manual of Mental Disorders, Fifth Edition (DSM 5), has divided substance-related disorders into two groups: (1) Substance-use disorders and (2) substance-induced disorders.

The DSM 5 no longer identifies substance-use disorder as abuse or dependence. The previous terminologies and categories of substance abuse and dependence are thus eliminated and discarded. The DSM 5 for substance-related disorders also has a new category of behavioral addictions, in which gambling is the sole disorder.

EPIDEMIOLOGY

The National Household Survey of Drug Use done in 2004 in India is the first organized and systematic effort to report pan India wide range of drug use. The current prevalence rates within the age group of 12–18 years were 21.4% for alcohol, the primary substance used apart from tobacco, followed by 3.0% for cannabis and 0.7% for opioids.

A meta-analysis (1998) revealed substance-use prevalence of approximately 6.9/1,000 population. The rates among male and female were 11.9 and 1.7%, respectively.

A Rapid Situation Assessment (RSA) by the United Nations Office on Drugs and Crime (UNODC) in 2002 of 4,648 drug users showed that cannabis (40%), alcohol (33%), and opioids (15%) were the major substances used.

In general, substance abuse among women has been studied and observed through Rapid Assessment Surveys. A survey of a total of 1,865 women by 110 nongovernmental organizations (NGOs) across the country revealed that 25% of these women currently were heroin users, whereas 18% used dextropropoxyphene. Around 11% of women used opioid-containing cough medicines and 7% used buprenorphine. It was also found that 87% of women used alcohol and 83% used tobacco concomitantly.

A Rapid Situation and Response Assessment (RSRA) was done by the United Nations among 5,800 men drug users in India, Nepal, Bhutan, Bangladesh, and Sri Lanka in 2009. This study revealed that 76% were injecting heroin, 70% were smoking heroin (chasing), and 64% were using propoxyphene. Majority of the drug users also used alcohol (80%).

The World Drug Report, which studied 81,802 treatment seekers in India in 2004–2005, reported that 61.3% used opioids whereas 15.5% of them used cannabis, 4.1% used sedatives, and very less percentage of them used cocaine, amphetamines, and solvents.

In the year 2019, the Ministry of Social Justice and Empowerment, Government of India, published a report titled "Magnitude of Substance Use in India, 2019." This research was carried out by the National Drug Dependence Treatment Centre, All India Institute of Medical Sciences, New Delhi. The key observation of this survey is that it found that there are wide variations in the extent and prevalence of use of various substances in different states of India. Alcohol was found to be the most common substance used followed by cannabis and opioids. The prevalence of alcohol use is around 4.6%, with the male:female ratio being 17:1. Next comes cannabis at 2.8% and opioids at 2.1%. Coming to potentially harmful and dependent use, 19% of alcohol users use it in a dependent manner, whereas in case of cannabis, only 0.25% of users use it in a dependent pattern.

ETIOPATHOGENESIS

Adolescence describes the psychosocial changes that occur as individuals leave childhood and develop into independent, contributing members of adult society. Various strategies employed to achieve these changes include exploration, experimentation, risk-taking, and questioning authority and established rules. These strategies may be functional in shaping normal adolescents, but they can also lead to serious illness and injury in the context of drug and alcohol use.

Addiction research focuses primarily on understanding two major aspects. Firstly, the underlying mechanisms of transition from occasional recreational drug use to an addicted state. Secondly, the mechanisms that are responsible for the persistence of drug-consuming behaviors even after prolonged drug abstinence.

This has become an area of genuine interest to identify the underlying mechanisms by which chronic drug exposure promotes strong and permanent changes in gene expression and thus regulates drug-consuming behavior. Drug-induced changes in gene expression in important brain regions that are associated with satisfaction and reward represent mechanisms thought to contribute to both factors. These regions are the nucleus accumbens (NAc), prefrontal cortex (PFC), and ventral tegmental area (VTA). The transcription factor ΔFosB is induced multiple fold in the NAc by chronic drug exposure and it has been implicated in the transition to an addicted state. Altered expression of specific genes, such as activator of G-protein signaling 3 (AGS3) and brain-derived neurotrophic factor (BDNF), has been reported even weeks after the last drug exposure.

Recent evidences have suggested that epigenetic mechanisms are the key cellular processes that integrate diverse environmental stimuli to exert potent and often permanent changes in gene expression through the regulation of chromatin structure contributing to these drug-induced transcriptional and behavioral changes. These transcriptional and epigenetic mechanisms of addiction offer novel insights for deaddiction therapy.

CLINICAL FEATURES

Clinical manifestations vary widely depending on the type of drugs but mostly present in the office without any physical manifestations. In majority of cases, substance abuse becomes an incidental finding where the adolescent presents with motor vehicle injuries, act of violence, or is in a debilitated and intoxicated state. As a rule of thumb, any adolescent presenting to the emergency with altered sensorium should be evaluated for substance use. In case of intravenous or intranasal substance abuse, some physical manifestation along the route of administration can be found such as multiple venous track and nasal mucosal injuries.

STAGES OF ADOLESCENT SUBSTANCE ABUSE

Stages of substance abuse as shown in **Table 1** need to be considered while recognizing the clinical manifestation and planning reversal. Knowledge of stages of substance abuse can also prevent serious life-threatening issues.

TABLE 1: Stages of substance-use disorder in adolescents.

Stage	Description
Stage 1: Initiation	Curiosity, peer pressure, emotional immaturity
Stage 2: Experimentation	Fun, euphoria, reward system activation, lack of awareness of consequences, only with friends
Stage 3: Regular use	Seeking euphoria, behavioral changes, uses drugs alone, can add other drugs as well
Stage 4: Problem use	Daily use, school performance hampers, not engaging with family and other friends, desperate and risk-taking behavior
Stage 5: Dependence	Drug use normalized, require higher doses to achieve the same "high," guilt, shame, depression, physical and mental deterioration, self-destructive or aggressive behaviors

SCREENING AND ASSESSMENT

The most effective method of screening is a good history, taken in the absence of parents or caregivers providing a confidential space. Additional information from family, peers, and school should be taken separately.

One very simple tool to screen an adolescent suspected of substance abuse is by CRAFFT questions as shown in **Box 1**. The adolescent is asked six simple questions mentioned below. Two or more answers as "*Yes*" indicate a need for further assessment and/or referral to specialty treatment.

Urine Drug Screening

Urine drug screening is a common and accepted method of drugs and performance-enhancing medication screening in athletes and sports persons. The person concerned is asked to drink plenty of water and then the urine is collected. The used and abused substances are excreted in the urine. Days that substance can be detected in urine after being last used are 1–2 days for opiates and amphetamines, 1–4 days for cocaine, 2–9 days for cannabinoids and benzodiazepine, and 3–14 days for barbiturates.

Urine drug screening in adolescents mainly shows evidence of marijuana use because cannabinoids last for almost 3–4 weeks after

BOX 1: CRAFFT questions for screening adolescents with suspected substance abuse.

> C—Have you ever ridden in a *car* driven by someone (including yourself) who was "high" or had been using alcohol or drugs?
> R—Do you ever use alcohol or drugs to *relax*, feel better about yourself, or fit in?
> A—Do you ever use alcohol or drugs while you are by yourself *alone*?
> F—Does your *family* or *friends* ever tell you that you should cut down on your drinking or drug use?
> F—Do you ever *forget* things you did while using alcohol or drugs?
> T—Have you ever gotten into *trouble* while you were using alcohol or drugs?

they are used on a regular basis. Most other drugs are only present for 1–2 days. Alcohol levels are determined from breath or blood testing.

DIAGNOSIS

Substance use-related disorders need formal diagnosis by a multidisciplinary team consisting of psychiatrists and psychologists. The DSM 5 criteria is the most common one to be used for diagnosis. It takes into account a total of four categories of a cluster of symptoms, i.e., impaired self-control, social impairment, increased risk related to substance use, and pharmacologic responses (tolerance/withdrawal). This criteria also considers the severity of symptoms in terms of mild, moderate, and severe along with specifiers or comorbidities.

The DSM 5 criteria has some limitations with adolescents because of differing patterns of use, developmental implications, and age-related consequences. So, adolescents who meet diagnostic criteria should be referred to the concerned specialist.

Intervention

Adolescent substance use is a complex condition that needs multidisciplinary interventions to approach it in a holistic way.

In order to deal with an adolescent with an addiction disorder, finding the stage of involvement is very important to determine the modality of intervention. In adolescents involved in recreational use, education about the detrimental effect of drugs and counseling is beneficial. Teenagers on regular use require the help of mental health professionals. Motivational interviewing by "FRAMES" as shown in **Box 2** is effective.

A detailed and complete psychiatric evaluation is always necessary because substance abuse often coexists with one or more psychiatric disorders like behavior disorders such as conduct disorder and attention deficit hyperactivity disorder (ADHD), anxiety disorder, mood disorder, and personality disorder. Hospitalization and rehabilitation may be required for more severe situations.

Adolescent Substance Abuse Intervention Workbook by Jaffe instructs adolescents to concretely explore how 12 areas of his or

BOX 2: Motivational interviewing by FRAMES.

F—*Feedback* on personal risk or impairment
R—Emphasis on personal *responsibility* for change
A—Clear *advice* to change
M—A *menu* of alternative change options
E—Therapist *empathy*
S—Facilitation of client *self-efficacy* or optimism

her life have been negatively affected by substance in an effort to move them to recognize a need to stop using the drug. The website of the National Institute of Drug Abuse (NIDA), www.drugabuse.gov, provides detailed information on the drugs, their abuse, diagnosis, treatment, and even prevention.

GUIDELINES FOR PARENTS

- Addiction is a disease, not a habit.
- Always have a suspicion if a sudden change in behavior or performance is noticed in an adolescent.
- Focus on the child, not at the source.
- Try to find out the cause, e.g., problem at school, family, or social level.
- Do not delay in taking the help of a professional in dealing with the situation.

BIBLIOGRAPHY

1. Ambekar A, Agrawal A, Rao R, Mishra AK, Khandelwal SK on behalf of the group of investigators for the National Survey on Extent and Pattern of Substance Use in India. Magnitude of substance use in India. New Delhi: Ministry of Social Justice and Empowerment, Government of India; 2019.
2. Bowers MS, McFarland K, Lake RW, Peterson YK, Lapish CC, Gregory ML, et al. Activator of G protein signaling 3: a gatekeeper of cocaine sensitization and drug seeking. Neuron. 2004;42:269-81.
3. CRAFFT questions. Two or more "YES" answers indicate a need for further assessment and/or referral to specialty treatment. (Adopted from Knight JR, Shrier LA Bravender TD, et al.: CRAFFT: a new brief screen for adolescent substance abuse. Abstract presented at Ambulatory Paediatric Association meeting. New Orleans, 1998).
4. Diagnostic and Statistical Manual of Mental Disorders, 5th edition. Washington DC: American Psychiatric Association; 2013.

5. Grimm JW, Lu L, Hayashi T, Hope BT, Su TP, Shaham Y. Time-dependent increases in brain-derived neurotrophic factor protein levels within the mesolimbic dopamine system after withdrawal from cocaine: implications for incubation of cocaine craving. J Neurosci. 2003;23:742-7.
6. Hope BT, Nye HE, Kelz MB, Self DW, Iadarola MJ, Nakabeppu Y, et al. Induction of a long-lasting AP-1 complex composed of altered Fos-like proteins in brain by chronic cocaine and other chronic treatments. Neuron. 1994;13:1235-44.
7. Hyman SE, Malenka RC, Nestler EJ. Neural mechanisms of addiction: the role of reward-related learning and memory. Annu Rev Neurosci. 2006;29:565-98.
8. Jaffe SL. Adolescent Substance Abuse Intervention Workbook: Taking a First Step. Washington DC: American Psychiatric Press; 2001.
9. Kalivas PW, Volkow N, Seamans J. Unmanageable motivation in addiction: a pathology in prefrontal-accumbens glutamate transmission. Neuron. 2005;45:647-50.
10. Kelz MB, Chen J, Carlezon Jr WA, Whisler K, Gilden L, Beckmann AM, et al. Expression of the transcription factor deltaFosB in the brain controls sensitivity to cocaine. Nature. 1999;401:272-6.
11. Koob G, Kreek MJ. Stress, dysregulation of drug reward pathways, and the transition to drug dependence. Am J Psychiatr. 2007;164:1149-59.
12. Kumar A, Choi KH, Renthal W, Tsankova NM, Theobald DEH, Truong HT, et al. Chromatin remodeling is a key mechanism underlying cocaine-induced plasticity in striatum. Neuron. 2005;48:303-14.
13. Kumar MS. Rapid assessment survey of drug abuse in India. Ministry of Social Justice and Empowerment, Government of India and United Nations Office on Drugs and Crime, Regional Office for South Asia. [online] Available from: https://www.unodc.org/pdf/india/RAS.pdf. [Last accessed August, 2023].
14. United Nations Office on Drugs and Crime. Rapid situation and response assessment of drugs and HIV in Bangladesh, Bhutan, India, Nepal and Sri Lanka: A regional report. [online] Available from: https://www.unodc.org/pdf/india/Presentation_RSRA_June_25_2008.pdf. [Last accessed August, 2023].
15. Levine AA, Guan Z, Barco A, Xu S, Kandel ER, Schwartz JH. CREB-binding protein controls response to cocaine by acetylating histones at the fosB promoter in the mouse striatum. Proc Natl Acad Sci U S A. 2005;102:19186-91.
16. McClung CA, Ulery PG, Perrotti LI, Zachariou V, Berton O, Nestler EJ. ΔFosB: a molecular switch for long-term adaptation in the brain. Brain Res Mol Brain Res. 2004;132:146-54.

17. Murthy P (Ed). (2008) Women and drug use in India. Substance, women and high risk assessment study. United Nations Office on Drugs and Crime, Ministry of Social Justice and Empowerment, Government of India and United Nations Development Fund for Women. [online] Available from: https://www.unodc.org/documents/southasia/reports/UNODC_Book_Women_and_Drug_Use_in_India_2008.pdf. [Last accessed August, 2023].
18. Ray R. (2004). The extent, pattern and trends of drug abuse in India, national survey. Ministry of Social Justice and Empowerment, Government of India and United Nations Office on Drugs and Crime, Regional Office for South Asia. [online] Available from: https://www.unodc.org/pdf/india/presentations/india_national_survey_2004.pdf. [Last accessed August, 2023].
19. Reddy MV, Chandrashekhar CR. Prevalence of mental and behavioural disorders in India: a meta-analysis. Indian J Psychiatr. 1998;40:149-57.
20. Renthal W, Maze I, Krishnan V, Covington 3rd HE, Xiao G, Kumar A, et al. Histone deacetylase 5 epigenetically controls behavioral adaptations to chronic emotional stimuli. Neuron. 2007;56:517-29.
21. The FRAMES mnemonic. (Data from Miller WR, Rollnick S: Motivational Interviewing. New York: Guilford Press; 1991).
22. United Nations Office on Drugs and Crime. World drug report 2009. [online] Available from: https://www.unodc.org/documents/wdr/WDR_2009/WDR2009_eng_web.pdf. [Last accessed August, 2023].

Mental Health of Children during Pandemic

Jaydeep Choudhury

INTRODUCTION

By nature, children are sensitive individuals. They do react to various life-changing events but in a different way. There is a major change in the lifestyle of children in pandemic situations. As adult members of the community, one must understand, address, and deal with the psychological changes in children.

Prolonged home confinement may provide an opportunity to enhance parent–child understanding, relationships, and bonding, but on the other hand, prolonged inactivity may adversely affect children's physical and mental health.

Evidence demonstrates that when children are out of school such as weekends and vacations, they are physically less active, have much longer screen time, have irregular sleep patterns, and have less balanced diets, resulting in weight gain and a loss of physical fitness.

Such negative effects on health are likely to be worse when children are confined to their homes without outdoor activities and interaction with the same age group friends during the outbreak. Under the circumstances of restriction of outdoor activities, they are less physically active, spend more time with social media and electronic devices, and eat an unbalanced poorer quality diet.

Following are the possible situations the children may face:
- The stress caused by a sharp change in the environment might be eased to some degree due to the presence of known faces if children are quarantined at home with their parents or relatives.
- Children whose parents are quarantined require special attention.

- Children who are infected or suspected of being infected, if quarantined in a local center, are in the high-risk group.

The last two groups of children might be more vulnerable to mental health problems. In an isolated situation, the mental health stressors include fear of infection, boredom, and social isolation. Separation from caregivers pushes children into a state of crisis and that might increase the risk of behavioral and psychiatric disorders.

Companionship is essential for children's normal psychological development and well-being. It has been observed that depression and anxiety are the main mental health issues. Children are likely to develop acute stress disorder, post-traumatic stress disorder, adjustment disorder, and grief. Prolonged separation from parents or parental loss during childhood also has long-term adverse effects on mental health, including a greater risk of developing mood disorders and psychosis. The age of the initial separation is known to be relevant to psychological development of the child. The parent–child separation in the first few years after birth might disrupt the attachment processes, which might be associated with poorer mental health development.

School closures related to health emergencies have been associated with an increased risk of violence and vulnerability at many homes which are already stressed or in foster care. Vulnerable children and adolescents are at particular risk for violence and adverse mental health effects.

CLINICIAN'S APPROACH

Adverse physical, mental, and emotional health effects in the children can be mitigated to a large extent and parent–child relations enhanced through parental role-modeling of staying calm, understanding behaviors, involving children in regular family activities, promotion of self-discipline and self-sufficiency skills, and having frank, developmentally appropriate conversations with children about the pandemic. The basic actions to be adopted by the parents are as follows:

- Regularly communicate well with children and families in hospital
- Be compassionate and precise with the language of communication

- Parents may believe that there is no treatment for situations such as COVID-19, but we must help them understand that supportive therapy is likely to be all that is needed.

As a clinician, it is of utmost importance to understand the mental state and concerns of the parents or caregiver along with the evaluation and assessment of the children. Clinicians should also consider the potential for violence to children and look for early signs of parental stress, irritability, depression, and/or harsh responses to child behaviors during each clinical encounter. They should try to indirectly inquire about parent stress levels, methods to manage stress, financial concern, social supports, and alcohol or substance use. Clinicians can also offer simple coping strategies such as deep breathing, recreational activities, and calling a friend or family member. If required, they can arrange resources and referrals to mental health providers to families who may benefit from these interventions.

ROLE OF PARENTS

- Stay calm, listen, and reassure.
- Parents are the role models. Children will respond and follow their reactions. They usually learn from example.
- Children must be aware of how the parents talk about a disease. Discussion about a disease can either increase or decrease a child's confusion and fear. If true, the child should be reminded that the family is healthy, and they are going to do everything with restrictions to keep loved ones safe and well. Children should be listened carefully with attention about their thoughts and feelings and responded to with truth and reassurance.
- Social distancing should be explained appropriately. Children probably do not clearly understand why parents/guardians are not allowing them to go to school or be with friends. Social distancing is a new concept to them. They should be explained that while we do not know how long it will take to control the infection to reduce the number of those infected, we do know that this is a critical time; hence, we must follow the guidelines of health experts to do our part. The older children should be allowed to connect with their friends virtually.

- The positive aspects should be focused upon. It is a time to celebrate having more time to spend as a family. A daily routine should be maintained, including fun time.
- Personal protective equipment (PPE) will look terrifying for children, many of whom will have heard about COVID-19 in the news or might even know of an adult with the disease.
- To reduce fear and other psychological discomfort, children who are quarantined or whose parents are quarantined can communicate with their parents via mobile devices at any time.
- During the phase when there is restricted outdoor activity, children may be allowed recreational activities with increased allowance of daily screen time, about 2–3 hours/day under supervision.
- Parents and guardians should monitor television, internet, and social media viewing for both themselves and their children. Watching continual updates on death and disease in the media may increase fear and anxiety.
- Rumors and inaccurate information should be clarified. Older children may be accessing a great deal of information online and from friends that contains various inaccuracies.
- Increase children's access to disease information via comic books and authentic videos; guide children to establish a regular activity schedule.
- Timely referrals to psychiatrists when children feel mental discomfort, such as worry, anxiety, difficulty sleeping, and loss of appetite, are required.
- Children who are not affected may feel confused that why they cannot go out to school or park and meet their friends. They must be explained the present scenario in a manner appropriate for their age.

MANAGEMENT

Most children can be managed well with the support of parents and other family members. Some children may show signs of some anxiety or concerns, such as difficulty in concentrating or sleeping. But these can be alleviated by parental support.

Few children may have risk factors for more intense reactions such as severe anxiety, depression, and sometimes suicidal behaviors.

Risk factors for such a serious turn may include a preexisting mental health issue, prior traumatic experiences or abuse, family instability, or the loss of a near one. Children should be managed by a professional if they exhibit significant changes in behavior or any of the following symptoms for >2 weeks.

Preschoolers: Excessive clinging to parents, sleep disturbances, loss of appetite, thumb-sucking, bed-wetting, fear of the dark, regression in behavior, and general withdrawal

School-going children: Excessive irritability, aggressiveness, nightmares, clinginess, school avoidance, poor concentration, and withdrawal from activities and friends

Adolescents: Sleeping and eating disturbances, agitation, increase in conflicts, physical complaints, delinquent behavior, and poor concentration

GUIDELINES FOR PARENTS

- Parents should remain calm and reassuring. Remind them that this is a temporary situation for the good of everybody.
- Children have to be told that they are safe. Let them know that it is okay to feel upset in the situation.
- Provide information that is realistic, truthful, and appropriate for the age and developmental level of the child so that he can understand.
- Children should be taught the basic safety actions in a pandemic situation, such as cough or sneeze hygiene. They have to be reminded to wash their hands frequently and stay away from people who are coughing or sneezing or are sick.

BIBLIOGRAPHY

1. Liu JJ, Bao Y, Huang X, Shi J, Lu L. Mental health considerations for children quarantined because of COVID-19. Lancet Child Adolesc Health. 2020;4(5):347-9.
2. World Health Organization. The Importance of Caregiver-Child Interactions for the Survival and Healthy Development of Young Children: A Review. Geneva: World Health Organization; 2004. [online] Available from: https://apps.who.int/iris/bitstream/handle/10665/42878/924159134X.pdf?sequence=1&isAllowed=yhttps://www.who.int/maternal_child_adolescent/documents/924159134X/en. [Last accessed August, 2023].

Index

Page numbers followed by *b* refer to box, *f* refer to figure, *fc* refer to flowchart, and *t* refer to table

A

Abdomen 14
Abuse 353
   alcohol 319, 357
   drug 319
   emotional 5
   physical 5, 319
   sexual 5
   substance 18, 351, 357, 364
Academic backwardness, causes of 26
Acceptable social behavior 333
Accidents 349
Accredited Social Health Activist workers 1
Acquired immunodeficiency syndrome 349
Acute food refusal 148
Adaptive behaviors 23
Addiction 349
Addictive behaviors 336
Addictive disorders 363
Adenovirus 277
Adequate nutrition, lack of 348
Adjustment disorder 266
Adolescent sexual offenders 314
Adolescent substance 368
Adrenocorticotropic hormone 86
Age-appropriate sexual behaviors 301*t*
Age-appropriate transitory anxieties 215
Aggression 90, 130, 360
Aggressive antisocial behavior 131
Aggressiveness 352
Agoraphobia 221

Airway 135
Akathisia 60
Alarm therapy 165
Alkaline phosphatase 285
Alpha-blocker therapy 157
Alternative communication system 89
Alternative therapy 167
American Academy of Pediatrics 92, 170, 338*b*
American Speech-Language-Hearing Association 67
Amphetamines 367
Amygdala-dominant emotional decision 330
Anemia 277
Angelman syndromes 9
Anger
   issues 217
   outbursts 361
Angry mood 125
Anorexia 135, 136
   early age 136
   infantile 143
   nervosa 137, 138, 283, 291, 299
Antecedents-behavior-consequences analysis 111
Anthropometry 13
Anticholinergics 166
   medication 160
Antidepressants 118
Antiepileptic drugs 235
Antioxidant 87
Antipsychotics, atypical 133
Antisocial behavior, isolated acts of 132
Antispasmodic 160

Anxiety 90, 223, 224, 266
   anticipatory 221
   degree of 224
   development of 216
   disorder 213, 214, 222, 227, 234, 362
      epidemiology 214
      etiopathogenesis 214
      important reasons for 217
      management 222
      types of 214, 218
   encompassing separation 266
   origin of 214
Anxious cognitive pattern 215
Argumentative behavior 125
Arthritis, juvenile 247
Articulation, disorders of 71
Aspirations, signs of 135
Asthma 277
Athletic skills 249
Atomoxetine 117, 118
Attention-deficit disorder 60, 169
Attention-deficit hyperactivity disorder 5, 10, 26, 29, 50, 62, 98, 100fc, 107, 119, 155, 182, 204, 209, 265, 362, 368
   clinical features 105
   developmental course of 110fc
   diagnosis 102
   differential diagnosis 107
   epidemiology 102
   etiology 99
   history and nomenclature 98
   investigations 106
   safety measures for 118
   schooling issues of 117
   treatment of 109, 118
Attention-seeking behaviors 267
Audiometry 18
Auditory impairment 12
Augmentative communication system 89
Authoritarian parenting 332, 334
Autism 69, 82, 91t, 94, 277
   biology of 87
   classical 82
   features of 90
   modified checklist for 92
   spectrum disorder 3, 5, 30, 60, 63, 69, 77, 108, 362
      clinical features 79, 88
      diagnostic criteria 81
      epidemiology 79
      etiology 85
      evolution 78
      history 79
      incidence 79
      laboratory tests and imaging 88
      management 88
      severity of 84t
Autonomy, disorders of 144

B

Bacteriuria 164
Bad dreams 217
Bar graph score 53f
Barbiturates 367
Barrett's esophagus 292
Barriers influencing eating behaviors 283
Behavioral disorders 1, 2
Behavioral dysregulation 200
Behavioral family interventions 210
Behavioral insomnia 199
Behavioral interventions 89, 90, 269
Behavioral management 111, 269
   strategies 113, 114
Behavioral modification 64, 112
Behavioral plan 177
Behavioral problems 1, 22, 203, 282, 337, 359
Behavioral signs 213
Behavioral therapy 127, 312
Behavioral treatments 149
Benzodiazepine 367
Beta-2 agonists 118
Beta-hemolytic streptococci 277
Bilateral motor coordination 53, 55f
Binge eating
   disorder 140, 287, 289
   recurrent episodes of 286, 290
Biofeedback therapy 239

Biological abnormalities 204
Biological treatment 312
Bipolar depression 212
Bipolar disorder 205, 206, 211, 362
  early onset 204
Bipolar mood disorder 108, 208*fc*
Birth weight, low 35
Bladder
  dysfunctions, treatment of 164
  filling, awareness of 153
  growth, normal 153
  urea nitrogen 209
  wall irritability 155
Bone marrow suppression 293
Botulinum toxin 191
Bowel patterns 279
Brain
  connecting muscular
    movement 183
  derived neurotrophic factor 365
  development, abnormal 277
  dysfunction 101
Breast
  shape 304
  size 304
Bruxism 198
Buddy system 43
Bulimia 288, 289
  nervosa 137, 139, 282, 286, 291,
    295, 299
Bullying in school 270
  evaluation 272
  management 272
  types of 271
Bupropion 118

C

Calcium, form of 252
Cardiac dysrhythmias, signs of 288
Cardiorespiratory system 233
Catatonia 61
Central nervous system 14, 209
  dysfunction 129
  tumors, survivors of 246
Cerebral palsy 9, 20, 69, 171
Cheilitis 282

Chest 14
Chromosomal microarray 21
Chronic illness
  diagnosis of 244
  psychological effects of 242
Chronic medical problems 26
Chronic motor tic disorder 184
Chronic pediatric illnesses 242
Circadian-based disorders 201
Classroom skills 259
Clinical linguistic and auditory
    milestone scale 68, 73
Clonazepam 108
Clonidine 116, 118, 191
Coarse facial features 19
Coexisting learning disability 117
Cognitive behavioral therapy 210,
    306, 323
Cognitive components 213
Cognitive function 37
  level of 67
Cognitive progress, milestone of 13
Communication 80, 249
  disorders 65, 67-69
  impairments, possible causes
    of 69
Complementary therapy 167
Complex biopsychosocial
    conditions 297
Complex chronic diseases 357
Conduct disorder 108, 128, 131,
    132, 265
  child abuse 129
  clinical features 131
  comorbid factors 129
  diagnosis 129
  differential diagnosis 132
  epidemiology 128
  etiology 128
  treatment 132
Confusional arousals 198
Conner's rating scales-revised
    version 105
Constipation 279
  treatment of 157
Constructional praxis 55*f*
Conversion disorder 227, 234

Coprolalia 187
Copropraxia 187
Cortico-amygdala circuit 216
COVID-19 375
 pandemic 1
Cow's milk
 free diet 280
 protein allergy 280
Cranial radiation therapy,
  high dose of 246
Crying 278
Cyberbullying 271
Cytomegalovirus 18

D

Dancing skills 249
Daytime frequency syndrome 157
Daytime sleepiness 200
Daytime urine incontinence
 clinical features 157
 etiology 154
 investigations 158
 management 159
 pathophysiology 154
Deceitfulness 130
Defensiveness 331
Delayed sleep phase disorder 198
Delinquents, juvenile 357
Dental
 enamel dysplasia 288
 erosion 282
Denver Congos study scale
  inventory 261
Denver model 89
Deoxyribonucleic acid 101
Depression 10, 90, 352, 362, 374
 maternal 107
 parental 224
Depressive disorder 266
 types of 208*fc*
Desmopressin 166
Detoxifier 87
Detrusor sphincter dyssynergia 156
Development disorders 85
Developmental articulation
  disorder 69

Developmental coordination
  disorder 48
 clinical features 50
 diagnosis 49
 epidemiology 49
 guidelines for parents 56
 management 55
 questionnaire 51
 treatment 51
Developmental delay 21, 337
Developmental dyspraxia 52
 diagnosis of 52
Developmental factors 215, 229
Developmental intervention 89
Developmental language
 delay 71
 disorder 69
Developmental quotient 68
Developmental theory 306
Deviant sexual behavior 300
 etiology of 306
Dextroamphetamine 118
Diabetes mellitus, gestational 35
Diagnostic and statistical manual of
  mental disorders 7, 123,
  235*b*
Dialectical behavior therapy 322
Diarrhea 350
Diet 177
Dietary intervention 90
Digital media 336, 337
 exposure 337
Digital rectal examination 173
Diphenhydramine 202
Disruptive behavior 123
Disruptive mood dysregulation
  disorder 206
Distress 215
 degree of 213
Diuretics 284
Dog bites 349
Dopamine 216
 antagonists 64
Double syndrome 82
Down syndrome 9, 18, 23
Drug dosage 211*t*
Dyscalculia 31, 50

Index

Dysfluency 70
Dysfunctional child-caregiver interactions 137
Dysgraphia 31, 34f, 50
Dyslexia 31, 50
Dysphoric feelings 337
Dyspraxia, types of 52
Dyssomnia 195
Dysuria 158

E

Ear 63, 233
   drainage 278
   infection 278
Early childhood disorder 135
Early language milestone scale 73
Eating difficulties 137
Eating disorders 135, 136, 142, 147, 147b, 282, 290, 297
   classical 138
   medical complications of 292
   moderate 147
   risk factors of 282
Eating disturbance 141, 142
Echolalia 187
Echopraxia 187
Education 11, 175
   street children, quality of 345
Electroencephalogram, abnormal 85
Electrolyte
   disturbances 148
   imbalance 292
Elimination disorders 142, 153
Emotional disorders 109
Emotional outbursts 331
Emotional stress 155
Emotions 80
Employment impairment 51
Encephalitis, postviral 185
Encephalopathy, evidence of 19
Encopresis 153, 168, 176f, 178
   classification 168
   clinical features 172
   etiology 169
   incidence 168
   investigation 175

   nonretentive 168
   pathophysiology 169
   treatment 175
Endocrine 205, 286, 293
Enemas 284
Enteral feeding 142
Enuresis 161
   classification 161
   clinical features 164
   genetics 162
   incidence 162
   investigations 164
   management 164
   monosymptomatic 163, 164
   pathogenesis 162
   pathophysiology 162
Epigenetic origin, etiology of diseases of 86
Epilepsy 26, 27, 235
   focal onset 20
   localization-related 27
Epileptic automatism 61
Epinephrine 216
Episodic illness 19
Esophageal reflux 140
Esophageal rupture 292
Eustress 214
Evaluation procedure 34
   birth history 35
   educational assessment 38
   family history 36
   medical history 34
   neurological examination 37
   physical examination 36
   school history 36
   social history 36
Evidence-based study strategies 249, 255
Exhibitionistic disorder 311
Exploitation 352
Expression study skills 259
Expressive language 65
Extrapyramidal symptoms 211
Eye
   blinking 182, 186
   hand coordination disorders 50
   rolling 186

F

Facial dysmorphism 21
Factitious disorder 227, 234
Failure to thrive 19, 21
Family focused
    cognitive-behavioral therapy 239
    psychoeducational treatment 211
Fear, development of 216
Fecal incontinence,
    causes of 174, 174t
Feeding
    difficulties 137
    disorders 10, 135, 142, 144, 147
    disturbance 141
    problems 11
Fetal alcohol syndrome 27, 87
Fetishistic disorder 309
Fiber supplement 177
Fibrinogen 285
Figurative language 70
Figure-ground perception 52, 55f
Finger identification 53, 55f
Flash cards 258
Fluid imbalance 292
Fluoxetine 133, 144
Fluphenazine 191
Focal neurological signs 20
Food
    refusal 143
    sensitivities 276, 280
Foster care home 358
Fragile X syndrome 18, 22, 28, 82
Frotteuristic disorder 311
Frustration 276
Functional neurologic
    disorder 233, 234
Functional voiding disorders 155

G

Gadgets, excessive use of 230
Gamma-aminobutyric acid 216
Gastric rupture 292
Gastroesophageal reflux 279
Gastrointestinal repair 86
Gastrointestinal system 232
Gender identity disorder 305
General physical examination 173
Generalized anxiety disorder 216, 218, 266
Genetic diseases 50
Genetic factors 86, 216, 231
Giggle incontinence 156
Glucosuria 164
Glutathione 87
Gonadotropin-releasing hormone, deficiency of 286
Graphesthesia 53f, 55f
Greenspan model 89
Guanfacine 191
Gynecomastia 304

H

Haemophilus influenzae 277
Haloperidol 191
Head and neck anomalies 135
Headache 278
Health problems 277, 348
Healthcare 355
    workers 338
Hearing
    deficit 69
    loss 9, 73
    problems 277
    senses of 258
Heart
    disease, congenital 9, 22
    rate reactivity 228
Hematemesis 296
Hemiplegia 20
Hemorrhage, antepartum 35
Herpes 18
Hinman syndrome 156
Hippocampus 216
Homelessness 348
Homeostasis, disorders of 143
Homework skills 259
Homosexuality 305
Hoover's test 237
Hospitalization, criteria for 148b
Human immunodeficiency
    virus 209, 349
Huntington's disease 185

Hyperactivity 98, 103
    disorder 50
Hyperkinetic disorder 98
Hypersomnia 195
Hypochondriasis disorder 226
Hypokalemia, signs of 288
Hypotension 288
Hypothyroidism 19
Hypotonia 19
Hypovolemia 287

I

Imipramine 167
Immune function 86
Immunologic problems 285
Impulsivity 90, 104
Inattention, persistent pattern of 103
Incontinence, pattern of 157
Indian Certificate of Secondary
    Education 43
Infections 164
    congenital 18
    fear of 373
Influenza 277
Insomnia 199, 200
    causes of 199
    idiopathic 199
Intellectual developmental
    disorder 7, 50, 107
Intellectual disability 7
    cause for 17
    clinical presentation 8
    definitive assessment for 15
    diagnosing 11
    functioning in domains 8
    guidelines for parents 24
    investigate child with 17
    long-term 23
    management 22
    prevalence 8
Intellectual function 16
Intelligence testing 34
Intensive outpatient psychiatric
    treatment 294
Intermittent explosive disorder 133
International Children's Continence
    Society 161

Interpersonal therapy 297
Intestinal illnesses 277
Intranasal substance abuse 366
Intravenous substance abuse 366
Iodine, form of 252
Iron, form of 252
Irregular sleep patterns 372
Irritability 278, 374
Irritable mood 125

J

Jigsaw puzzle 253

K

Kinesthesia 53, 53*f*, 55*f*

L

Lamotrigine 108
Lancet psychiatry 3
Landau–Kleffner syndrome 20
Language
    components of 65
    delay 73*fc*
    development 35, 66, 66*t*, 253
    pathologist 74
    skills 249
Laxative 168
    diuretic abuse 289
    misuse of 284, 291
Learned behavior, unlearning of 351
Learning 249
    celebration of 260
    disability 10, 21, 39, 43, 62, 265
    disorders 26, 108
        etiology 26
        higher chance of 27
        investigations 38
        management 39
    early foundations of 252
    essentials for 250
    problems 26
    strategies, use of 261
Lesbianism 304
Lethality 320
Leukopenia 286

Lip smacking 182
Logical intelligence 251
Love and affection 330
Low luteinizing hormone 286

M

Macrocephaly 20
Magnesium 90
Magnetic resonance imaging 204, 209
Major paraphilias, clinical features of 309
Maladaptive behavior, development of 129
Male gender identity variants, categorization of 307t
Mallory–Weiss tears 292
Malnutrition
  acute medical complications of 148
  severe 148
Mannerisms 63
Marriage, consanguinity of 12
Masturbation 304
Maturation 86
M-chat table 93t
Medical disorders 26
Memory 255
  enhancing skills 257
Menstruation, physical changes of 284
Mental
  disorder 200
  distress 307
  health 372
    issues 41, 228, 372
    problems 51
    management 375
  illness, parental 5
  retardation 24, 39, 60, 69, 73, 87, 135, 362
    diagnosis of 7
  rituals 222
Metabolic abnormalities 296
Metabolic disorders 19
Metacognitive skills 260
Metallization-based therapy 322
Methylphenidate 116, 118

Microcephaly 20
Minimal brain dysfunction, concept of 101
Mitochondrial dysfunction 87
Mood disorder 132, 203, 204, 266, 362
  classification of 207fc
  clinical features 205
  diagnosis 206
  differential diagnosis 209
  epidemiology 203
  etiology 204
  neuropathology of 205
  prognosis and outcome 212
  treatment 210
Mood disturbance, self-esteem 295
Morphology 65
Motivation 250, 320
Motor accuracy 53
Motor movements 83
Motor skill deficit 49
Motor tic 182
Movement
  coordination of 48
  disorders 10, 188
    features of 189t
Multiple intelligences 251
Multiple nutritional deficiency 142
Multisensory learning 259
Multisystemic therapy 322
Murmur heart rate, heart for 14
Muscle tone 14
Muscular dystrophy 20
Musculoskeletal disorders 135
Myelination, essential for 252

N

Nasal block 277
Nasal congestion 277
National Institute of Drug Abuse 369
Neophobia 145
Nephropathy, hypokalemic 287
Nervous system 233
Neuroacanthocytosis 60
Neurobiological factors 129, 216
Neurochemical research 86
Neuroinflammations 87
Neurologic factors 171

Neurologic signs 161
Neurological diseases 50
Neurological disorders 26
Neuronal growth 252
    essential for 252
Neutral stimuli 215
Night eating syndrome 146, 291
Night time fears 197
Night waking, painful bursts of 279
Nightmares 197
Nighttime eating, recurrent episodes of 146
Nocturnal calciuria 163
Nocturnal continence, physiology of 162
Nocturnal emission 304
Nocturnal enuresis 158
Nocturnal incontinence 161
Nonfunctional motor behavior 60
Nonnutritive substances, persistent eating of 141
Nonverbal communication 77
    behaviors 83
Noradrenaline reuptake inhibitors 118
Normal language development 66
Nose 73, 233
Nucleus accumbens 365
Nutrition 349
Nutritional counseling 297
Nutritious food 354

O

Obesity 337
Obsessive-compulsive disorder 61, 183, 216, 221, 222, 266, 362
Obstructive sleep apnea 163
    syndrome 200
Occupational therapist 40
    evaluation 34
Ocular abnormalities 19
Olanzapine 133
Omega-3 fatty acids, form of 252
Oppositional defiant disorder 109, 124, 362
    clinical features 126
    diagnosis 125
    differential diagnosis 127
    early warning signs 126
    epidemiology 124
    etiology 124
    specify current severity 126
    treatment 127
Oral nutritional supplements 142
Oral praxis 53
Organomegaly 19
Otitis media, acute 278
Overstimulation 276
Overt parental conflict 5
Overtiredness 276
Oxidative stress 87
Oxybutynin 160

P

Pain
    abdominal 217, 280
    disorder 226, 233
Pancreatitis, acute 292
Panic attacks 221
Panic disorder 221
Paradoxical insomnia 200
Parainfluenza 277
Paraphilia, treatment of 312
Paraphilic disorders 308, 309
    characteristics of 308
Parasomnias 195
Parathyroid hormone 286
Parental stress, signs of 374
Paroxysmal dyskinesia 63
Pediatric autoimmune neuropsychiatric disorders 183
Pediatric sleep clinic 201
Pediatric unstable bladder 156
Pediatrician, role of 119
Pedophilic disorder 311
Peer pressure 304
Pemoline 118
Perianal region, examination of 173
Periodontitis 282
Peripheral neuropathies 154
Persistent depressive disorder 206
Personal protective equipment 375

Pervasive developmental disorder 78
Pharmacologic therapy 297
Pharmacotherapeutic agents 210
Phenobarbitone 108
Phenothiazines 64
Phonology 65
  disorders of 71
Physical disability 243
Physical health 372
Physical problems 337, 348
Picky eating 145, 146
Pimozide 191
Poor academic performance 337
Poor sleep hygiene 199
Positron emission tomography 101
Postrotary nystagmus 53
Post-traumatic eating
    disturbances 144
Post-traumatic stress
  disorder 217, 221, 362
  symptoms 246
Postural praxis 53
Prader–Willi syndrome 9, 18
Prealbumin 285
Predominantly hyperactivity-
    impulsivity
    presentation 104
Predominantly inattentive
    presentation 104
Prefrontal cortex 365
Pregnancy 349
  unwanted 349
Prelinguistic period 66
Premenstrual dysphoric disorder 206
Prodromal behavioral symptoms 185
Progressive supranuclear palsy 39
Proteins, form of 252
Pseudo-Bartter syndrome 289
Psychiatric comorbidity 229
Psychiatric disorders 26, 29, 266
Psychiatric emergencies, acute 148
Psychiatric morbidity 266
Psychiatrist 294
  role of 41
Psychodynamic therapy 296
Psychoeducation 222
Psychogenic nonepileptic seizure 233

Psychogenic symptoms, diagnosis
    of 237
Psychological adaptability 245
Psychological factors 129, 234, 344
Psychological maladjustment 242
Psychological problems 224, 245, 350
Psychological reaction 245
Psychologist 294
Psychophysiological insomnia 199
Psychosis risk syndrome 317
Psychosocial factors 229
Psychosocial maladjustment 247
Psychosomatic conditions 240
Psychotherapeutic interventions 269
Psychotherapy 127
  interpersonal 210
Psychotropic medication 91*t*
Puberty, onset of 304
Pubic hair 285
Pudendal nerve injury 154
Purging disorder 291
Pyorrhea 288
Pyuria 164

R

Rapid eye movement sleep 194
Reactive attachment disorder 360, 362
Rectal biopsy, abnormal 280
Recurrent inappropriate
    compensatory behavior 287
Reflex
  bladder contraction 153
  evidence of 11
Relaxation
  exercises 252
  training 223
Repetitive speech 83
Respiratory dysregulation 228
Respiratory infections 350
Respiratory syncytial virus 277
Restless legs syndrome 61
Restrictive food intake disorder 141
Retentive encopresis 168
Rett's syndrome 18, 60, 62, 82, 87
Rhinovirus 277

Index

Risperidone 133, 191
Rubella 18
Rumination disorder 140

S

Salivary glands 288
  hypertrophy of 282
Savant skills 87
Schizophrenia 61
  manifestation of 78
School
  environment 231
  phobia 265
  problems 265
  refusal 265
    clinical features 266
    etiology 266
    evaluation 268
    management 269
    short-term sequelae of 267
Seizures 19, 87
  myoclonic 20
Selective mutism 69
Selective serotonin reuptake
        inhibitor 210
  drugs 144, 269
Self-esteem 56
Self-harm 318, 321
  prevalence of 316f, 320
Self-injurious behaviors 10, 317
Sense organ 253
  deficits 108
Sensitive periods 145
Sensitivities problems 87
Sensitization 306
Sensory deficits 26, 38
Sensory integration 52
  and praxis tests 52
  theory of 52
Sensory neural hearing loss 73
Separation anxiety disorder 217, 218
Serotonin 216
  reuptake inhibitors 133
  transporter gene 204
Sertraline 133
Severe failure to thrive 135

Sexual abuse 346
Sexual behaviors 301
  types of 300
Sexual dysfunction
  management of 312
  treatment of 312
Sexual identity development,
        troiden's model of 306
Sexual masochism 310t
  disorder 310
Sexual sadism disorder 311
Sexuality 300
  development of 331
Sexually transmitted diseases 349
Single photon emission computed
        tomography 101
Single-gene disorders 22
Skills, progressive loss of 19
Skin infections 349
Sleep 337
  difficulties 90
  disorder 9, 10, 163
    breathing 200
  medicine behavioral specialist 201
  problem 194, 196, 217
    evaluation 196
    general management 201
    types of 195
  terror 196
Sleepiness
  behavioral manifestations of 200
  excessive 195
Sleeplessness 278
Sleepwalking 197
Smooth muscle contractions 228
Social
  anxiety disorder 219
  communication 83
  domain 8, 16
  emotional reciprocity 83
  factors 344
  impairment 51
  interactions, impairment of 77
  isolation 319
  learning theory 306
  skills 56, 247, 298
Socialization 79

Somatic symptom and related
        disorders 226, 227
    assessment 236
    clinical features 232
    diagnosis 234
    epidemiology 228
    etiology 228
    treatment 238
Somatization 226
Somatodyspraxia 52
Somatoform 226
    disorders 226, 227
Somnambulism 197
Somniloquy 198
Southern California Sensory
        Integration Test 52
Spasms, infantile 87
Specific disorders, testing for 18, 21
Specific language impairment 69
Specific learning disabilities 26, 30,
        39, 50
    clinical presentation 33
    epidemiology 31
    genetic basis 32
    neurobiological basis 31
    outcome of 45
    pathophysiology 31
    phonologic basis 32
    types 31
Specific learning disorder 108, 209
Specific phobia 220, 266
    typical signs of 220
Speech 73*fc*
    development 35
    difficulties 50
    evaluation 34
    language, and communication
            needs 50
    pathologist 74
    problems 277
    therapy 73
Sphincter dysfunction 161
Spillover 252
Spinal cord lesions 154
Standard deviation scores 53
Start bed-wetting 278
Stereotypic behavior 61

Stereotypic movements
    clinical features 61
    course and outcome 63
    diagnostic criteria 61
    disorder 60
    epidemiology 60
    treatment 64
Stigmatization 354
Stimulant medication 116
    like methylphenidate 182
Stream, quality of 158
Street children 341
    age 343
    broken homes 346
    categories 342
    cruelty and abuse 346
    economic causes 345
    gender 343
    influence of media 347
    location 343
    natural calamities 346
    neglect 347
    number 342
    peer group influence 347
Streptococcal infection 183
Stress 235
    disorder, acute 217
Structural brain malformation 19
Study skills 249, 260
    classification of 256
    inventory 261
    objective assessment of 261
Substance abuse 18, 351, 364
    stages of 366
Substance-use disorder 363, 368
    stages of 366*t*
Substitute care 357, 360
    types of 358
Sudden mood change 331
Suicidal behavior 315
Suicide 315, 318, 321
    crisis and intervention 324
    prevalence of 316*f*, 320, 324
    risk, assessment for 316
Superior mesenteric artery
        syndrome 293
Sweaty palms 213

Synaptogenesis 252
Syntax 65

T

Tactile defensiveness 146
Tactile stimuli, localization of 53, 53f
Tardive dyskinesia 60
Three-dimensional language acquisition test 73
Throat 73, 233
Thyroid
 function studies 175, 205
 stimulating hormone 286
Thyroxine 286
Tic disorders 5, 63, 182
 clinical features 183
 diagnosis 188
 differential diagnosis 188
 epidemiology 182
 etiology 183
 prognosis 191
 treatment 188
Tone, abnormal 21
Tongue thrusting 182
Toothache 279
Topical estrogen creams 155
Tourette's syndrome 27, 28, 61, 184-186
Toxins 18
Transient autism 82
Transient lactase deficiency 280
Transient stereotypic movements 60
Transient tic disorder 184
Transvestic disorder 310
Tricyclic 118
 antidepressants 116, 269
Tri-iodothyronine 286
Trousseau sign 288
Tuberous sclerosis 87
Turner syndrome 9

U

Ulcers, aphthous 280
Unique disability identity card 40
Unwitnessed head injury 277

Upper respiratory infection 277
Urinalysis 158
Urinary incontinence 153
Urinary tract infection 155, 278
 recurrent 10
Urine
 drug screening 367
 production, excessive 155

V

Vaginal reflux 155
Valproic acid 18
Varicella 18
Ventral tegmental area 365
Verbal ability 67
Verbal communication 77
Vesicoureteral reflux 278
Victims 270
Vigabatrin 108
Vindictiveness 125
Viral infections 277
Visiodyspraxia 52
Vision impairment 9
Visual devices 336
Visual imagery 165
Visual impairment 12
Vitamin 90
 form of 252
Vocal tic disorder 184
Voiding cystourethrography 156
Voluntary muscles 48
Vomiting 288, 289
 self-induced 284, 291
Voyeuristic disorder 311
 characteristics of 311

W

Walking balance 53
Weight loss 141
Whole exome sequencing 21
Williams syndrome 60
Worm infestation 279

Z

Ziprasidone 191

www.ingramcontent.com/pod-product-compliance
Ingram Content Group UK Ltd.
Pitfield, Milton Keynes, MK11 3LW, UK
UKHW022119120525
458461UK00001B/8